T0359096

Precision ACL Reconstruction

Editors

VOLKER MUSAHL
ALAN M.J. GETGOOD

CLINICS IN SPORTS MEDICINE

www.sportsmed.theclinics.com

Consulting Editor
F. WINSTON GWATHMEY

July 2024 • Volume 43 • Number 3

ELSEVIER

1600 John F. Kennedy Boulevard • Suite 1800 • Philadelphia, Pennsylvania, 19103-2899

http://www.theclinics.com

CLINICS IN SPORTS MEDICINE Volume 43, Number 3
July 2024 ISSN 0278-5919, ISBN-13: 978-0-443-18398-0

Editor: Megan Ashdown
Developmental Editor: Malvika Shah

Clinics in Sports Medicine (ISSN 0278-5919) is published quarterly by Elsevier Inc., 360 Park Avenue South, New York, NY 10010-1710. Months of issue are January, April, July, and October. Business and Editorial Offices: 1600 John F. Kennedy Blvd., Ste. 1800, Philadelphia, PA 19103-2899. Customer Service Office: 3251 Riverport Lane, Maryland Heights, MO 63043. Periodicals postage paid at New York, NY and additional mailing offices. Subscription prices are $390.00 per year (US individuals), $100.00 per year (US students), $430.00 per year (Canadian individuals), $100.00 (Canadian students), $504.00 per year (foreign individuals), and $235.00 per year (foreign students). For institutional access pricing please contact Customer Service via the contact information below. Foreign air speed delivery is included in all *Clinics* subscription prices. All prices are subject to change without notice. **POSTMASTER:** Send address changes to *Clinics in Sports Medicine*, Elsevier Health Sciences Division, Subscription Customer Service, 3251 Riverport Lane, Maryland Heights, MO 63043. Customer Service (orders, claims, online, change of address): Elsevier Health Sciences Division, Subscription Customer Service, 3251 Riverport Lane, Maryland Heights, MO 63043. **Tel: 1-800-654-2452 (U.S. and Canada); 314-447-8871 (outside U.S. and Canada). Fax: 314-447-8029. E-mail: journalscustomerservice-usa@elsevier.com (for print support); journalsonlinesupport-usa@elsevier.com (for online support).**

Reprints. For copies of 100 or more of articles in this publication, please contact the Commercial Reprints Department, Elsevier Inc., 360 Park Avenue South, New York, NY 10010-1710. Tel.: 212-633-3874; Fax: 212-633-3820; E-mail: reprints@elsevier.com.

Clinics in Sports Medicine is covered in *MEDLINE/PubMed (Index Medicus) Current Contents/Clinical Medicine, Excerpta Medica,* and *ISI/Biomed.*

Contributors

CONSULTING EDITOR

F. WINSTON GWATHMEY, MD
Associate Professor of Orthopaedic Surgery, University of Virginia Health System, Vice Chair for Orthopaedic Education and Residency Program Director, Team Physician, UVA Athletics, Charlottesville, Virginia, USA

EDITORS

VOLKER MUSAHL, MD
Assistant Professor, Department of Orthopaedic Surgery, UPMC Freddie Fu Sports Medicine Center, University of Pittsburgh, Pittsburgh, Pennsylvania, USA; Department of Orthopaedics, Institute of Clinical Sciences, Sahlgrenska Academy, University of Gothenburg, Gothenburg, Sweden

ALAN M.J. GETGOOD, MPhil, MD, FRCS(Tr&Orth)
Department of Orthopaedic Surgery, London Health Sciences Centre, University Hospital, Associate Professor, Department of Surgery, Western University, Consultant Orthopaedic Surgeon, Fowler Kennedy Sport Medicine Clinic, Western's Bone and Joint Institute, University Hospital, London, Ontario, Canada

AUTHORS

NEILEN BENVEGNU, MD
Orthopedic Surgeon, Department of Orthopaedic Surgery, UPMC Freddie Fu Sports Medicine Center, University of Pittsburgh, Pittsburgh, Pennsylvania, USA

BERTE BØE, MD, PhD
Consultant orthopaedic surgeon Division of Orthopaedics, Oslo University Hospital, Ullevål Sykehus, Nydalen, Oslo

CORTEZ BROWN, MD
Resident, Department of Orthopaedic Surgery, University of Pittsburgh, Pittsburgh, Pennsylvania, USA

DIANNE M. BRYANT, MSc, PhD
Faculty of Health Sciences, Fowler Kennedy Sport Medicine Clinic, Bone and Joint Institute, Lawson Research, London Health Sciences Centre, Schulich School of Medicine and Dentistry, Western University, Department of Health Research Methods, Evidence and Impact, McMaster University, Hamilton, Ontario, Canada

JACOB G. CALCEI, MD
Orthopaedic Surgeon University Hospitals Drusinsky Sports Medicine Institute, Assistant Professor of Orthopaedic Surgery, Case Western Reserve University School of Medicine, Cleveland, Ohio, USA

ALESSANDRO CARROZZO, MD
Orthopedic Surgeon, Orthopedic Unit, Sant'Andrea University Hospital, La Sapienza University, Rome, Italy

ALEXIS COLVIN, MD
Professor, Department of Orthopedics, The Mount Sinai Hospital, New York, New York, USA

ANDREW J. CURLEY, MD
UPMC Freddie Fu Sports Medicine Center, University of Pittsburgh, Pittsburgh, Pennsylvania, USA

SAHIL DADOO, BS
Research Assistant, Department of Orthopaedic Surgery, UPMC Freddie Fu Sports Medicine Center, University of Pittsburgh, Pittsburgh, Pennsylvania, USA

IAN D. ENGLER, MD
Orthopaedic Surgeon Central Maine Healthcare Orthopedics, Central Maine Medical Center, Auburn, Maine, USA; UPMC Freddie Fu Sports Medicine Center, University of Pittsburgh, Pittsburgh, Pennsylvania, USA

GABRIELLE FATORA, MD
Resident, Department of Orthopaedic Surgery, University of Pittsburgh, Pittsburgh, Pennsylvania, USA

MICHAEL A. FOX, MD
Resident Physician, Department of Orthopaedic Surgery, UPMC Freddie Fu Sports Medicine Center, University of Pittsburgh, Pittsburgh, Pennsylvania, USA

SIMON GÖRTZ, MD
Department of Orthopaedic Surgery, Center for Cartilage Repair and Sports Medicine, Brigham and Women's Hospital, Assistant Professor of Orthopedic Surgery, Harvard Medical School, Boston, Massachusetts, USA

ALAN M.J. GETGOOD, MPhil, MD, FRCS(Tr&Orth)
Department of Orthopaedic Surgery, London Health Sciences Centre, University Hospital, Assistant Professor, Department of Surgery, Western University, Consultant Orthopaedic Surgeon, Fowler Kennedy Sport Medicine Clinic, Western's Bone and Joint Institute, University Hospital, London, Ontario, Canada

JOHAN HÖGBERG, PT, MSc
Sportrehab Sports Medicine Clinic, Sahlgrenska Sports Medicine Center, Unit of Physiotherapy, Department of Health and Rehabilitation, Institute of Neuroscience and Physiology, Sahlgrenska Academy, University of Gothenburg, Gothenburg, Sweden

ERIC HAMRIN SENORSKI, PT, PhD
Sportrehab Sports Medicine Clinic, Sahlgrenska Sports Medicine Center, Unit of Physiotherapy, Visiting Research Fellow Department of Health and Rehabilitation, Institute of Neuroscience and Physiology, Sahlgrenska Academy, University of Gothenburg, Gothenburg, Sweden; Swedish Olympic Committee, Stockholm, Sweden

ZACHARY J. HERMAN, MD
Resident, Department of Orthopaedic Surgery, UPMC Freddie Fu Sports Medicine Center, University of Pittsburgh, Pittsburgh, Pennsylvania, USA

JONATHAN D. HUGHES, MD
Assistant Professor, Department of Orthopaedic Surgery, UPMC Freddie Fu Sports Medicine Center, University of Pittsburgh, Pittsburgh, Pennsylvania, USA; Department of Orthopaedics, Institute of Clinical Sciences, Sahlgrenska Academy, University of Gothenburg, Gothenburg, Sweden

JANINA KAARRE, MD, MSc
Department of Orthopaedic Surgery, UPMC Freddie Fu Sports Medicine Center, University of Pittsburgh, Pittsburgh, Pennsylvania, USA; Department of Orthopaedics, Institute of Clinical Sciences, Sahlgrenska Academy, University of Gothenburg, Gothenburg, Sweden

DAVID E. KANTROWITZ, MD
Resident Department of Orthopaedics, The Mount Sinai Hospital, New York, New York, USA

LAURA E. KEELING, MD
Department of Orthopaedic Surgery, UPMC Freddie Fu Sports Medicine Center, University of Pittsburgh, Pittsburgh, Pennsylvania, USA

FRANCES L. KOBACK, BS
Medical Student, Geisel School of Medicine at Dartmouth, Dartmouth College, Hanover, New Hampshire, USA

CHRISTIAN LATTERMANN, MD
Department of Orthopaedic Surgery, Center for Cartilage Repair and Sports Medicine, Brigham and Women's Hospital, Harvard Medical School, Boston, Massachusetts, USA

OPHELIE Z. LAVOIE-GAGNE, MD
Department of Orthopaedic Surgery, Director of Research Center for Cartilage Repair and Sports Medicine, Brigham and Women's Hospital, Harvard Medical School, Boston, Massachusetts, USA

CHILAN B.G. LEITE, MD
Research fellow, Department of Orthopaedic Surgery, Center for Cartilage Repair and Sports Medicine, Brigham and Women's Hospital, Harvard Medical School, Boston, Massachusetts, USA

BRYSON P. LESNIAK, MD
Associate professor Department of Orthopaedic Surgery, University of Pittsburgh, Pittsburgh, Pennsylvania, USA

HANA MARMURA, BSc, MPT, PhD (Candidate)
Faculty of Health Sciences, Fowler Kennedy Sport Medicine Clinic, Bone and Joint Institute, Western University, Lawson Research, London Health Sciences Centre, Ontario, Canada

VOLKER MUSAHL, MD
Assistant Professor, Department of Orthopaedic Surgery, UPMC Freddie Fu Sports Medicine Center, University of Pittsburgh, Pittsburgh, Pennsylvania, USA; Department of Orthopaedics, Institute of Clinical Sciences, Sahlgrenska Academy, University of Gothenburg, Gothenburg, Sweden

ERIC NARUP, MD, MSc
Department of Orthopaedics, Institute of Clinical Sciences, Sahlgrenska Academy, University of Gothenburg, Gothenburg, Sweden

RAMANA PIUSSI, PT, MSc
Sportrehab Sports Medicine Clinic, Sahlgrenska Sports Medicine Center, Unit of Physiotherapy, Doctoral Student Department of Health and Rehabilitation, Institute of Neuroscience and Physiology, Sahlgrenska Academy, University of Gothenburg, Gothenburg, Sweden

YAZDAN RAJI, MD
Fellow, Department of Orthopaedic Surgery, Stanford University School of Medicine, Redwood City, California, USA

KRISTIAN SAMUELSSON, MD, PhD, MSc
Professor, Department of Orthopaedics, Institute of Clinical Sciences, Sahlgrenska Academy, University of Gothenburg, Gothenburg, Sweden; Department of Orthopaedics, Sahlgrenska University Hospital, Mölndal, Sweden

MARK F. SHERMAN, MD
Orthopedics Surgeon, Department of Orthopedics Surgery Richmond University Medical Center, Staten Island, New York, USA

SETH L. SHERMAN, MD
Associate Professor, Fellowship Director, Division of Sports Medicine, Head Team Physician, Stanford Cardinal Football, Associate Professor, Department of Orthopaedic Surgery, Stanford University School of Medicine, Redwood City, California, USA

REBECCA SIMONSSON, PT, MSc
Sportrehab Sports Medicine Clinic, Sahlgrenska Sports Medicine Center, Unit of Physiotherapy, Department of Health and Rehabilitation, Institute of Neuroscience and Physiology, Sahlgrenska Academy, University of Gothenburg, Gothenburg, Sweden

RICHARD SMITH, MD, DPhil
Department of Orthopaedic Surgery, Center for Cartilage Repair and Sports Medicine, Brigham and Women's Hospital, Harvard Medical School, Boston, Massachusetts, USA

BERTRAND SONNERY-COTTET, MD, PhD
Orthopaedic Surgery, Centre Orthopédique Santy, FIFA Medical Centre of Excellence, Groupe Ramsay-Générale de Santé, Hôpital Privé Jean Mermoz, Lyon, France

AXEL SUNDBERG, PT, MSc
Sahlgrenska Sports Medicine Center, Unit of Physiotherapy, Department of Health and Rehabilitation, Institute of Neuroscience and Physiology, Sahlgrenska Academy, University of Gothenburg, Capio Ortho Center, Gothenburg, Sweden

NYALUMA N. WAGALA, MD
Resident Department of Orthopaedic Surgery, University of Pittsburgh, Pittsburgh, Pennsylvania, USA

TETSUYA YAMAMOTO, MD
Professor, Department of Orthopaedic Surgery, UPMC Freddie Fu Sports Medicine Center, University of Pittsburgh, Pittsburgh, Pennsylvania, USA; Department of Orthopaedic Surgery, Kobe University Graduate School of Medicine, Kobe, Japan

BÁLINT ZSIDAI, MD
Department of Orthopaedics, Institute of Clinical Sciences, Sahlgrenska Academy, University of Gothenburg, Gothenburg, Sweden

Contents

Foreword: Precision Anterior Cruciate Ligament Reconstruction xiii

F. Winston Gwathmey

Preface: Precision Anterior Cruciate Ligament Reconstruction xv

Volker Musahl and Alan M.J. Getgood

Preoperative

Comprehensive Clinical Examination of ACL Injuries 311

David E. Kantrowitz and Alexis Colvin

Video content accompanies this article at http://www.sportsmed.theclinics.com.

A comprehensive clinical examination of the potentially anterior cruciate ligament (ACL)-deficient knee should proceed as follows: inspection; palpation; range of motion; varus and valgus stress; neurovascular status; and finally provocative maneuvers. The Lachman, anterior drawer, Lever, and pivot shift tests are all greater than 90% specific for ACL pathology. Due to the relatively high coincidence of ACL injuries and those to the posterior cruciate ligament, posterolateral corner , posteromedial corner , and menisci, it is critical that the examiner perform provocative maneuvers to evaluate the integrity of these structures as well.

Timing of Anterior Cruciate Ligament Surgery 331

Bálint Zsidai, Janina Kaarre, Eric Narup, and Kristian Samuelsson

This narrative review examines the current literature for the influence of the surgical timing in the setting of anterior cruciate ligament (ACL) reconstruction on various outcomes. Although the exact definition of early and delayed ACL reconstruction (ACLR) is a subject of controversy, surgical timing influences arthrofibrosis and postoperative stiffness, quadriceps strength, postoperative knee function, and the incidence of intra-articular injuries to the menisci and cartilage. Additionally, there is a shortage of evidence regarding the role of ACLR timing in the setting of multiligament knee injury and when concurrent procedures are performed during the operative treatment of the ACL-injured knee.

Nonoperative Anterior Cruciate Ligament Injury Treatment 343

Berte Bøe

This article outlines the key points in the nonoperative treatment of an anterior cruciate ligament (ACL) injury. Initial evaluation and treatment of an acute knee injury, often performed by a physician with limited experience in the treatment of an ACL injury, follow the basic diagnostic workup that lead to the diagnosis. The principles of rehabilitation after ACL injury have

changed from time based to criteria based, and the different phases based on physical criteria are described.

Perioperative

Value-Based, Environmentally Sustainable Anterior Cruciate Ligament Surgery 355

Ian D. Engler, Frances L. Koback, and Andrew J. Curley

Orthopedic surgeons are increasingly recognizing the broader societal impact of their clinical decisions, which includes value-based and environmentally sustainable care. Within anterior cruciate ligament reconstruction, value-based care—or most cost-effective care—includes an outpatient surgical setting with regional anesthesia, use of autograft, meniscus repair when indicated, and use of traditional metal implants such as interference screws and staples. Environmentally sustainable care includes slimming down surgical packs and trays to avoid opening unnecessary equipment, avoiding desflurane as an inhaled anesthetic agent, and minimizing waste in the operating room—a priority that addresses both cost and environmental impact.

Avoiding Graft Failure: Lessons Learned from the Stability Trial 367

Alan M.J. Getgood

The Stability Study was a multicenter, pragmatic, parallel groups, randomized clinical trial comparing hamstring tendon autograft anterior cruciate ligament reconstruction with or without the addition of lateral extra-articular tenodesis in young patients at high risk of graft failure. Having recruited 618 patients with a 5% loss to follow up, we were able to demonstrate a clinically and statistically significant reduction in clinical failure and graft rupture at 2 years postoperative. No differences in patient-reported outcomes (PROs) were demonstrated between groups; however, patients who experienced an adverse event had significantly worse PROs than those who did not.

The Role of Osteotomy in Anterior Cruciate Ligament Reconstruction 383

Zachary J. Herman, Laura E. Keeling, Michael A. Fox, Sahil Dadoo, and Volker Musahl

Coronal and sagittal plane knee malalignments have been shown to increase the forces on anterior cruciate ligament (ACL) grafts after ACL reconstruction (ACLR). Studies have shown the benefit of high tibial osteotomy to address coronal and sagittal imbalance in revision ACLR. The purpose of this article is to further describe the use of osteotomy by reviewing preoperative planning, indications, techniques, and outcomes of high tibial opening and closing wedge as well as anterior tibial closing wedge osteotomies in the setting of ACLR.

Surgical Techniques in Primary ACL Reconstruction: Getting It Right the First Time 399

Sahil Dadoo, Zachary J. Herman, and Jonathan D. Hughes

The ideal anterior cruciate ligament reconstruction (ACLR) is an individualized anatomic approach aimed at restoring the native structure and function of the knee. Surgeons are tasked with difficult decisions during operative planning, including the optimal graft choice for the patient and appropriate anatomic tunnel placement. Special considerations should additionally be given for skeletally immature patients and those at high-risk for failure, including younger, active patients participating in pivoting sports. The purpose of this review is to provide an overview of the individualized approach to ACLR, including the necessary preoperative and operative considerations to optimize patient outcomes.

Lateral Extra-Articular Tenodesis and Anterolateral Procedures **413**

Bertrand Sonnery-Cottet and Alessandro Carrozzo

The treatment of rotational instability has been an intriguing challenge since the era of modern anterior cruciate ligament (ACL) surgery. Lateral extra-articular procedures (LEAPs) have emerged as a solution to this problem, particularly in high-risk populations. Several studies have shown significant benefits of combining LEAPs with ACL reconstruction, including reduced graft failure rates, improved knee stability, improved rotational stability, and higher return-to-play rates. These findings have led to an in-depth evaluation of LEAPs as lateral extra-articular tenodesis and anterolateral ligament reconstruction and their potential role in improving outcomes after ACL reconstruction.

Anterior Cruciate Ligament Repair—Here to Stay or History Repeating Itself? **433**

Seth L. Sherman, Yazdan Raji, Jacob G. Calcei, and Mark F. Sherman

Anterior cruciate ligament (ACL) injuries continue to be a prevalent concern among athletes and individuals with an active lifestyle. Traditionally, the standard of care for ACL tears has involved surgical reconstruction using autograft or allograft. This article aims to provide an overview of the evolving landscape of primary ACL repair, examining the current evidence, surgical techniques, patient selection criteria, outcomes, and potential future directions in this field.

Revision Anterior Cruciate Ligament Reconstruction and Associated Procedures **449**

Sahil Dadoo, Neilen Benvegnu, Zachary J. Herman, Tetsuya Yamamoto, Jonathan D. Hughes, and Volker Musahl

Failure of anterior cruciate ligament reconstruction (ACLR) is a common yet devastating complication due to inferior clinical outcomes associated with revision ACLR. Identifying the cause and associated risk factors for failure is the most important consideration during preoperative planning. Special attention to tunnel quality, concomitant injuries, and modifiable risk factors will help determine the optimal approach and staging for revision ACLR. Additional procedures including lateral extra-articular tenodesis and osteotomy may be considered for at-risk populations. The purpose of this review is to explore causes of ACLR failure, clinical indications and appropriate patient evaluation, and technical considerations when performing revision ACLR.

Complications in Anterior Cruciate Ligament Surgery and How to Avoid Them **465**

Nyaluma N. Wagala, Gabrielle Fatora, Cortez Brown, and Bryson P. Lesniak

Complications following anterior cruciate ligament (ACL) reconstruction can be detrimental to a patient's recovery and limit their ability to successfully return to sport. Arthrofibrosis, graft failure, and infection are a few examples of complications that can arise. Therefore, it is important for surgeons to recognize that each step during perioperative surgical decision making can impact patients' risk for such complications. The purpose of this paper is to discuss common complications following ACL reconstruction and how surgeons can avoid or reduce the risk of complications.

Postoperative

Evaluation of Outcomes After Anterior Cruciate Ligament Reconstruction: What We Know, What We Have, and What to Consider **479**

Hana Marmura and Dianne M. Bryant

Measurement of success following anterior cruciate ligament reconstruction (ACLR) hinges on the appropriate use of high quality and meaningful outcome measures. We identified and categorized over 100 outcome measures for ACLR using the International Classification of Functioning, Disability and Health (ICF) model. The ICF model is a useful framework to facilitate decisions about outcome selection and describe recovery following ACL injury. We outline key considerations when selecting outcome measures during study design (purpose, measurement properties, sample size, global assessment) or evaluating reported outcomes (measurement properties, sample size, magnitude/precision, clinical relevance, applicability), and discuss challenges in outcome measurement following ACLR.

Biologic Impact of Anterior Cruciate Ligament Injury and Reconstruction **501**

Chilan B.G. Leite, Richard Smith, Ophelie Z. Lavoie-Gagne, Simon Görtz, and Christian Lattermann

Surgical intervention after anterior cruciate ligament (ACL) tears is typically required because of the limited healing capacity of the ACL. However, mechanical factors and the inflammatory response triggered by the injury and surgery can impact patient outcomes. This review explores key aspects of ACL injury and reconstruction biology, including the inflammatory response, limited spontaneous healing, secondary inflammation after reconstruction, and graft healing processes. Understanding these biologic mechanisms is crucial for developing new treatment strategies and enhancing patient well-being. By shedding light on these aspects, clinicians and researchers can work toward improving quality of life for individuals affected by ACL tears.

Rehabilitation and Return to Sport After Anterior Cruciate Ligament Reconstruction **513**

Rebecca Simonsson, Ramana Piussi, Johan Högberg, Axel Sundberg, and Eric Hamrin Senorski

Rehabilitation after an anterior cruciate ligament (ACL) reconstruction requires patience, devotion, and discipline. Rehabilitation should be individualized to each patient's specific need and sport. Return to sport is a continuum throughout the rehabilitation, and patients should not return to performance before passing a battery of muscle function tests and patient-reported outcomes, as well as change of direction-specific tests. Return to full participation should be an agreement between the patient, physical therapist, surgeon, and coach. For minimal risk for second ACL injury, patients should continue with maintenance and prevention training even after returning to sport.

Precision Anterior Cruciate Ligament Reconstruction **535**

Zachary J. Herman, Janina Kaarre, Alan M.J. Getgood, and Volker Musahl

Precision anterior cruciate ligament reconstruction (ACLR) refers to the individualized approach to prerehabilitation, surgery (including anatomy, bony morphology, and repair/reconstruction of concomitant injuries), postrehabilitation, and functional recovery. This individualized approach is poised to revolutionize orthopedic sports medicine, aiming to improve patient outcomes. The purpose of this article is to provide a summary of precision ACLR, from the time of diagnosis to the time of return to play, with additional insight into the future of ACLR.

CLINICS IN SPORTS MEDICINE

FORTHCOMING ISSUES

October 2024
Shoulder Instability
Jonathan F. Dickens and Brian C. Lau, *Editors*

January 2025
Building a Sports Medicine Practice: Guide to Navigating the First Five Years
James B. Carr II, *Editor*

April 2025
The Baseball Athlete
Steven Cohen, *Editor*

RECENT ISSUES

April 2024
Equality, Diversity, and Inclusion in Sports Medicine
Constance Chu, Erica Taylor and Joel Boyd, *Editors*

January 2024
Mental Health Considerations in the Athlete
Siobhán M. Statuta, Editor

October 2023
Acromioclavicular, Clavicle, and Sternoclavicular Injuries in Athletes
Katherine J. Coyner, *Editor*

SERIES OF RELATED INTERESTED

Orthopedic Clinics
https://www.orthopedic.theclinics.com/
Foot and Ankle Clinics
https://www.foot.theclinics.com/
Hand Clinics
https://www.hand.theclinics.com/
Physical Medicine and Rehabilitation Clinics
https://www.pmr.theclinics.com/

Foreword
Precision Anterior Cruciate Ligament Reconstruction

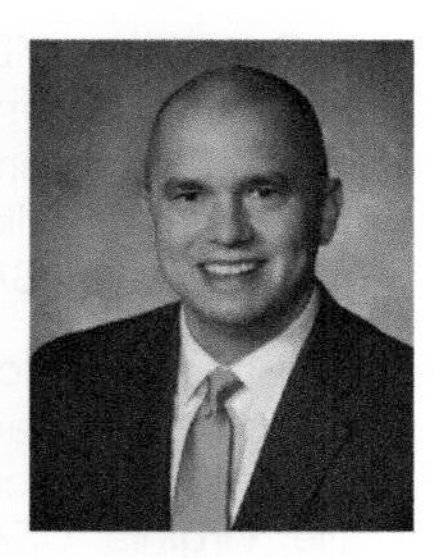

F. Winston Gwathmey, MD
Consulting Editor

The anterior cruciate ligament (ACL) is *the* ligament of sports medicine knee surgery. No structure in the human body has generated as much intrigue, investigation, debate, and controversy among knee surgeons as the ACL. No structure has been responsible for as many devastating season-ending injuries among elite athletes and weekend warriors as the ACL. The physical, psychological, and financial implications of ACL injury are immense. With so much on the line, the sports medicine knee surgeon performing ACL reconstruction needs to understand how to "get it right" and be able to execute the best surgical procedure.

The great Freddie Fu taught us so much about the importance of anatomy in ACL reconstruction, and the great Peter Fowler elucidated essential technical aspects. Building off their contributions, clinician scientists over the past decade have pushed the continued advancement in the understanding of the pathomechanics of ACL injury and the ACL deficient knee. Likewise, there has been considerable evolution in the optimal surgical strategy to restore normal knee kinematics. Now, ancillary procedures, such as anterolateral ligament reconstruction, lateral extraarticular tenodesis, and slope correcting osteotomy, have become staples of the ACL treatment lexicon. Improvements in rehabilitation protocols and a better understanding of return-to-play criteria have allowed surgeons to return patients to their activities and sports with more confidence. ACL reconstruction in 2024 looks very different than it did ten years ago.

In this issue of *Clinics in Sports Medicine* on "Precision Anterior Cruciate Ligament Reconstruction," Drs Volker Musahl and Alan M.J. Getgood carry on the outstanding legacy of their legendary predecessors, Drs Fu and Fowler, showcasing the significant advancements in ACL surgery. Every aspect of the treatment of ACL injury from the preoperative evaluation to precision primary and revision surgical reconstruction to

Clin Sports Med 43 (2024) xiii–xiv
https://doi.org/10.1016/j.csm.2024.02.002
0278-5919/24/

postoperative rehabilitation is covered by world experts. Ancillary procedures and complications are reviewed in detail as well as the financial implications of ACL surgery. The article in this issue, "Precision Anterior Cruciate Ligament Reconstruction," provides extraordinary insights from two masters in knee surgery, Drs Musahl and Getgood. Ultimately, this issue will help the knee surgeon "get it right" when managing ACL injury.

Sincerely,

F. Winston Gwathmey, MD
Associate Professor of Orthopaedic Surgery
University of Virginia Health System
Charlottesville
Virginia, USA

Vice Chair for Orthopaedic Education and Residency Program Director
Team Physician
UVA and JMU Athletics
Charlottesville, Virginia, USA

E-mail address:
FWG7D@uvahealth.org

Preface

Precision Anterior Cruciate Ligament Reconstruction

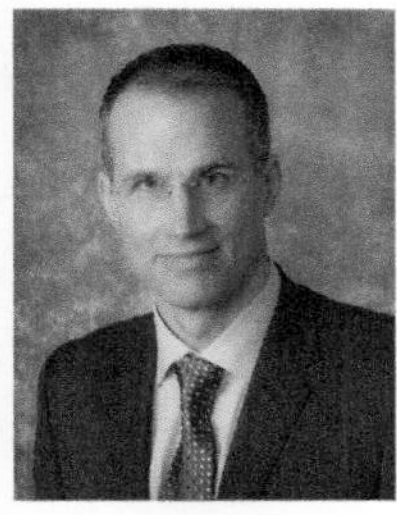

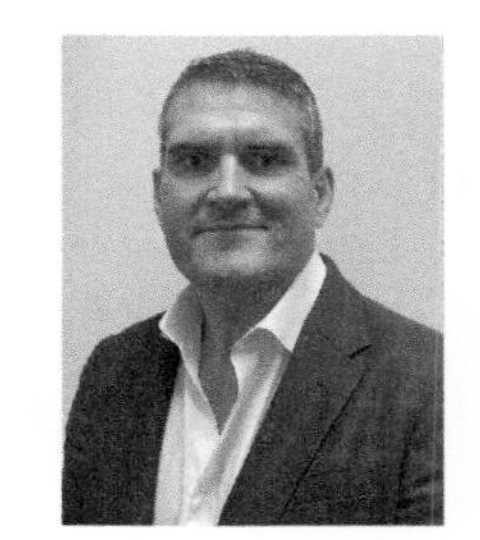

Volker Musahl, MD Alan M.J. Getgood, MD
Editors

In this publication of *Clinics in Sports Medicine*, the reader will find the most relevant topics in anterior cruciate ligament (ACL) and ACL reconstruction. Many world experts are part of this project, which covers a wide array of topics ranging from diagnosis and timing of decision making to treatment options for patients with ACL injury. We would like to thank Sahil Dadoo, BS and Zachary Herrman, MD for their valuable work in editing this fantastic special issue. In particular, the reader will find six articles on surgical techniques for ACL and associated procedures addressing the anteromedial and anterolateral complexes and other soft tissue and bony procedures in primary and revision ACL reconstruction. There is a special focus on tibial osteotomy addressing the tibial slope, a current hot topic of interest to sports medicine surgeons and knee preservation surgeons alike. This special issue will also address sustainability of ACL surgery, which will become more important with time as conservation efforts are being made to preserve the planet. Finally, the reader will be able to find helpful information on complications of ACL surgery and how to avoid them, clinical outcomes, the biological effects of ACL injury, and posttraumatic arthritis. The editors hope that this theme issue of *Clinics in Sports Medicine* will add not only to a complete library in ACL surgery but also to improved treatment for patients. We would like to dedicate this special issue to our mentors, Freddie Fu and Peter Fowler, who were pioneers in ACL and knee surgery.

Conflict of interest/disclosures: V. Musahl: Smith and Nephew, consultant; Newclip, consultant; Ostesys Robotics, stock; NIH, DOD, grant/research support; Ipad Technology, patent, currently not licensed, no royalties. A. Getgood: Smith and

Clin Sports Med 43 (2024) xv–xvi
https://doi.org/10.1016/j.csm.2023.09.002
0278-5919/24/© 2023 Published by Elsevier Inc.

Nephew, consultant and research support; Precision OS, stock; LinkX Robotics, stock; Ostesys Robotics, stock; Spring Loaded Technologies, advisory board and stock.

Volker Musahl, MD
UPMC Freddie Fu Sports Medicine Center
Department of Orthopaedic Surgery
University of Pittsburgh
3200 South Water Street
Pittsburgh, PA 15203, USA

Alan M.J. Getgood, MPhil, MD, FRCS(Tr&Orth)
Fowler Kennedy Sport Medicine Clinic
Western University
3M Centre
London, Ontario N6A 3K7, Canada

E-mail addresses:
musahlv@upmc.edu (V. Musahl)
agetgoo@uwo.ca (A.M.J. Getgood)

Preoperative

Comprehensive Clinical Examination of ACL Injuries

David E. Kantrowitz, MD*, Alexis Colvin, MD

KEYWORDS

• ACL • Knee exam • Anterolateral instability • Lachman • Pivot-shift

KEY POINTS

- A comprehensive clinical examination of the potentially anterior cruciate ligament (ACL)-deficient knee is needed to prompt advanced imaging orders and identify anterior and/or anterolateral rotary instability of the knee, which help inform surgical indications.
- Examination maneuvers vary widely in their accuracy, sensitivity, and specificity. The Lever test, pivot shift, heel height test, and palpation of the anterolateral ligament insertion are all greater than 90% specific for ACL pathology.
- Due to the relatively high coincidence of ACL injuries and those to the posterior cruciate ligament, posterolateral corner, posteromedial corner, and menisci, and the ability of these injuries to alter knee kinematics and increase future graft stress, it is critical that the examiner perform provocative maneuvers to evaluate the integrity of these structures as well.

Video content accompanies this article at http://www.sportsmed.theclinics.com.

INTRODUCTION

Composed of anteromedial and posterolateral bundles, the anterior cruciate ligament (ACL) is the primary restraint to anterior translation of the tibia relative to the femur, and a secondary restraint to tibial rotation and varus and valgus stress. With increasing sports participation, injury awareness, and diagnostic capabilities, the incidence of ACL ruptures has risen to nearly 1 in 1000 people, with up to a quarter-million ACL ruptures occurring annually.[1] Across all age groups, the rate of rupture is nearly 50% greater in males than females, with the peak incidence occurring in males between 19 and 25 years of age, and in females between 14 and 18.[2] During adolescence, female athletes are 1.5 times more likely to sustain an ACL rupture compared to their male counterparts, with multisport female athletes estimated to have as high as a 10%

Department of Orthopedics, The Mount Sinai Hospital, 5 E 98th Street, 9th floor, New York, NY 10029, USA
* Corresponding author.
E-mail address: david.kantrowitz@mountsinai.org

Clin Sports Med 43 (2024) 311–330
https://doi.org/10.1016/j.csm.2023.08.001
0278-5919/24/

risk of ACL rupture during their high school careers.[3] As the number of ACL injuries occurring annually has grown, so concordantly has the rate of ACL reconstruction. Over 130,000 procedures are performed in the United States each year,[4] with a recent increase in the rate of surgical intervention in patients over the age of 40.[5] ACL reconstruction is typically indicated for complete ruptures in young patients and in those with persistent instability, which can lead to knee dysfunction, progressive injury, and osteoarthritis.[6–11] Timely diagnosis of ACL injuries is critical—a process which begins with a comprehensive history and physical examination.

HISTORY TAKING

A patient with an ACL rupture may present acutely, subacutely, or even chronically, and typically recounts a moment of injury during which they heard a "pop," followed by significant swelling and pain. Depending on chronicity, they may complain of instability, which is commonly gesticulated as the "double fist sign," or the patient rubbing their clenched fists together in a circular motion.[12] Elucidating the mechanism of injury can also help guide the differential diagnosis toward ACL pathology. A total of 70% of isolated ACL ruptures occur secondary to noncontact injuries,[13] at the moment when the foot meets the ground during attempted deceleration with the knee extended or minimally flexed, the quadriceps maximally contracted and the hamstrings relaxed, often with the addition of knee valgus, and internal or external rotation.[14] The other 30% that are due to contact injuries typically occur via excessive valgus force applied to the knee.[15]

CLINICAL EXAMINATION

The following subsections represent the authors' recommended approach to examining a knee with suspicion for ACL pathology.

INSPECTION

A thorough clinical examination begins the moment the patient walks into the examination room. ACL ruptures are associated with an antalgic, but specifically quad avoidant, gait, whereby knee flexion is maintained throughout the swing phase of the gait cycle. Increased knee flexion confers greater joint stability in the ACL-deficient knee.[16] The quadriceps and gastrocnemius act as ACL antagonists, as they pull the tibia anteriorly and the femur posteriorly, respectively, which exacerbate the sensation of anterior instability of the tibia. Conversely, the hamstring is an ACL agonist, as it pulls the tibia posteriorly. Patients may have preferentially less quadriceps function and more hamstring function during their gait. In the axial plane, ACL-deficient knee kinematics in the subacute setting also include excessive internal rotation of the tibia during the stance phase.[17] In addition to gait, the knee should be inspected for effusions and evidence of hemarthrosis, which can manifest as a lack of patellar contour, a ballotable knee, or a fluid wave.[12] This examination finding is important, as between 72% and 77% of all acute knee injuries presenting with hemarthrosis and disability are associated with an ACL tear, even in the absence of clinical ligamentous laxity.[18,19] Finally, gross knee alignment can be noted if the patient is able to weightbear.

PALPATION

Following inspection, careful palpation of the knee is recommended. Meniscus tears occur in up to 80% of knees with a concomitant acute ACL rupture and are even higher in frequency in chronic ACL tears. Tears of the lateral meniscus are found in 70% of acute

ACL tears.[20] As a test for isolated lateral meniscus tears, lateral joint line tenderness (LJT) is both highly sensitive (89%) and specific (97%).[21] However, in ACL-deficient knees, LJT is only 46% sensitive and 52% specific for lateral meniscus tears.[22] LJT can also be suggestive of lateral collateral ligament injury, posterolateral corner injury, and lateral bony contusions or cartilage injuries. While less common in ACL tears, medial joint line tenderness can be indicative of medial meniscal tears, medial collateral ligament injury, posteromedial corner injury, and medial bony contusions or cartilage injuries. Tenderness to palpation of the quadriceps tendon, patella, or patellar tendon could indicate extensor mechanism injury. One study of patients with patellar tendon ruptures found an 18% association with ACL rupture.[23] Finally, pain on palpation of the anterolateral ligament (ALL) could be a useful predictor of anterolateral rotatory instability to be discovered later in the examination. Commonly injured in ACL ruptures, the ALL is part of the anterolateral complex of the knee and is a contributor to anterolateral rotatory stability.[24] Injuries to the ALL occur unanimously at the tibial insertion,[25] which is located halfway between the fibular head and Gerdy's tubercle.[26] In a 2020 study of 130 patients with complete, isolated ACL ruptures, pain with palpation of the ALL insertion was 88% sensitive and 97% specific for a positive pivot shift performed under anesthesia.[27]

RANGE OF MOTION

After palpation, the knee should be taken through a range of motion, both actively and passively, measured with a goniometer. Physiologically normal range of motion of the knee is 0° to 140° of flexion, with a 3° to 5° difference attributable to increased age.[28] Patients with acute ACL ruptures may lack flexion due to pain, effusion, and hemarthrosis. A loss of extension is more suggestive of possible ACL pathology due to the torn ACL stump impinging between the tibia and femur thereby blocking full extension and eliciting pain.[29,30] A displaced bucket handle meniscus tear may also limit range of motion.

STRESS TESTING

Varus and valgus stress testing assesses the competency of the collateral ligaments and should be performed as part of every comprehensive physical examination of the knee. Collateral ligament injuries are common in ACL ruptures, with ACL-*medial collateral ligament* (MCL) being the most common multi-ligamentous knee injury pattern. In a recent study of 100 patients with presumed isolated ACL ruptures, the MCL complex was found to be injured in 67%, specifically the superficial MCL in 62%.[31] Conversely, injuries to the lateral collateral ligament (LCL) in the setting of ACL rupture are rare (5%).[32] Of note, collateral ligament injuries concomitant with ACL tears are much less common in patients under the age of 18. In a study of over 500 pediatric patients with ACL tears, 20% were found to have a concomitant MCL tear and 4.5% had an LCL tear.[33] To properly stress the collateral ligaments, the patient should be supine with the examiner stabilizing the knee with one hand and manipulating the lower leg with the other hand at the ankle. The LCL should be stressed by applying a varus force and the MCL by applying a valgus force. Both tests should be conducted in full extension and then again in 30° of flexion. Valgus stress testing has demonstrated a sensitivity between 86% and 96%[34,35] for identifying MCL tears, but varus stress testing only 25% for the diagnosis of LCL tears.[35]

NEUROVASCULAR EXAMINATION

ACL injuries can occur secondary to a variety of mechanisms and levels of energy. High-energy injuries can be associated with multi-ligamentous pathology, dislocations, or neurovascular compromise. ACL ruptures concomitant with other ligamentous injuries are associated with a 14% rate of peroneal nerve injury and a 4% rate of vascular injury. These rates increase to 38% and 18%, respectively, in multiligamentous knee injuries with a dislocation.[36] A careful neurovascular evaluation should therefore be performed during every examination of the knee. Any abnormal findings should be documented pre-operatively and additional workup, such as MRI, electromyography/nerve conduction studies, or computed tomography angiography, ordered as needed.

PROVOCATIVE MANEUVERS

The following sections describe examination maneuvers to test for ACL and concomitant injuries. These maneuvers are often less sensitive and reliable in the office setting acutely following injury, and should be repeated in the operating room under anesthesia. They should also always be compared to the contralateral, uninjured side.

TESTS FOR ACL RUPTURE

Lachman

The ACL is the primary restraint to anterior translation, contributing its greatest strength in partial knee flexion. When the knee is flexed to 30°, the ACL resists 87% of the applied anterior load.[37] First described by Dr Joseph Torg in 1976 and named after Dr John Lachman who famously taught it, the Lachman test capitalizes on the ACL's maximal resistance against anterior translation in slight knee flexion. The test was originally described with the knee in no more than 15° of flexion, pulling the tibia anteriorly while applying posteriorly directed pressure on the femur. A positive result was visual or proprioceptive translation and a "mushy" endpoint.[38] We recommend positioning the patient supine, holding the leg in neutral rotation, flexing the knee to 30°, placing the proximal hand on the femur anteriorly and the distal hand on the tibia posteriorly, and attempting to manually translate the tibia anteriorly (Video 1). Maintaining neutral rotation of the leg is critical to avoid recruitment of other ligamentous stabilizers and place maximum translational burden solely on the ACL.[39] The widely used grading system for this test estimates translation as either less than 5 mm, 5 to 10 mm, or more than 10 mm to give a designation of grade 1, 2, or 3, respectively, and assesses the endpoint as "firm" or "soft," to provide a designation of A or B, respectively. Often considered the most accurate test for ACL injuries, a large 2022 meta-analysis of literature reporting sensitivity and specificity for ACL examination maneuvers demonstrated it is more modest, with sensitivity of 81% and specificity of 85%.[40] Like many of the following provocative maneuvers, the Lachman test is more accurate when performed under anesthesia, being positive in 100% of anesthetized ACL-deficient patients in one classical series.[18] Examiners should beware of potential false-negative and positive results of the Lachman test: bucket handle meniscal tears causing impingement or scarred, chronic ACL or Posterior cruciate ligament (PCL) lesions can limit anterior translation; conversely, PCL rupture resulting in initial posterior subluxation of the tibia can cause a false sense of anterior translation.

Anterior Drawer

Similar to the Lachman test, the anterior drawer stresses the ACL with the knee in flexion, but at 90° rather than 30°. The ACL is a slightly weaker restraint to anterior translation at 90° of flexion, resisting 85% of the applied load.[37] In addition, 90° of flexion allows more engagement of the MCL. In cadaveric studies, sacrificing the

MCL increased anterior translation at 90° of flexion but not at 30°.[41] Despite these biomechanical handicaps, the anterior drawer has advantages over the Lachman test in that it is more feasible to perform on patients with larger thighs, and it has a marginally higher sensitivity of 83%, with equal specificity of 85%.[40] The authors recommend performing the test with the patient supine, the knee flexed to 90°, and the foot flat on the table. The examiner should sit on the foot and wrap both hands around the proximal tibia and attempt to translate it anteriorly (**Fig. 1**), while assessing for translation and the presence of a firm endpoint. Prior to applying an anterior force on the tibia, the authors recommend checking the starting position of the tibia relative to the femur to avoid a false-positive result from preexisting posterior sag. In a normal knee flexed to 90°, the medial tibial plateau should be palpable 1 cm anterior to the femoral condyles.[42] The patient should also be encouraged to relax their hamstrings as much as possible to avoid posterior counter force on the tibia during testing. False negatives of the anterior drawer can be due to hamstring spasm or MCL contribution against anterior translation at 90°. One limitation of the anterior drawer is that it may be difficult to perform in an acutely injured patient with hemarthrosis who has pain and difficulty with flexion to 90°.

Lever Test

Described in 2005 by Dr Alessando Lelli, the lever test is a relatively new clinical maneuver for assessing anterior instability. The test utilizes the extensor mechanism to expose a nonintact ACL. It is performed with the patient supine, the affected leg fully extended and in neutral rotation. The examiner's distal hand is made into a closed fist and placed under the center of the proximal third of the calf. This creates a fulcrum about which the tibia can lever. The examiner's proximal hand is then placed on the quadriceps tendon and downward pressure is applied. This is demonstrated in Video 2. With an intact ACL, the quadriceps force will extend the leg against gravity and the heel will rise off of the examination table. This is a negative test. With a deficient ACL, the proximal tibia will translate anteriorly and the heel will remain on the table. This is a positive result. Multiple studies investigating the efficacy of the lever test for diagnosing ACL rupture have demonstrated sensitivity between 64% and 83% and high specificity between 90% and 100%.[40,43,44] In anesthetized patients, the sensitivity improved to 86%.[43] Advantages of the lever test include the ability to easily perform it regardless of thigh to hand size mismatch, an objective and binary grading

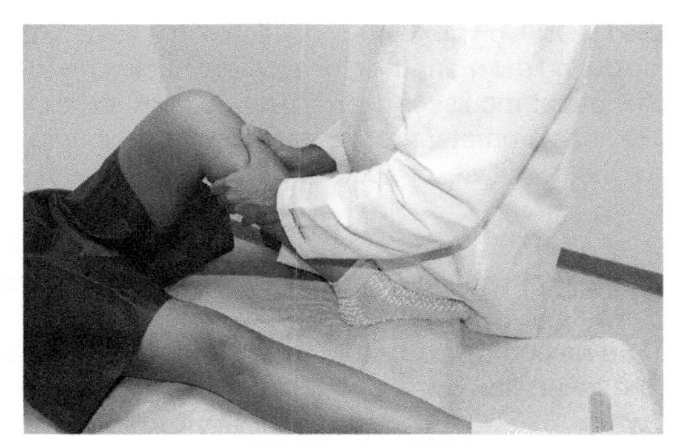

Fig. 1. A demonstration of the anterior drawer. With the patient supine, the knee flexed to 90°, and the foot flat on the table, the examiner sits on the patient's foot and places both hands around the proximal tibia and attempts to translate it anteriorly.

system, and the lack of painful positioning such as deep flexion or knee valgus. One particular limitation of the test is its reliance on an intact extensor mechanism, rendering it nonviable for patients with concurrent quadricep, patellar, or patellar tendon pathology.

Pivot Shift

The pivot shift test demonstrates clinically meaningful anterolateral instability of the tibia with the knee in extension, internal rotation, and valgus, which is subsequently reduced by the iliotibial band (ITB) as the knee moves from extension to flexion. At 30° to 40° of knee flexion, the IT band converts from a knee extensor to a knee flexor and reduces the subluxated anterolateral tibia plateau.[45,46] A positive test is one during which the patient notes a perceptible "clunk" when the tibia moves from a subluxated to reduced position. Notably, the rate of tibial acceleration during the pivot shift is greater in patients more than 1 year post-injury and in those with concomitant lateral meniscus tears.[47] Under anesthesia, the pivot shift test is 81.8% sensitive and 98.4% specific.[48] However, in an awake patient, the test becomes much less sensitive at 55% sensitivity, but similarly specific at 94%.[40] In a series of 37 knees with isolated ACL tears, the pivot shift was positive in only 35% when initially examined at the time of presentation, but 98% positive when the same patients were examined under anesthesia.[49] The large discrepancy in sensitivity of the pivot shift in awake versus anesthetized patients is most likely secondary to discomfort generated by the maneuver which elicits guarding by the patient. A recent 2022 publication aimed at improving the sensitivity of the pivot shift in awake patients recommended 4 modifications to the classic technique, which were "minimizing the sagittal plane arc of motion, avoiding applying valgus force to the knee, application of gentle anteriorly directed force to the lateral tibia, and performing the examination on the patient's non-injured knee first." With these modifications, the pivot shift had a 95.5% accuracy and 94.7% sensitivity in 353 knees examined by 71 clinicians.[50] Our recommendations for the pivot shift is to position the patient supine, place the injured leg in abduction, full extension, and internal rotation, place both hands on the tibia, apply a very slight valgus force to the knee as well as an anterior force to the lower leg when the knee is in initial extension, then slowly flex the knee from 0° to 40° and assess for a "clunk" as the tibia reduces during flexion as the ITB tensions. This technique is demonstrated in Video 3. Maintaining hip abduction results in statistically significantly higher pivot shift grades compared to a neutral or adducted hip, likely due to maintaining ITB relaxation such that the tibia can subluxate anteriorly until knee flexion occurs.[51] False positives of the pivot shift may be secondary to generalized ligamentous laxity, while false negatives can arise with a ruptured ITB which prevents reduction of the tibia, a ruptured MCL which precludes valgus force during the maneuver, or a locked bucket handle meniscus tear or a posterior horn of the lateral meniscus tear.[46] The authors do not recommend using commercially available accelerometers to measure tibial acceleration as they have not been found to improve the sensitivity or accuracy of the pivot shift test.[52]

Jerk Test

Anterolateral rotary instability produced by an incompetent ACL can also be assessed using the Jerk test. Developed by Hughston, this maneuver is similar to the pivot shift, but instead moves from flexion to extension. The examiner stands at the side of the supine patient with the knee flexed to 90° and internally rotates the leg as the knee is slowly extended while an abduction stress is applied. This is demonstrated in Video 4. A positive result is instability perceived by the patient at roughly 30° of knee flexion as the proximal tibia subluxates anteriorly as the ITB converts to a knee extensor.[53]

Losee Test

The test for anterolateral rotary instability is another useful maneuver for examining the possibly ACL-deficient knee. The Losee test is performed with the examiner at the supine patient's side with the foot in the examiner's distal hand, the leg initially in external rotation, and the knee flexed to 30°. A valgus force is applied using the examiner's abdomen as a fulcrum, and the knee is slowly extended and internally rotated while the examiner's proximal hand is placed palm down over the patella and the thumb is used to drive the fibula anteriorly. This is demonstrated in Video 5. A positive result is the recognition of anterior instability of the tibia by the patient as the knee comes just short of full extension.[54]

KT-1000 and Other Instrumented Examinations

Manual clinical tests for anterior translation such as the Lachman and anterior drawer have inherent variability in the magnitude, direction, and rate of anterior force applied by the examiner, which decrease their generalizability and standardization.[55] For this reason, instrumented manual tests, such as the KT-1000 and KT-2000 were invented to help objectively measure anterior translation. These devices are highly sensitive to increases in anterior translation, however, they too suffer from inter-examiner variability (inter-tester ICC 81%–86%). Adding the use of a rotational laximeter, or torque application device, to the KT-1000 to control for secondary ligament tension when in external or internal rotation can increase the inter-rater ICC to as high as 98%.[56] While their precision is noteworthy, the authors do not recommend the routine use of instrumented tests in the standard examination of a suspected ACL injury.

TESTS FOR PCL RUPTURE

PCL tears can occur in up to 44% of acute knee injuries.[57] PCL injury concomitant with ACL rupture is a rare phenomenon, typically occurring in the setting of high-energy trauma with or without a knee dislocation. In more than 100 patients presenting to a level 1 trauma center with multi-ligamentous knee injuries, the most common pattern—seen in nearly 50% of patients—involved simultaneous ACL, PCL, and posterolateral corner pathologies. For this reason, it is important for the orthopedic clinician to assess the integrity of the PCL when examining a patient in whom an ACL rupture is suspected.

Posterior Drawer

The PCL resists 85% of posterior-directed force with the knee flexed to 30°, and 100% at 90°.[58] With the leg in neutral rotation, the knee should be flexed to 90° and the examiner should begin by assessing the starting point of the tibia relative to the femur from the lateral perspective. The medial tibial plateau should be roughly 1 cm anterior to the medial femoral condyle.[42] If the proximal tibia of the affected side lies more posterior to the femur than on the unaffected side, this is deemed a positive "posterior sag sign." The posterior sag sign is 79% sensitive and 100% specific for diagnosing chronic PCL-deficient knees.[59] Following inspection, the examiner sits on the patient's foot and grasps the proximal tibia with both hands to apply a posteriorly directed force (**Fig. 2**), while assessing for endpoint and degree of translation. The posterior drawer is 90% sensitive and 99% specific for the diagnosis of isolated posterior laxity.[59] However, intact secondary stabilizers have the potential to obscure a soft end point.

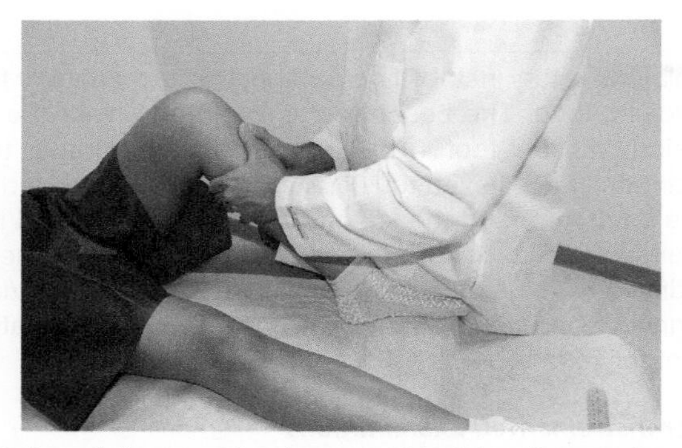

Fig. 2. A demonstration of the posterior drawer. With the patient supine, the knee flexed to 90°, and the foot flat on the table, the examiner sits on the patient's foot and places both hands around the proximal tibia and attempts to translate it posteriorly.

Posterior Lachman

The posterior variant of the classic Lachman maneuver can be used as an alternative to the posterior drawer test. While the PCL resists less posterior force at 30° of knee flexion, the test has the advantage of requiring less knee flexion which can often be uncomfortable, or even impossible, for patients with acute ligamentous knee injuries. The test begins the same as the Lachman test (Video 1), with the patient supine, the leg in neutral rotation, and the examiner with one hand on the distal femur and one on the proximal tibia. The tibia is then translated posteriorly and its excursion and end point is assessed. The sensitivity and specificity of the test for posterior laxity is 62% and 89%, respectively.[59] It is important to note the difference in translation between the posterior Lachman and the posterior drawer, as increased laxity in 30° of flexion compared to 90° can indicate the presence of a posterolateral corner (PLC) injury.

Quadriceps Active Test

The quadriceps active test utilizes the extensor mechanism to produce anterior translation that is apparent in a PCL-deficient knee due to the initial posterior subluxation of the tibia. With the patient supine on the examination table, the examiner flexes the knee to 90° and places the foot flat on the table. The examiner places a hand on the anterior distal tibia and applies counter force as the patient attempts to slide their foot forward; the proximal tibia is observed for anterior translation (**Fig. 3**). The test is considered positive if the proximal tibia demonstrates visible anterior translation, originally quantified as 2 mm or more.[60] The test is 98% sensitive in an unrandomized and unblinded study of 42 knees with PCL tears.[59,60]

POSTEROLATERAL CORNER INJURY

The PLC includes the LCL, popliteofibular ligament, popliteus tendon, fabellofibular ligament, arcuate ligament, lateral joint capsule, anterolateral ligament, lateral coronary ligament, biceps femoris, lateral gastrocnemius tendon, and the distal iliotibial band. Isolated posterolateral corner injuries are rare, occurring in only a quarter of all PLC injuries.[61] However, the PLC is often concomitantly injured with the ACL. In a retrospective review of patients with PLC injuries, 60% also had an injury to the ACL.[62] Given that untreated high-grade PLC injuries yield poor outcomes and the coincidence of PLC and ACL pathologies is significant, it is imperative that the examiner be familiar with the maneuvers for posterolateral instability.

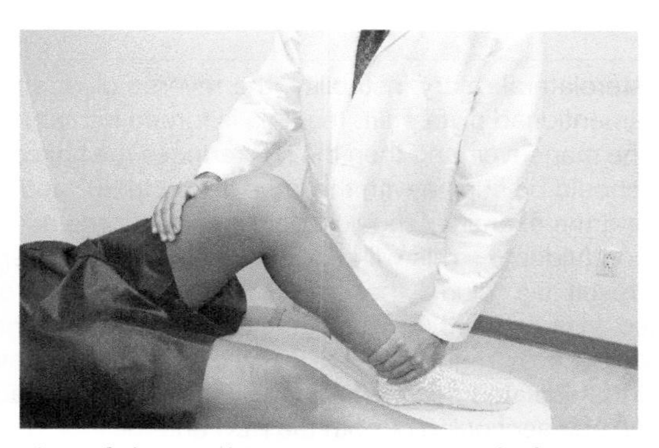

Fig. 3. A demonstration of the quadriceps active test. With the patient supine, the knee flexed to 90°, and the foot flat on the examination table, the examiner places a hand on the anterior distal tibia and applies counter force as the patient attempts to slide their foot forward; the proximal tibia is observed for anterior translation.

Dial Test

The dial test evaluates rotational instability in the setting of a PLC injury.[63] The test is conducted with the patient either supine or prone and the knees together in full adduction. Both knees are flexed to 30° initially, then to 90°. The examiner holds both feet and the lower leg is maximally externally rotated and the thigh foot angle of each leg is measured (**Fig. 4**). A positive result is increased side-to-side difference (SSD) in external rotation between the affected leg and the contralateral side; grade I is 0° to 5°, grade II is 5° to 10°, and grade III is greater than 10°.[64] A positive result at 30° of knee flexion implies a PLC injury, while an additionally positive result at 90° implies combined PLC and PCL pathologies.[65] For diagnosing isolated PLC injuries, the dial test with an SSD cutoff of 10° has modest sensitivity of 20% but robust specificity of 100%.[66] The positive predictive value (PPV) of the test for an isolated PLC injury is 100%. In non-isolated PLC disruptions with concomitant PCL rupture, the accuracy of the test can be improved by applying an anterior force on the tibia to maintain reduction while external rotation is assessed.[67]

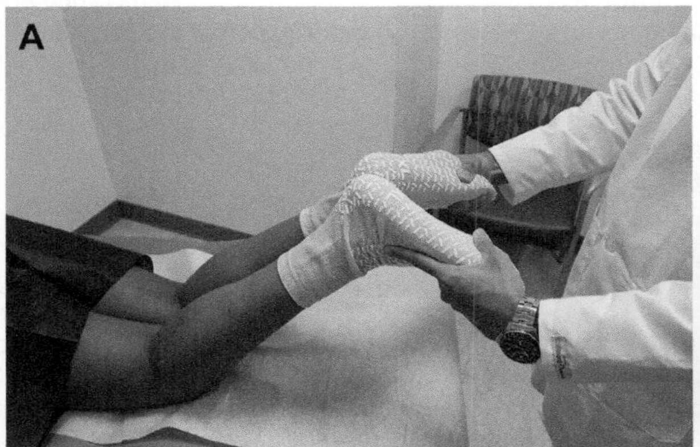

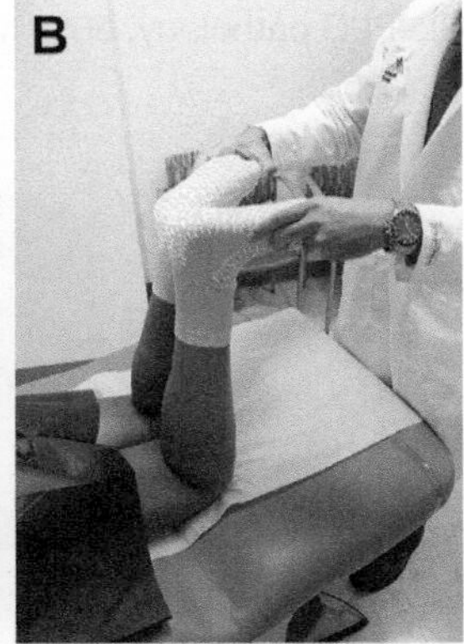

Fig. 4. A demonstration of the dial test. With the patient prone and the knees together in full adduction, the examiner holds both feet and maximally externally rotates the lower leg and measures the thigh foot angle of each leg. This is done at 30° (*A*) and then 90° (*B*).

Reverse Pivot Shift

Another test for posterolateral rotary instability, the reverse pivot shift is conceptually identical to the aforementioned pivot shift: the tibia is forced into a position of subluxation at the onset of the maneuver, and then the ITB reduces the tibia at the 30° to 40° of flexion. The patient should be supine with the knee flexed to 90° and the leg maximally externally rotated, and the examiner should apply a valgus force as the knee is slowly brought into extension (Video 6). This will exacerbate the posterolateral subluxation of the tibia. A positive result is a "clunk" that occurs with the reduction of the tibia during extension of the knee. In isolated PLC injuries, the reverse pivot shift has demonstrated a PPV of 68% and a negative predictive value (NPV) of 89%.[68] A cadaveric study, however, demonstrated that isolated sectioning of the PLC had no impact on the reverse pivot shift. Only combined sectioning of both the PLC and the PCL produced a positive result on the reverse pivot shift test.[69] Of note, the test can also be positive in as much as 35% of physiologically normal knees when examined under anesthesia,[70] highlighting the importance of examining the unaffected side.

POSTEROLATERAL DRAWER

The posterolateral drawer is another test which identifies posterolateral rotary instability, with a PPV of 69% and NPV of 100%.[68] The test begins with the same set up as the anterior/posterior drawer maneuvers, with the patient supine, the knee flexed to 90°, and the examiner sitting on the patient's foot. The lower leg is then maximally externally rotated, and a posteriorly directed force is applied to the proximal tibia (**Fig. 5**). The test is considered positive if the degree of external rotation increases as posterior force is applied.

External Rotation Recurvatum

The external rotation recurvatum (ERR) test is conducted with the patient supine, the legs adducted, and the examiner at the end of the table elevating both legs by grasping the patient's great toes (**Fig. 6**). The test is positive if the knee falls into varus, external rotation and recurvatum. Previous studies had reported good sensitivity of the test near 80%,[71] and a PPV and NPV of 71% and 94%, respectively.[68] However, in a more recent series of 134 patients with PLC injuries, the test was positive in only 7.5%, and all of these patients had concomitant ACL tears. Of the patients in the study with combined ACL–PLC pathology, 30% had a positive ERR test.[71] A modification of the ERR test is

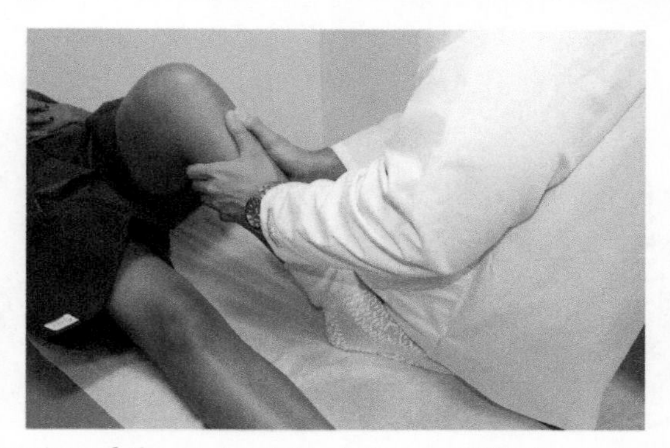

Fig. 5. A demonstration of the posterolateral drawer. With the patient supine, the knee flexed to 90°, and the lower leg is maximally externally rotated, the examiner sits on the patient's foot and applies a posteriorly directed force to the proximal tibia.

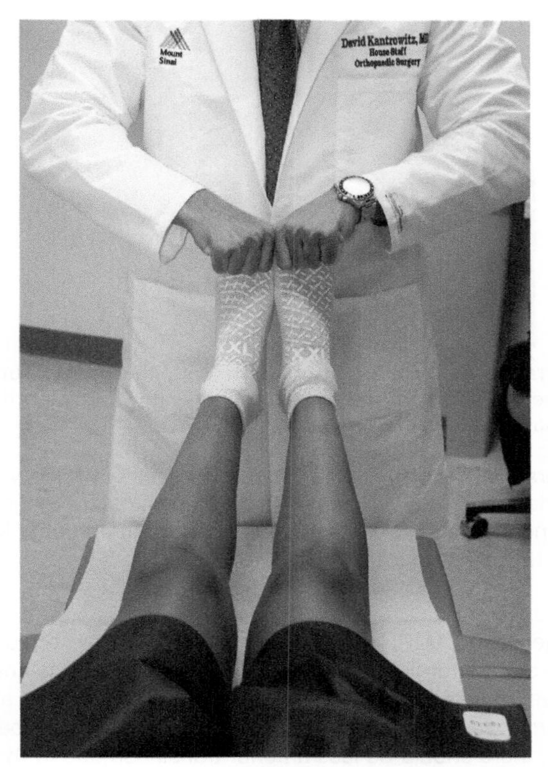

Fig. 6. A demonstration of the external rotation recurvatum test. With the patient supine and the legs adducted, the examiner elevates both legs by grasping the patient's great toes from the end of the table.

the heel height test, in which the patient is supine with the leg extended and stabilized in neutral rotation with the examiner's proximal hand pushing downward on the thigh, while the examiner's distal hand lifts the foot off the table via the great toe (**Fig. 7**). A positive result is a greater height between the table and the heel on the affected side compared to the contralateral side. A recent study examining this test in a large series of patients found that a SSD in heel height of 3 cm or greater was present in 8.2% of the patients with an isolated ACL tear and 72% of the patients with combined ACL–PLC pathology. The sensitivity and specificity of this test for diagnosing combined ACL–PLC injuries are 72% and 92%, respectively.[72] For this reason, the authors highly recommend performing the heel height test in addition to the classic ERR maneuver.

POSTEROMEDIAL CORNER INJURY

The posteromedial corner (PMC) is composed of 5 principle components: the semimembranosus tendon and its expansion, oblique popliteal ligament, posterior oblique ligament, posteromedial joint capsule (which contains the deep MCL), and posterior horn of medial meniscus. Disruption of the PMC can result in anteromedial rotatory instability (AMRI) which is excessive external rotation and anterior translation of the medial tibia plateau relative to the femur, and medial joint space laxity.[73] While ACL ruptures with simultaneous PMC injuries are rare, it is important to recognize the presence of a PMC injury in ACL-deficient patients as the PMC is a secondary stabilizer

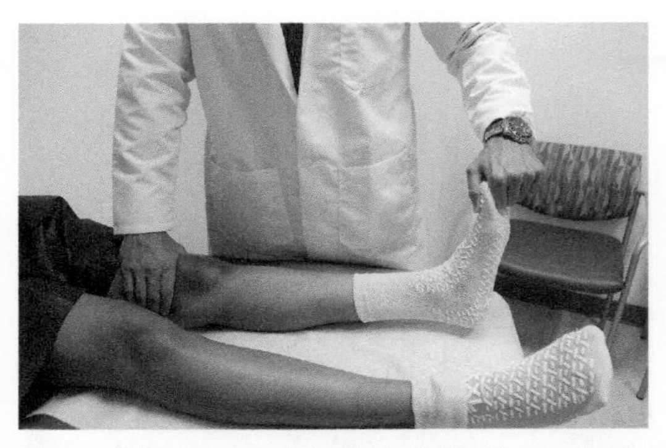

Fig. 7. A demonstration of the heel height test. With the patient supine and the leg extended and in neutral rotation, the examiner pushes downward on the thigh and lifts the foot off the examination table via the great toe.

against anterior translation of the tibia in an ACL-deficient knee when the knee is flexed and externally rotated.[74] Moreover, untreated posteromedial corner injuries biomechanically increase the force seen by the ACL graft and alter knee kinematics, which could lead to increased rates of graft rupture.[75]

Slocum Test

The key test for identifying AMRI is the Slocum test. The test is conducted in the same positioning as the anterior drawer, with the patient supine and the knee flexed to 90°. The anterior drawer is first conducted (Video 1), and translation is appreciated. The tibia is then externally rotated 30° and the anterior drawer is repeated (**Fig. 8**). If the PMC is intact, there should be less anterior translation due to the restraint of the PMC when the tibia is in external rotation. Lack of diminished anterior translation indicates PMC injury. In ACL-deficient knees, the Slocum test is 90% sensitive and 100% specific for diagnosing a PMC injury.[76]

MENISCUS INJURY

Meniscal tears are found in up to 79% of knees with an acute ACL rupture, and 85% of chronically ACL-deficient knees.[20] In addition to palpation of the joint line, the

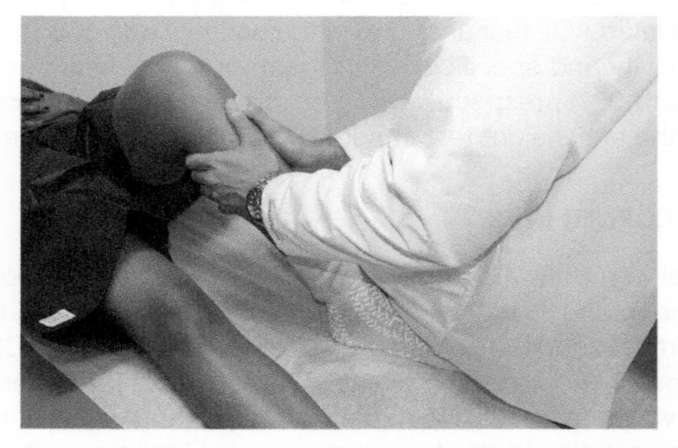

Fig. 8. A demonstration of the Slocum test. With the patient supine, the knee flexed to 90°, and the tibia externally rotated 30°, the examiner sits on the patient's foot and attempts to translate the tibia anteriorly.

following tests are also clinically useful for identifying meniscal injuries and should be performed by the examiner.

McMurray

McMurray's test uses varus and valgus stress along with rotation of the tibia to compress the menisci between the tibial plateau and the femoral condyles and elicit pain. The patient should be positioned supine with the examiner at the patient's affected side. The patient's knee is hyper-flexed past 90° at the onset. With one hand controlling the knee and the other hand on the foot, the examiner slowly extends the knee while externally rotating the tibia and applying a valgus force to evaluate for medial meniscus tears. The knee is then brought back to the hyper-flexed starting position and extension is repeated but with internal tibial rotation and varus force to test the lateral meniscus. This is demonstrated in Video 7. A positive test is the presence of pain or a clicking sound. The test has modest sensitivity, ranging between 34.3% and 71.9% in several studies, and robust specificity, between 86.4% and 93.4%.[77–79]

Apley

The Apley test utilizes compression and rotation to induce meniscal impingement. The patient is positioned prone with the bilateral knees flexed to 90°. The examiner stabilizes the thigh by placing his or her knee on the patient's posterior thigh. The ankle is held with both hands just above the malleoli and the lower leg is internally and externally rotated while simultaneously distracting the knee joint; this process is then repeated with compression of the joint (Video 8). If pain is greater with compression compared to distraction, the test is considered positive. The Apley test has demonstrated sensitivity between 68.7% and 83.7% and specificity between 70.4% and 71.4%.[77,80] The test is not statistically significantly more accurate than McMurray's test.[77]

Thessaly

The Thessaly test requires the patient to weight bear on the affected extremity, which may be difficult in the setting of acute rupture. The patient stands on 1 leg with the examiner holding their outstretched hands for support. The patient flexes the knee first to 5° (**Fig. 9**A), and then to 20° (**Fig. 9**B), and rotates their torso and knee internally and externally 3 times each (Video 9). The test is considered positive if the patient experiences pain, catching, or locking. In its initial description, the test demonstrated diagnostic accuracy of 90% and 96% for the diagnosis of a lateral meniscus tear at 5° and 20° of flexion, respectively.[81] In subsequent validations of the Thessaly test at 20° of knee flexion, it has demonstrated sensitivity of roughly 90% and specificity between 90.7% and 97.7%.[77,82] In one study, the maneuver was statistically significantly more accurate than the McMurray and Apley tests, and statistically equivocal to MRI for the diagnosis of meniscus tears confirmed arthroscopically.[77]

DISCUSSION

A comprehensive clinical examination for a potential ACL injury includes the following: inspection of the knee, particularly for effusion and quad avoidance gait; palpation, particularly of the lateral joint line and anterolateral ligament insertion; range of motion; varus and valgus stress testing; neurovascular examination; and finally provocative maneuvers. To evaluate the competency of the ACL, the authors recommend performing the Lachman, anterior drawer, and lever test to assess for anterior translation, with the lever test being the most highly specific of these maneuvers.

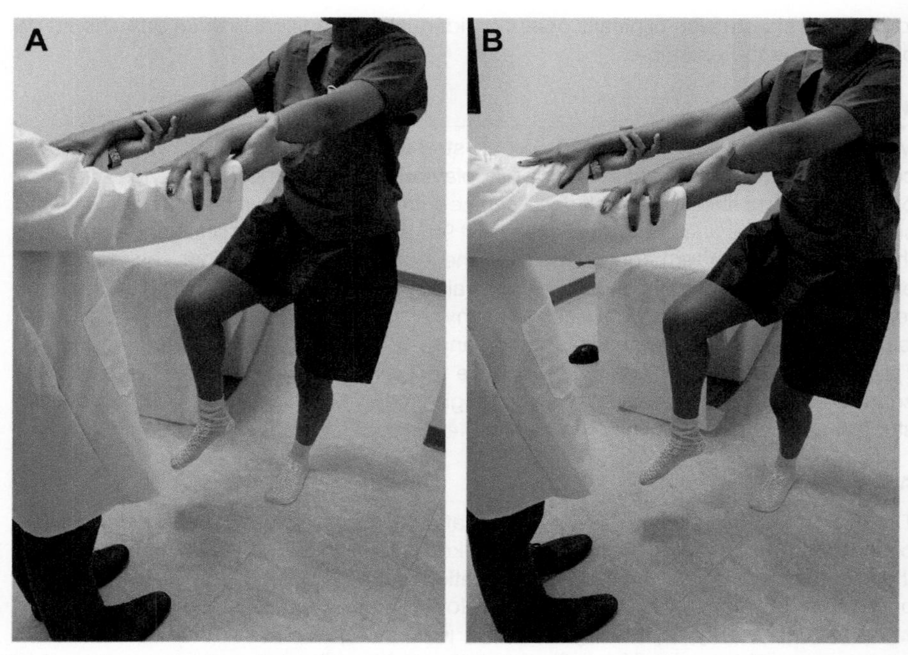

Fig. 9. A demonstration of the Thessaly test. With the patient standing on 1 leg and holding the examiner's outstretched hands for support, the knee is flexed first to 5° (*A*) and then to 20° (*B*).

The authors recommend performing the pivot shift to elucidate anterolateral rotary instability. Bates and colleagues' low-profile modifications to the pivot shift, which include limiting the flexion-extension arc of motion, eliminating painful valgus stress, and applying an anterior force on the proximal tibia to encourage initial subluxation have the ability to significantly enhance the pivot shift's sensitivity in awake patients, which is a classical shortcoming of the maneuver.[50] Accelerometers and the KT-1000 and 2000 are useful adjuncts, but are not standardly recommended in the routine examination of possible ACL injuries.

Due to the relatively high coincidence of ACL injuries and those to the PCL, PLC, PMC, and menisci, and the ability of these injuries to alter knee kinematics and graft stress, it is critical that the examiner perform provocative maneuvers to evaluate the integrity of these structures as well. Of these additional tests, the heel height test is particularly useful, as it is highly specific for combined ACL–PLC injuries.[72] When examining for meniscal injuries, the authors encourage the use of the Thessaly test as it is statistically significantly more accurate than the McMurray and Apley, and statistically equivocal to MRI for the diagnosis of meniscus tears.[77]

SUMMARY

A comprehensive clinical examination of the potentially ACL-deficient knee includes examination of the contralateral healthy knee and should proceed as follows: inspection; palpation; range of motion; varus and valgus stress; neurovascular status; and finally provocative maneuvers. The Lachman, anterior drawer, Lever, and pivot shift tests are all greater than 90% specific for ACL pathology. Due to the relatively high coincidence of ACL injuries and those to the PCL, PLC, PMC, and menisci, it is critical that the examiner perform provocative maneuvers to evaluate the integrity of these structures as well.

CLINICS CARE POINTS

- Elicit a thorough history from the patient, specifically regarding the mechanism and moment of injury.
- Non-contact pivoting injuries and valgus blows are classic for ACL injuries.
- Assess the patient's gait for a quad-avoidant pattern, which is common in ACL-deficient knees.
- Inspect the knee carefully for effusion or hemarthrosis. Three out of four acute knee injuries associated with hemarthrosis and disability will have an ACL rupture.
- Palpate all bony landmarks, specifically the lateral joint line and the ALL insertion.
- The ALL inserts halfway between the fibular head and Gerdy's tubercle; pain on palpation is 97% specific for anterolateral rotary instability.
- Conduct a complete neurovascular examination. ACL ruptures in the setting of multi-ligamentous injuries or dislocations are often associated with peroneal nerve injury.
- Bucket handle meniscal tears or ACL or PCL cyclops lesions can create a false- negative result of the Lachman test.
- PCL rupture causing initial posterior subluxation of the tibia can cause a false positive.
- Always check the resting starting position of the tibia relative to the femur prior to conducting an anterior or posterior drawer.
- In a normal knee flexed to 90°, the medial tibial plateau should be 1 cm anterior to the femoral condyles.
- The Lever test has excellent sensitivity and specificity for ACL ruptures in awake patients.
- The pivot shift test is classically insensitive for diagnosing anterolateral instability in awake patients due to the discomfort associated with the maneuver.
- Minimizing sagittal plane arc of motion, avoiding excessive valgus force, applying gentle anteriorly directed force to the lateral tibia. and performing the test on the uninjured side first can improve its sensitivity to greater than 90%.
- Sixty% of all posterolateral corner injuries occur with a concomitant ACL injury.
- The heel height test is 92% specific for diagnosing combined ACL–PCL pathology.
- The Slocum test is 90% sensitive and 100% specific for diagnosing a PMC injury in the setting of an ACL rupture.
- Meniscal tears can be found in 80% or more of ACL-deficient knees.
- Lateral joint line tenderness is highly sensitive and specific for isolated lateral meniscal tears but decreases in accuracy in the setting of ACL rupture.
- The McMurray and Apley tests are statistically equivocal to one another.
- The Thessaly test is greater than 90% sensitive and specific for meniscal tears and should be performed if the patient is able to weightbear on the affected extremity.

ACKNOWLEDGMENTS

The authors would like to acknowledge Thomas Boucher, MD, and Hulaimatu Jalloh, MD for their contributions.

DISCLOSURE

The authors have nothing to disclose.

SUPPLEMENTARY DATA

Supplementary data related to this article can be found online at https://doi.org/10.1016/j.csm.2023.08.001.

REFERENCES

1. Carbone A, Rodeo S. Review of current understanding of post-traumatic osteoarthritis resulting from sports injuries: REVIEW OF UNDERSTANDING OF PTOA FROM SPORTS INJURIES. J Orthop Res 2017;35(3):397–405.
2. Sanders TL, Maradit Kremers H, Bryan AJ, et al. Incidence of Anterior Cruciate Ligament Tears and Reconstruction: A 21-Year Population-Based Study. Am J Sports Med 2016;44(6):1502–7.
3. Bram JT, Magee LC, Mehta NN, et al. Anterior Cruciate Ligament Injury Incidence in Adolescent Athletes: A Systematic Review and Meta-analysis. Am J Sports Med 2021;49(7):1962–72.
4. Buller LT, Best MJ, Baraga MG, et al. Trends in Anterior Cruciate Ligament Reconstruction in the United States. Orthop J Sports Med 2015;3(1). 2325967114563664.
5. Mall NA, Chalmers PN, Moric M, et al. Incidence and trends of anterior cruciate ligament reconstruction in the United States. Am J Sports Med 2014;42(10):2363–70.
6. Segawa H, Omori G, Koga Y. Long-term results of non-operative treatment of anterior cruciate ligament injury. Knee 2001;8(1):5–11.
7. Barenius B, Ponzer S, Shalabi A, et al. Increased risk of osteoarthritis after anterior cruciate ligament reconstruction: a 14-year follow-up study of a randomized controlled trial. Am J Sports Med 2014;42(5):1049–57.
8. Lohmander LS, Ostenberg A, Englund M, et al. High prevalence of knee osteoarthritis, pain, and functional limitations in female soccer players twelve years after anterior cruciate ligament injury. Arthritis Rheum 2004;50(10):3145–52.
9. Kessler MA, Behrend H, Henz S, et al. Function, osteoarthritis and activity after ACL-rupture: 11 years follow-up results of conservative versus reconstructive treatment. Knee Surg Sports Traumatol Arthrosc Off J ESSKA 2008;16(5):442–8.
10. Mihelic R, Jurdana H, Jotanovic Z, et al. Long-term results of anterior cruciate ligament reconstruction: a comparison with non-operative treatment with a follow-up of 17–20 years. Int Orthop 2011;35(7):1093–7.
11. Cheung EC, DiLallo M, Feeley BT, et al. Osteoarthritis and ACL Reconstruction—Myths and Risks. Curr Rev Musculoskelet Med 2020;13(1):115–22.
12. Cimino F, Volk BS, Setter D. Anterior Cruciate Ligament Injury: Diagnosis, Management, and Prevention. Am Fam Physician 2010;82(8):917–22.
13. McNair PJ, Marshall RN, Matheson JA. Important features associated with acute anterior cruciate ligament injury. N Z Med J 1990;103(901):537–9.
14. Shimokochi Y, Shultz SJ. Mechanisms of Noncontact Anterior Cruciate Ligament Injury. J Athl Train 2008;43(4):396–408.
15. Boden BP, Dean GS, Feagin JA, et al. Mechanisms of Anterior Cruciate Ligament Injury. Orthopedics 2000;23(6):573–8.
16. Sharifi M, Shirazi-Adl A. Knee flexion angle and muscle activations control the stability of an anterior cruciate ligament deficient joint in gait. J Biomech 2021;117. 110258.

17. Shabani B, Bytyqi D, Lustig S, et al. Gait changes of the ACL-deficient knee 3D kinematic assessment. Knee Surg Sports Traumatol Arthrosc 2015;23(11):3259–65.
18. Dehaven KE. Diagnosis of acute knee injuries with hemarthrosis. Am J Sports Med 1980;8(1):9–14.
19. Hardaker WT, Garrett WE, Bassett FH. Evaluation of acute traumatic hemarthrosis of the knee joint. South Med J 1990;83(6):640–4.
20. Hagino T, Ochiai S, Senga S, et al. Meniscal tears associated with anterior cruciate ligament injury. Arch Orthop Trauma Surg 2015;135(12):1701–6.
21. Eren OT. The accuracy of joint line tenderness by physical examination in the diagnosis of meniscal tears. Arthrosc J Arthrosc Relat Surg 2003;19(8):850–4.
22. Shelbourne KD, Benner RW. Correlation of Joint Line Tenderness and Meniscus Pathology in Patients with Subacute and Chronic Anterior Cruciate Ligament Injuries. J Knee Surg 2009;22(3):187–90.
23. McKinney B, Cherney S, Penna J. Intra-articular knee injuries in patients with knee extensor mechanism ruptures. Knee Surg Sports Traumatol Arthrosc 2008;16(7):633–8.
24. Murgier J, Devitt B, Sevre J, et al. The Origin of the Knee Anterolateral Ligament Discovery. A Translation of Segond's Original Work With Commentary. Arthrosc J Arthrosc Relat Surg 2019;35. https://doi.org/10.1016/j.arthro.2018.10.003.
25. Faruch Bilfeld M, Cavaignac E, Wytrykowski K, et al. Anterolateral ligament injuries in knees with an anterior cruciate ligament tear: Contribution of ultrasonography and MRI. Eur Radiol 2018;28(1):58–65.
26. Claes S, Vereecke E, Maes M, et al. Anatomy of the anterolateral ligament of the knee. J Anat 2013;223(4):321–8.
27. Murgier J, Thomas P, Reina N, et al. Painful Palpation of the Tibial Insertion of the Anterolateral Ligament Is Concordant With Acute Anterolateral Ligament Injury. Orthop J Sports Med 2020;8(6). 2325967120930200.
28. Roach KE, Miles TP. Normal Hip and Knee Active Range of Motion: The Relationship to Age. Phys Ther 1991;71(9):656–65.
29. Shelbourne KD, Rowdon GA. Anterior Cruciate Ligament Injury. Sports Med 1994;17(2):132–40.
30. McMahon PJ, Dettling JR, Yocum LA, et al. The Cyclops Lesion: A Cause of Diminished Knee Extension After Rupture of the Anterior Cruciate Ligament. Arthrosc J Arthrosc Relat Surg 1999;15(7):757–61.
31. Willinger L, Balendra G, Pai V, et al. High incidence of superficial and deep medial collateral ligament injuries in 'isolated' anterior cruciate ligament ruptures: a long overlooked injury. Knee Surg Sports Traumatol Arthrosc 2022;30(1):167–75.
32. Temponi EF, de Carvalho Júnior LH, Saithna A, et al. Incidence and MRI characterization of the spectrum of posterolateral corner injuries occurring in association with ACL rupture. Skeletal Radiol 2017;46(8):1063–70.
33. Lee RJ, Margalit A, Nduaguba A, et al. Risk Factors for Concomitant Collateral Ligament Injuries in Children and Adolescents With Anterior Cruciate Ligament Tears. Orthop J Sports Med 2018;6(11). 2325967118810389.
34. Garvin GJ, Munk PL, Vellet AD. Tears of the medial collateral ligament: magnetic resonance imaging findings and associated injuries. Can Assoc Radiol J J Assoc Can Radiol 1993;44(3):199–204.
35. Harilainen A. Evaluation of knee instability in acute ligamentous injuries. Ann Chir Gynaecol 1987;76(5):269–73.

36. Kahan JB, Schneble CA, Li D, et al. Increased Neurovascular Morbidity Is Seen in Documented Knee Dislocation Versus Multiligamentous Knee Injury. JBJS 2021; 103(10):921.
37. Butler DL, Noyes FR, Grood ES. Ligamentous restraints to anterior-posterior drawer in the human knee. A biomechanical study. JBJS 1980;62(2):259.
38. Torg JS, Conrad W, Kalen V. Clinical I diagnosis of anterior cruciate ligament instability in the athlete. Am J Sports Med 1976;4(2):84–93.
39. Markolf KL, Burchfield DM, Shapiro MM, et al. Biomechanical Consequences of Replacement of the Anterior Cruciate Ligament with a Patellar Ligament Allograft. Part I: Insertion of the Graft and Anterior-Posterior Testing. JBJS 1996;78(11): 1720.
40. Sokal PA, Norris R, Maddox TW, et al. The diagnostic accuracy of clinical tests for anterior cruciate ligament tears are comparable but the Lachman test has been previously overestimated: a systematic review and meta-analysis. Knee Surg Sports Traumatol Arthrosc 2022;30(10):3287–303.
41. Haimes JL, Wroble RR, Grood ES, et al. Role of the Medial Structures in the intact and Anterior Cruciate Ligament-Deficient Knee: Limits of Motion in the Human Knee. Am J Sports Med 1994;22(3):402–9.
42. Malanga GA, Andrus S, Nadler SF, et al. Physical examination of the knee: A review of the original test description and scientific validity of common orthopedic tests. Arch Phys Med Rehabil 2003;84(4):592–603.
43. Jarbo KA, Hartigan DE, Scott KL, et al. Accuracy of the Lever Sign Test in the Diagnosis of Anterior Cruciate Ligament Injuries. Orthop J Sports Med 2017; 5(10). 2325967117729809.
44. Sobrado MF, Bonadio MB, Ribeiro GF, et al. LEVER SIGN TEST FOR CHRONIC ACL INJURY: A COMPARISON WITH LACHMAN AND ANTERIOR DRAWER TESTS. Acta Ortopédica Bras 2021;29:132–6.
45. Galway HR, Macintosh DL. The Lateral Pivot Shift: A Symptom and Sign of Anterior Cruciate Ligament Insufficiency. Clin Orthop Relat Res 1980;147:45.
46. Lubowitz JH, Bernardini BJ, Reid JB. Current Concepts Review: Comprehensive Physical Examination for Instability of the Knee. Am J Sports Med 2008;36(3): 577–94.
47. Nishida K, Matsushita T, Hoshino Y, et al. The Influences of Chronicity and Meniscal Injuries on Pivot Shift in Anterior Cruciate Ligament–Deficient Knees: Quantitative Evaluation Using an Electromagnetic Measurement System. Arthrosc J Arthrosc Relat Surg 2020;36(5):1398–406.
48. Katz JW, Fingeroth RJ. The diagnostic accuracy of ruptures of the anterior cruciate ligament comparing the Lachman test, the anterior drawer sign, and the pivot shift test in acute and chronic knee injuries. Am J Sports Med 1986;14(1):88–91.
49. Donaldson WF, Warren RF, Wickiewicz T. A comparison of acute anterior cruciate ligament examinations. Initial versus examination under anesthesia. Am J Sports Med 1985;13(1):5–10.
50. Bates B, Albright J, Methenitis A, et al. Low-Profile Modifications of the Losee Pivot Shift Test for Assessment of an ACL-Deficient Knee in the Awake Patient. Video J Sports Med 2022;2(6). 263502542211225.
51. Bach BR, Warren RF, Wickiewicz TL. The pivot shift phenomenon: Results and description of a modified clinical test for anterior cruciate ligament insufficiency. Am J Sports Med 1988;16(6):571–6.
52. Napier RJ, Feller JA, Devitt BM, et al. Is the KiRA Device Useful in Quantifying the Pivot Shift in Anterior Cruciate Ligament–Deficient Knees? Orthop J Sports Med 2021;9(1). 232596712097786.

53. Hughston JC, Andrews JR, Cross MJ, et al. Classification of knee ligament instabilities. Part II. The lateral compartment. JBJS 1976;58(2):173.
54. Losee RE, Johnson TR, Southwick WO. Anterior subluxation of the lateral tibial plateau. A diagnostic test and operative repair. JBJS 1978;60(8):1015.
55. Branch TP, Mayr HO, Browne JE, et al. Instrumented Examination of Anterior Cruciate Ligament Injuries: Minimizing Flaws of the Manual Clinical Examination. Arthrosc J Arthrosc Relat Surg 2010;26(7):997–1004.
56. Mayr H. Manual measurement of rotational stability with new KT device. Int ATOS-Live Summit Heidelb Ger. 2009.
57. Shelbourne KD, Davis TJ, Patel DV. The Natural History of Acute, Isolated, Nonoperatively Treated Posterior Cruciate Ligament Injuries. Am J Sports Med 1999; 27(3):276–83.
58. Cosgarea AJ, Jay PR. Posterior Cruciate Ligament Injuries: Evaluation and Management. JAAOS - J Am Acad Orthop Surg. 2001;9(5):297.
59. Rubinstein RA, Shelbourne KD, McCarroll JR, et al. The Accuracy of the Clinical Examination in the Setting of Posterior Cruciate Ligament Injuries. Am J Sports Med 1994;22(4):550–7.
60. Daniel DM, Stone ML, Barnett P, et al. Use of the quadriceps active test to diagnose posterior cruciate-ligament disruption and measure posterior laxity of the knee. JBJS 1988;70(3):386.
61. Dean RS, LaPrade RF. ACL and Posterolateral Corner Injuries. Curr Rev Musculoskelet Med 2020;13(1):123–32.
62. Pacheco RJ, Ayre CA, Bollen SR. Posterolateral corner injuries of the knee: A SERIOUS INJURY COMMONLY MISSED. J Bone Joint Surg Br 2011;93-B(2): 194–7.
63. Cooper D, Warren R, Warner J. The posterior cruciate ligament and posterolateral structures of the knee: anatomy, function, and patterns of injury. Presented at: Instructional Course Lecture 40; 1991.
64. Jacobsen K. Gonylaxometry: Stress Radiographic Measurement of Passive Stability in the Knee Joints of Normal Subjects and Patients with Ligament Injuries: Accuracy and Range of Application. Acta Orthop Scand 1981;52(sup194):9–263.
65. LaPrade RF, Floyd ER, Carlson GB, et al. The Posterolateral Corner: Explanations and Outcomes. J Arthrosc Surg Sports Med 2021;2(2):108–18.
66. Norris R, Kopkow C, McNicholas MJ. Interpretations of the dial test should be reconsidered. A diagnostic accuracy study reporting sensitivity, specificity, predictive values and likelihood ratios. J ISAKOS 2018;3(4):198–204.
67. Jung YB, Nam CH, Jung HJ, et al. The Influence of Tibial Positioning on the Diagnostic Accuracy of Combined Posterior Cruciate Ligament and Posterolateral Rotatory Instability of the Knee. Clin Orthop Surg 2009;1(2):68–73.
68. LaPrade RF, Terry GC. Injuries to the Posterolateral Aspect of the Knee: Association of Anatomic Injury Patterns with Clinical Instability. Am J Sports Med 1997; 25(4):433–8.
69. Petrigliano FA, Lane CG, Suero EM, et al. Posterior Cruciate Ligament and Posterolateral Corner Deficiency Results in a Reverse Pivot Shift. Clin Orthop 2012;470(3):815–23.
70. Cooper DE. Tests for posterolateral instability of the knee in normal subjects. Results of examination under anesthesia. JBJS 1991;73(1):30.
71. Swinford ST, LaPrade R, Engebretsen L, et al. Biomechanics and physical examination of the posteromedial and posterolateral knee: state of the art. J ISAKOS 2020;5(6):378–88.

72. Cinque ME, Geeslin AG, Chahla J, et al. The Heel Height Test: A Novel Tool for the Detection of Combined Anterior Cruciate Ligament and Fibular Collateral Ligament Tears. Arthrosc J Arthrosc Relat Surg 2017;33(12):2177–81.
73. Lundquist RB, Matcuk GR, Schein AJ, et al. Posteromedial Corner of the Knee: The Neglected Corner. Radiographics 2015;35(4):1123–37.
74. Slocum DB, Larson RL, James SL. Late Reconstruction of Ligamentous Injuries of the Medial Compartment of the Knee. Clin Orthop Relat Res 1974;100:23.
75. Van der Wal WA, Meijer DT, Hoogeslag RAG, et al. Meniscal Tears, Posterolateral and Posteromedial Corner Injuries, Increased Coronal Plane, and Increased Sagittal Plane Tibial Slope All Influence Anterior Cruciate Ligament–Related Knee Kinematics and Increase Forces on the Native and Reconstructed Anterior Cruciate Ligament: A Systematic Review of Cadaveric Studies. Arthrosc J Arthrosc Relat Surg 2022;38(5):1664–88.e1.
76. Dong J, Wang XF, Men X, et al. Surgical Treatment of Acute Grade III Medial Collateral Ligament Injury Combined With Anterior Cruciate Ligament Injury: Anatomic Ligament Repair Versus Triangular Ligament Reconstruction. Arthrosc J Arthrosc Relat Surg 2015;31(6):1108–16.
77. Hashemi SA, Ranjbar MR, Tahami M, et al. Comparison of Accuracy in Expert Clinical Examination versus Magnetic Resonance Imaging and Arthroscopic Exam in Diagnosis of Meniscal Tear. Adv Orthop 2020;2020. e1895852.
78. Galli M, Ciriello V, Menghi A, et al. Joint Line Tenderness and McMurray Tests for the Detection of Meniscal Lesions: What Is Their Real Diagnostic Value? Arch Phys Med Rehabil 2013;94(6):1126–31.
79. Corea JR, Moussa M, Othman AA. McMurray's test tested. Knee Surg Sports Traumatol Arthrosc 1994;2(2):70–2.
80. Rinonapoli G, Carraro A, Delcogliano A. The Clinical Diagnosis of Meniscal Tear is Not Easy. Reliability of Two Clinical Meniscal Tests and Magnetic Resonance Imaging. Int J Immunopathol Pharmacol 2011;24(1_suppl2):39–44.
81. Karachalios T, Hantes M, Zibis AH, et al. Diagnostic Accuracy of a New Clinical Test (the Thessaly Test) for Early Detection of Meniscal Tears. JBJS 2005;87(5):955.
82. Harrison BK, Abell BE, Gibson TW. The Thessaly Test for Detection of Meniscal Tears: Validation of a New Physical Examination Technique for Primary Care Medicine. Clin J Sport Med 2009;19(1):9.

Timing of Anterior Cruciate Ligament Surgery

Bálint Zsidai, MD[a,*], Janina Kaarre, MD, MSc[a,b],
Eric Narup, MD, MSc[a], Kristian Samuelsson, MD, PhD, MSc[a,c]

KEYWORDS

- Anterior cruciate ligament • ACL • Reconstruction • Timing • Knee ligament surgery • Knee injuries • Arthroscopy • Sports medicine

KEY POINTS

- There is considerable uncertainty surrounding the definition of early and delayed anterior cruciate ligament reconstruction (ACLR), with the definition for early surgery ranging from days to months and for delayed surgery ranging from weeks to years in the current literature.
- Modern arthroscopic surgical techniques and early rehabilitation have mitigated the risk of arthrofibrosis and postoperative stiffness with early ACLR.
- Early ACLR is shown to be equivalent or superior to delayed ACLR in terms of clinical outcomes, subjective postoperative knee function, the incidence of intra-articular injury within the timeframe between injury and surgery, as well as cost-effectiveness.
- Concomitant surgical procedures addressing anterolateral instability, anteromedial instability, and meniscus injury may be more advantageous when performed in conjunction with early ACLR.

INTRODUCTION

Anterior cruciate ligament (ACL) tears are one of the most frequent injuries to the ligamentous structures of the knee. Although arthroscopic ACL reconstruction (ACLR) is the gold standard for the surgical treatment of ACL tears, the ACL surgeon needs to be aware of the wide range of patient-related, injury-related, and surgery-related factors influencing treatment outcomes. Although the timing of ACLR is one such factor, there currently is no clear consensus about the definition of early and delayed ACLR or the optimal timing of surgery following ACL tears. Surgical treatment is generally

[a] Department of Orthopaedics, Institute of Clinical Sciences, Sahlgrenska Academy, University of Gothenburg, Gothenburg, Sweden; [b] Department of Orthopaedic Surgery, UPMC Freddie Fu Sports Medicine Center, University of Pittsburgh, 3200 South Water Street, Pittsburgh, PA, USA; [c] Department of Orthopaedics, Sahlgrenska University Hospital, Göteborgsvägen 31, 431 30 Mölndal, Sweden
* Corresponding author. Göteborgsvägen 31, Mölndal 431 80, Sweden.
E-mail address: balint.zsidai@gu.se

Clin Sports Med 43 (2024) 331–341
https://doi.org/10.1016/j.csm.2023.08.002
sportsmed.theclinics.com

recommended to restore knee stability in patients with high demand for knee-strenuous activity but the decision of when to perform ACLR varies among surgeons and may be influenced by factors such as patient age, activity level, and associated injuries.

Acute knee ligament injuries were historically treated with open repair followed by postoperative immobilization with a cast. Because early surgery often resulted in a high incidence of knee stiffness and arthrofibrosis, delayed surgical treatment was proposed as an alternative, which provides time for joint inflammation to subside, recovery in knee range of motion (ROM), and restoration of muscle strength, potentially diminishing the rate of postoperative joint stiffness. However, a greater incidence of secondary intra-articular damage and potential quadriceps atrophy were proposed as drawbacks inherent to delayed ACL surgery. As a result, the complex interplay between the risk of timing-associated complications, economic factors, surgeon preference, and patient motivation to return to preinjury activity level ultimately determines surgical timing in ACLR.

Despite the growing awareness of the role of surgical timing, consensus surrounding the definition of the cutoff time interval from injury distinguishing early and delayed ACLR is currently lacking. Cutoff time intervals ranging between 8 days and[1] 12 months[2] have been reported for early isolated ACLR, whereas a cutoff as early as 3 weeks was used for delayed isolated ACLR in a recent meta-analysis,[3] emphasizing the heterogeneity with respect to timing among existing studies.

The setting of multiligament knee injury (MLKI) may also influence the decision of the operating surgeon to opt for early or delayed ACLR. Although several studies investigated outcomes following ACLR combined with the surgical or nonsurgical treatment of concomitant knee ligament injuries, evidence is currently inconclusive regarding the optimal timing of surgical treatment of MLKIs where ACLR is performed.[4]

The aim of this review is to critically assess the current literature regarding the impact of surgical timing in the setting of ACL injury treatment on a broad range of postoperative outcomes. A thorough analysis of the inconsistencies surrounding the definition of early and delayed ACLR, the influence of early versus delayed surgery on the prevalence of associated knee injuries and the influence of surgical timing on functional and clinical patient outcomes may facilitate evidence-based decision-making for surgeons performing isolated ACLR and ACLR in the setting of MLKI (**Fig. 1**).

A RATIONALE FOR THE NEED OF CLEARER DEFINITIONS OF EARLY AND DELAYED ANTERIOR CRUCIATE LIGAMENT RECONSTRUCTION

During the recent years, several systematic reviews and meta-analyses attempted to clarify the association between ACLR timing relative to the incidence of ACL injury and postoperative outcomes.[3,5–10] Although most of these studies did not determine clear differences in outcomes related to early or delayed surgery, there is unanimous agreement that conclusions are hampered by the heterogeneity of existing studies concerning the definition of early and delayed surgical timing. One systematic review considering the definitions of acute and chronic orthopedic conditions determined early ACL tears to be less than 6 week old with respect to the time of injury, whereas chronic ACL tears were defined as more than 6 month old relative to the time of injury. However, a large proportion of studies in the existing literature define ACLR as delayed even when performed before 6 weeks of ACL injury, which decreases the reliability of the currently available evidence.[10,11] Furthermore, the role of the time interval between 6 weeks and 6 months relative to the incidence of ACL injury remains unaddressed and the current definition of early and delayed ACLR remains arbitrary rather than explicit. Ain improved understanding of the inflammatory state of the knee joint in

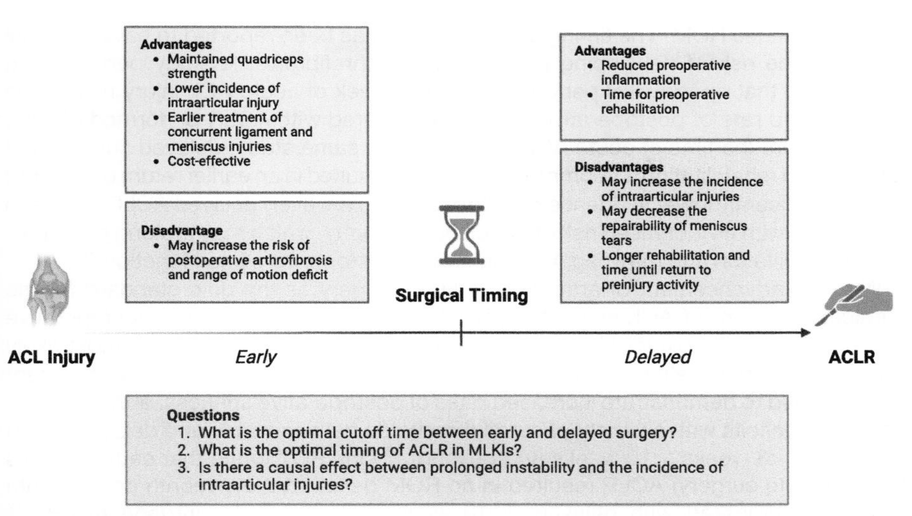

Fig. 1. The potential advantages and disadvantages of early versus delayed ACLR. ACLR, anterior cruciate ligament reconstruction; MLKI, multiple knee ligament injury.

the setting of ACL injury was also proposed to help define early and delayed surgical timing for ACLR. Synovial proinflammatory cytokine levels have been shown to increase within 24 to 72 hours of ACL injury, followed by decreasing levels during a 1-month interval before surgery.[12] However, the clinical utility of synovial biomarkers in determining the timing of ACLR remains unclear.

Despite the lack of clarity surrounding early and delayed ACLR, a recent study from the Swedish National Knee Ligament Registry determined that patients with early ACLR (<1 year from injury) reported a superior rate of acceptable knee-related symptom state and improved overall knee function compared with patients initial nonoperative treatment followed by delayed ACLR.[13] However, the time from injury to surgery was on average 6 months (standard deviation = 2.4 months) in the early ACLR group (n = 20,352) with the appropriate threshold for early ACLR remaining inconclusive.[13] In a recent systematic review and meta-analysis, comparison of 5 randomized controlled trials (RCTs) determined that patients with early isolated ACLR were on average treated 44 days earlier compared with patients who underwent delayed ACLR, with no difference in postoperative outcomes.[10] This broad time interval makes it difficult to define a clear cutoff for early and delayed ACLR and suggests that the context of surgical timing should be considered on a spectrum of months rather than a few weeks to show an impact on postoperative outcomes. Importantly, there is a lack of RCTs assessing the role of ACLR timing in the context of surgically treated MLKIs. One recent multicenter RCT reported that a complete tear of the ACL was involved in 56.5% of MLKIs and that the average time from injury to primary multiligament knee surgery was 64 days (interquartile range = 29–190 days).[4] Consequently, further high-level studies are required to determine the impact of ACLR timing in the setting of both surgically treated isolated ACL injuries and MLKIs.

THE INCIDENCE OF POSTOPERATIVE STIFFNESS AND ARTHROFIBROSIS WITH ANTERIOR CRUCIATE LIGAMENT RECONSTRUCTION TIMING

Arthrofibrosis of the knee joint is caused by excessive scar tissue formation, resulting in pain and limited potential for the patient to regain the terminal 5° of extension throughout knee ROM. The timing of ACL surgery has been reported to have a crucial effect on the risk of developing postoperative arthrofibrosis. A study performed in 1991 found that open ACLR performed within a week of acute ACL injury resulted in an increased rate of postoperative stiffness compared with ACLR performed at least 3 weeks from the time of acute ACL injury.[14] In the same study, delayed surgery and accelerated rehabilitation (uncommon at the time) resulted in an earlier return of strength and a significantly lower incidence of arthrofibrosis. However, delayed ACLR has been associated with an increased risk of quadriceps atrophy, which may prolong postoperative rehabilitation and may negatively influence postoperative knee function.[15]

With the advancement of arthroscopic knee surgery as the gold standard for the surgical treatment of ACL injury, the prevalence of arthrofibrosis and postoperative stiffness showed a diminishing tendency in patients undergoing ACLR, most likely due to early rehabilitation programs and improved surgical techniques.[6] More recent studies failed to demonstrate increased rates of postoperative stiffness, arthrofibrosis, and ROM deficits with a variety of cutoff thresholds between early and delayed ACLR (<2 weeks, <3 weeks, <10 weeks and beyond).[16] One RCT found that early (<8 days from injury to surgery) ACLR resulted in no ROM deficit at the 6-month or 24-month follow-up compared with delayed (6–10 weeks from injury to surgery) ACLR.[1,17] Additionally, early (<8 days from injury to surgery) surgery resulted in superior isokinetic knee flexion strength at the 24-month follow-up compared with delayed (6–10 weeks from injury to surgery) treatment.[17] Furthermore, a case series of early patellar tendon ACLRs (n = 25) performed 9 days or lesser from injury to surgery did not identify any patients with a postoperative knee extension deficit greater than 3° and knee flexion deficit greater than 5° compared with the contralateral knee at the final follow-up.[18] Authors of the referenced studies highlight the prominent role of modern arthroscopic techniques and accelerated rehabilitation protocols to facilitate early restoration of knee ROM during the postoperative period.[17,18] In contrast, one recent retrospective study of 29,888 patients found that a 6 week or longer delay of ACLR reduces the 2-year likelihood of surgical treatment of arthrofibrosis by 65% in patients aged younger than 40 years.[19] Although the timing of ACL surgery may affect the likelihood of postoperative arthrofibrosis, existing evidence suggests that early surgery combined with accelerated rehabilitation can lead to earlier return of strength and an infrequent incidence of arthrofibrosis. Conversely, delayed surgery may increase the risk of quadriceps atrophy and negatively influence postoperative knee function, especially problematic for high-level athletes who aim for rapid return to preinjury activity levels.

COMPARISON OF CLINICAL OUTCOMES AFTER EARLY AND DELAYED ANTERIOR CRUCIATE LIGAMENT RECONSTRUCTION

During the years, surgical timing was determined as an influential factor on clinical outcomes after ACLR. Several studies compared the effects of early and delayed ACLR on the risk of graft failure and revision surgery. Economic and decision analysis using registry-based patient data from the Knee Anterior Cruciate Ligament Nonsurgical versus Surgical Treatment trial and Multicenter Orthopedic Outcomes Network cohort determined that early isolated ACLR results in less sick-leave days (on average −31.6 days) and superior gains in Quality Adjusted Life Years compared with rehabilitation with optional delayed ACLR. However, findings are conflicting regarding the association between ACLR timing and the risk of revision ACLR. One study of 11,867 patients reported an increased risk of revision ACLR with delayed ACLR (performed at least 6 months after injury) compared with early ACLR (performed within 2 months of injury).[20] Conversely, an increased revision risk (relative risk = 2.07) was reported in patients undergoing early isolated ACLR (defined as surgery performed within 3 months of injury).[21] Furthermore, a 2 to 3-fold revision ACLR rate was found in patients undergoing ACLR within 90 days of injury compared with patients undergoing surgery after 365 days from injury.[22] However, it is worth noting that the likelihood of revision after early and delayed ACLR is likely influenced by factors such as activity level after surgery and patient age, rather than the timing of surgery itself.[23] Therefore, the risk of revision should be considered multifactorial and should not solely rely on the timing of surgery.

COMPARISON OF FUNCTIONAL OUTCOMES AFTER EARLY AND DELAYED ANTERIOR CRUCIATE LIGAMENT RECONSTRUCTION

Another major controversy in ACL surgery is whether early or delayed ACLR leads to superior objective and subjective outcomes for patients. Several studies report comparable clinical outcomes and superior knee stability because of both early and delayed ACLR.[24,25] One systematic review found similar tibiofemoral laxity, assessed with the KT-1000 arthrometer, Lachman test, and the pivot shift test, in patients who underwent early ACLR (performed within 1 month of injury) versus those who underwent delayed ACLR (performed >8 weeks after injury).[26] No significant differences in postoperative knee ROM were found between the 2 groups.[26] Additionally, one recent study showed comparable patient-reported outcomes, with significant improvements in all subscales of the Knee Injury and Osteoarthritis Outcome Score (KOOS) and favorable return rate to preinjury Tegner activity level after both early and delayed ACLR.[17] Notably, a high proportion of patients in both the early and delayed ACLR groups were able to return to Tegner activity level 6 or higher, suggesting surgical timing may have a limited influence on the rate of return to sport.[17] Furthermore, objective IKDC scores were shown to be similar among patient groups, with the majority of (82% vs 71%, respectively) patients having grade AB pivot shift at the 12-month postoperative follow-up, indicative of restored knee laxity because of both early and delayed ACLR.[17]

Further research showed that patients with early hamstring tendon ACLR achieve superior outcomes in terms of postoperative isokinetic knee flexion strength after 2 years compared with patients who underwent delayed ACLR.[27] Specifically, patients with early surgery achieved significantly greater improvement in flexor strength at 180° (8.1% improvement) and 240° (9.4% improvement) per second, without significant improvement in extensor strength.[27] In the same study, early ACLR was associated with fewer sick-leave days and decreased socioeconomic costs compared with delayed ACLR.[27] Consequently, while both early and delayed surgery seem to yield good to excellent functional outcomes, a combination of functional outcomes should be assessed to determine the optimal timing of isolated ACLR.

The Impact of Anterior Cruciate Ligament Reconstruction Timing on the Incidence of Secondary Intra-articular Injury

Due to conflicting results in the current literature, the influence of ACLR timing on the incidence of secondary intra-articular injury remains a topic of debate. Delayed surgery was proposed to lead to meniscal[8] and chondral[7] damage secondary to knee instability because of prolonged ACL deficiency.[28]

One retrospective study of 226 patients who underwent primary ACLR found that surgery delayed beyond 7 months of injury was associated with 4.1-fold odds of the presence of medial meniscus injury recoded at surgery compared with ACLR performed within 6 months of injury.[29] Furthermore, patients with primary ACLR beyond 5 months from injury had 1.9-fold odds for lateral meniscus injury compared with surgery performed within 4 months of injury.[29] A systematic review performed in 2018 found that 6 of the 7 included studies implicated the role of prolonged knee instability with delayed primary ACLR in the development of medial meniscus injury (odds ratio [OR] range 3.46–11.56), despite an inconclusive association of prolonged instability with lateral meniscus injury rate.[30] The more predominant role of chronic ACL deficiency on the prevalence of subsequent medial meniscus injury is further supported by additional recent studies from the literature, which also highlight inferior rates of repairability of these lesions with time.[23,31–34] A recent systematic review and meta-analysis concluded that primary ACLR delayed beyond 3 months of ACL injury results in a 2.24-fold odds of medical meniscus injury compared with surgery performed earlier than 3 months, whereas the causal effect of timing on the prevalence of meniscal injuries remains unclear.[8] Consequently, early ACLR may be recommended to protect the integrity of the medial meniscus from prolonged knee instability.

During the last 20 years, several studies corroborated the negative influence of delayed ACL surgery on chondral wear.[2,35,36] One systematic review of 40 articles found a positive correlation between the rate of cartilage injury and ACLR delayed beyond 12 months (risk ratio = 0.42).[31] Furthermore, retrospective analysis of 3976 patients undergoing isolated primary ACLR at a single institution determined that surgery performed 12 months from injury resulted in a 1.20 OR of cartilage injury rate.[32] Additionally, one United States integrated health-care registry study found that 24.8% of patients with early (<3 weeks from injury to surgery) ACLR presented with cartilage injury at the time of surgery, whereas patients with delayed (≥9 months) ACLR had a 40.0% rate of concurrent cartilage injury.[23] One recent systematic review and meta-analysis compared cartilage injury rates as a function of 3-month, 6-month, and 12-month time intervals from ACL injury to ACLR with ACLR performed within 3 months of injury.[7] The analysis of 14 studies included in the final synthesis found an increase of the prevalence of chondral injury at each time interval compared with early surgery (<3 months), with low-grade cartilage injuries becoming prevalent after the 3-month interval (OR = 1.91) and high-grade cartilage injuries becoming more prominent after 12 months (OR = 3.06).[7] In contrast, another recent meta-analysis found no difference in the rate of cartilage injury between early (<3 weeks) and delayed (>6 weeks) ACLR is prevalent in the setting of MLKI but not in isolated ligamentous injury only involving the ACL.[10] However, heterogeneity between different syntheses performed on the available literature is likely due to different interpretations of cutoff values for early and delayed surgery. Despite the difficulty to determine the causality between surgical timing and the development of intra-articular injuries due to the inability to obtain baseline MRIs at the time of injury, current evidence predominantly suggests that early ACLR has a protective effect on the development of further intra-articular pathology with time. Prevention of chondral damage in patients with ACL injury is essential because patients with concomitant partial-thickness and full-thickness cartilage lesions at the time of ACLR report inferior 5-year subjective knee function measured with the KOOS.[37]

INTERPLAY BETWEEN ANTERIOR CRUCIATE LIGAMENT RECONSTRUCTION TIMING AND CONCURRENT SURGICAL INTERVENTIONS

Injury to the ACL is frequently accompanied by concomitant injuries and adequate treatment consists of addressing concurrent pathologic condition with concurrent surgical interventions. However, the interplay between additional surgical interventions concurrent with ACLR and surgical timing remains to be clarified. Patients with high-grade rotatory knee instability may benefit from additional lateral extra-articular interventions concurrent to ACLR to restore rotatory knee stability.[38,39] One recent study compared postoperative outcomes among a cohort of patients with early (<8 weeks from injury to surgery) combined ACLR and anterolateral ligament (ALL) reconstruction and a cohort with delayed (>8 weeks from injury to surgery) combined ACLR and ALL reconstruction, with no differences in objective knee stability, subjective knee function, and graft failure rates (2.9% and 2.1%, respectively).[40] Furthermore, patients with ACL injury often present with concomitant injury to the medial collateral ligament (MCL).[4,41] Although the choice between surgical or nonoperative treatment of MCL injuries concomitant to ACLR remains a controversial topic, it was recently reported that as few as 10% of patients nonoperatively treated for MCL injury concurrent with ACLR return to preinjury activity level.[42] Due to the detrimental effect of persistent valgus laxity on the integrity of intra-articular soft-tissue, prolonged rehabilitation with incomplete healing and stress on the ACL graft, early combined ACLR and MCL reconstruction is increasingly favored.[43] Consequently, patients with anterolateral and anteromedial instability in the setting of surgically treated ACL injury may benefit from early ACLR with concurrent lateral extra-articular tenodesis and MCL reconstruction. Repair of treatable meniscus pathologic condition in conjunction with ACLR is also considered advantageous in patients with ACL injury. It was reported that 77.6% of meniscus injuries were repaired concomitant to early (<6 months from injury to surgery) ACLR, whereas only 46.7% of meniscus injuries were repaired with delayed (>6 months from injury to surgery) ACLR. Additionally, meniscus repair performed in the setting of early (<48 hours from injury) ACLR resulted in lower rates of extension deficit between 3° and 5° at the 12-month postoperative follow-up compared with delayed (performed in the inflammation-free period) ACLR and meniscus repair (3.7% vs 22.2%, respectively).[11] Therefore, early surgical timing for ACLR may be preferred in highly active patients with concurrent repairable meniscus injury to prevent the incidence of downstream chondral wear and posttraumatic OA.

SUMMARY

In light of the current evidence, an improved understanding of surgical timing is warranted to optimize patient outcomes with ACLR in the setting of isolated ACL and MLKIs. Although interpretation of the existing data is hampered by inconsistent definitions of surgical timing, early ACLR performed within weeks of injury may result in equivalent to superior clinical and functional outcomes. Importantly, early ACLR seems to be beneficial for decreasing the incidence of medial meniscus and chondral injury by avoiding prolonged knee instability, with excellent clinical and functional outcomes and no marked increase in the risk of postoperative arthrofibrosis compared with delayed surgery. Future studies are required to clarify the cutoff between early and delayed surgeries to determine the influence of concurrent surgical procedures on optimal surgical timing and to explore the role of surgical timing in the treatment of patients with MLKIs.

CLINICS CARE POINTS

- Delayed ACLR may increase the incidence of secondary intraarticular injuries and quadriceps atrophy, with a potentially negative impact on postoperative outcomes.
- Inconsistent definitions of early and delayed ACLR may lead to ambiguity and hinder evidence-based decision-making.

- The timing of ACLR in the setting of MLKI can be challenging due to the complex nature of these injuries.
- Both early and delayed ACLR yield good to excellent functional outcomes, with patients often returning to preinjury activity levels.
- Patients with ACL injuries may benefit from concurrent surgical treatment for associated pathologies, such as lateral extraarticular tenodesis, MCL reconstruction, and meniscus repair.

DISCLOSURE

K. Samuelsson is a member of the board of directors of Getinge AB (publ.). All other authors have no disclosures.

REFERENCES

1. Eriksson K, von Essen C, Jönhagen S, et al. No risk of arthrofibrosis after acute anterior cruciate ligament reconstruction. Knee Surg Sports Traumatol Arthrosc 2018;26(10):2875–82.
2. Fok AW, Yau WP. Delay in ACL reconstruction is associated with more severe and painful meniscal and chondral injuries. Knee Surg Sports Traumatol Arthrosc 2013;21(4):928–33.
3. Ferguson D, Palmer A, Khan S, et al. Early or delayed anterior cruciate ligament reconstruction: Is one superior? A systematic review and meta-analysis. Eur J Orthop Surg Traumatol 2019;29(6):1277–89.
4. Poploski KM, Lynch AD, Burns TC, et al. Presentation and Surgical Management of Multiple Ligament Knee Injuries: A Multicenter Study from the Surgical Timing and Rehabilitation (STaR) Trial for MLKIs Network. J Bone Joint Surg Am 2023; 105(8):607–13.
5. Andernord D, Karlsson J, Musahl V, et al. Timing of surgery of the anterior cruciate ligament. Arthroscopy 2013;29(11):1863–71.
6. Deabate L, Previtali D, Grassi A, et al. Anterior Cruciate Ligament Reconstruction Within 3 Weeks Does Not Increase Stiffness and Complications Compared With Delayed Reconstruction: A Meta-analysis of Randomized Controlled Trials. Am J Sports Med 2020;48(5):1263–72.
7. Prodromidis AD, Drosatou C, Mourikis A, et al. Relationship Between Timing of Anterior Cruciate Ligament Reconstruction and Chondral Injuries: A Systematic Review and Meta-analysis. Am J Sports Med 2022;50(13):3719–31.
8. Prodromidis AD, Drosatou C, Thivaios GC, et al. Timing of Anterior Cruciate Ligament Reconstruction and Relationship With Meniscal Tears: A Systematic Review and Meta-analysis. Am J Sports Med 2021;49(9):2551–62.
9. Shen X, Liu T, Xu S, et al. Optimal Timing of Anterior Cruciate Ligament Reconstruction in Patients With Anterior Cruciate Ligament Tear: A Systematic Review and Meta-analysis. JAMA Netw Open 2022;5(11). e2242742.
10. Vermeijden HD, Yang XA, Rademakers MV, et al. Early and Delayed Surgery for Isolated ACL and Multiligamentous Knee Injuries Have Equivalent Results: A Systematic Review and Meta-analysis. Am J Sports Med 2023;51(4):1106–16.
11. Herbst E, Hoser C, Gföller P, et al. Impact of surgical timing on the outcome of anterior cruciate ligament reconstruction. Knee Surg Sports Traumatol Arthrosc 2017;25(2):569–77.

12. Bigoni M, Turati M, Gandolla M, et al. Effects of ACL Reconstructive Surgery on Temporal Variations of Cytokine Levels in Synovial Fluid. Mediators Inflamm 2016; 2016. 8243601.
13. Bergerson E, Persson K, Svantesson E, et al. Superior Outcome of Early ACL Reconstruction versus Initial Non-reconstructive Treatment With Late Crossover to Surgery: A Study From the Swedish National Knee Ligament Registry. Am J Sports Med 2022;50(4):896–903.
14. Shelbourne KD, Wilckens JH, Mollabashy A, et al. Arthrofibrosis in acute anterior cruciate ligament reconstruction. The effect of timing of reconstruction and rehabilitation. Am J Sports Med 1991;19(4):332–6.
15. Thomas AC, Villwock M, Wojtys EM, et al. Lower extremity muscle strength after anterior cruciate ligament injury and reconstruction. J Athl Train 2013;48(5): 610–20.
16. Kwok CS, Harrison T, Servant C. The optimal timing for anterior cruciate ligament reconstruction with respect to the risk of postoperative stiffness. Arthroscopy 2013;29(3):556–65.
17. von Essen C, Eriksson K, Barenius B. Acute ACL reconstruction shows superior clinical results and can be performed safely without an increased risk of developing arthrofibrosis. Knee Surg Sports Traumatol Arthrosc 2020;28(7):2036–43.
18. Harris MC, Venrick C, Hines AC, et al. Prospective Evaluation of Range of Motion in Acute ACL Reconstruction Using Patellar Tendon Autograft. Orthop J Sports Med 2019;7(10). 2325967119875415.
19. Agarwal AR, Harris AB, Tarawneh O, et al. Delay of Timing of Anterior Cruciate Ligament Reconstruction Is Associated With Lower Risk of Arthrofibrosis Requiring Intervention. Arthrosc J Arthrosc Relat Surg 2023;39(7):1682–9.
20. Freshman RD, Truong NM, Cevallos N, et al. Delayed ACL reconstruction increases rates of concomitant procedures and risk of subsequent surgery. Knee Surg Sports Traumatol Arthrosc 2022;31(7):2897–905.
21. Snaebjörnsson T, Hamrin Senorski E, Svantesson E, et al. Graft Fixation and Timing of Surgery Are Predictors of Early Anterior Cruciate Ligament Revision: A Cohort Study from the Swedish and Norwegian Knee Ligament Registries Based on 18,425 Patients. JB JS Open Access 2019;4(4). e0037.
22. Fältström A, Hägglund M, Magnusson H, et al. Predictors for additional anterior cruciate ligament reconstruction: data from the Swedish national ACL register. Knee Surg Sports Traumatol Arthrosc 2016;24(3):885–94.
23. Ding DY, Chang RN, Allahabadi S, et al. Acute and subacute anterior cruciate ligament reconstructions are associated with a higher risk of revision and reoperation. Knee Surg Sports Traumatol Arthrosc 2022;30(10):3311–21.
24. Lee YS, Lee OS, Lee SH, et al. Effect of the Timing of Anterior Cruciate Ligament Reconstruction on Clinical and Stability Outcomes: A Systematic Review and Meta-analysis. Arthroscopy 2018;34(2):592–602.
25. James EW, Dawkins BJ, Schachne JM, et al. Early Operative Versus Delayed Operative Versus Nonoperative Treatment of Pediatric and Adolescent Anterior Cruciate Ligament Injuries: A Systematic Review and Meta-analysis. Am J Sports Med 2021;49(14):4008–17.
26. Smith TO, Davies L, Hing CB. Early versus delayed surgery for anterior cruciate ligament reconstruction: a systematic review and meta-analysis. Knee Surg Sports Traumatol Arthrosc 2010;18(3):304–11.
27. von Essen C, McCallum S, Barenius B, et al. Acute reconstruction results in less sick-leave days and as such fewer indirect costs to the individual and society

compared to delayed reconstruction for ACL injuries. Knee Surg Sports Traumatol Arthrosc 2020;28(7):2044–52.
28. Granan LP, Bahr R, Lie SA, et al. Timing of anterior cruciate ligament reconstructive surgery and risk of cartilage lesions and meniscal tears: A cohort study based on the norwegian national knee ligament registry. Am J Sports Med 2009;37(5):955–61.
29. Taketomi S, Inui H, Yamagami R, et al. Surgical timing of anterior cruciate ligament reconstruction to prevent associated meniscal and cartilage lesions. J Orthop Sci 2018;23(3):546–51.
30. Sommerfeldt M, Raheem A, Whittaker J, et al. Recurrent Instability Episodes and Meniscal or Cartilage Damage After Anterior Cruciate Ligament Injury: A Systematic Review. Orthop J Sports Med 2018;6(7). 2325967118786507.
31. Mehl J, Otto A, Baldino JB, et al. The ACL-deficient knee and the prevalence of meniscus and cartilage lesions: a systematic review and meta-analysis (CRD42017076897). Arch Orthop Trauma Surg 2019;139(6):819–41.
32. Cristiani R, Janarv PM, Engström B, et al. Delayed Anterior Cruciate Ligament Reconstruction Increases the Risk of Abnormal Prereconstruction Laxity, Cartilage, and Medial Meniscus Injuries. Arthroscopy 2021;37(4):1214–20.
33. Giordano L, Maffulli N, Carimati G, et al. Increased Time to Surgery After Anterior Cruciate Ligament Tear in Female Patients Results in Greater Risk of Medial Meniscus Tear: A Study of 489 Female Patients. Arthrosc J Arthrosc Relat Surg 2023;39(3):613–22.
34. Shamrock AG, Hall JR, Hajewski CJ, et al. Cartilage and Meniscus Injuries Are More Common in Patients Undergoing Delayed Multiligament Reconstruction. J Knee Surg 2022;35(5):560–5.
35. Chen G, Tang X, Li Q, et al. The evaluation of patient-specific factors associated with meniscal and chondral injuries accompanying ACL rupture in young adult patients. Knee Surg Sports Traumatol Arthrosc 2015;23(3):792–8.
36. Church S, Keating JF. Reconstruction of the anterior cruciate ligament: timing of surgery and the incidence of meniscal tears and degenerative change. J Bone Joint Surg Br 2005;87(12):1639–42.
37. Ulstein S, Årøen A, Engebretsen L, et al. Effect of Concomitant Cartilage Lesions on Patient-Reported Outcomes After Anterior Cruciate Ligament Reconstruction: A Nationwide Cohort Study From Norway and Sweden of 8470 Patients With 5-Year Follow-up. Orthop J Sports Med 2018;6(7). 2325967118786219.
38. Firth AD, Bryant DM, Litchfield R, et al. Predictors of Graft Failure in Young Active Patients Undergoing Hamstring Autograft Anterior Cruciate Ligament Reconstruction With or Without a Lateral Extra-articular Tenodesis: The Stability Experience. Am J Sports Med 2022;50(2):384–95.
39. Getgood AMJ, Bryant DM, Litchfield R, et al. Lateral Extra-articular Tenodesis Reduces Failure of Hamstring Tendon Autograft Anterior Cruciate Ligament Reconstruction: 2-Year Outcomes From the STABILITY Study Randomized Clinical Trial. Am J Sports Med 2020;48(2):285–97.
40. Helito CP, Sobrado MF, Giglio PN, et al. Surgical Timing Does Not Interfere on Clinical Outcomes in Combined Reconstruction of the Anterior Cruciate Ligament and Anterolateral Ligament: A Comparative Study With Minimum 2-Year Follow-Up. Arthroscopy 2021;37(6):1909–17.
41. Willinger L, Balendra G, Pai V, et al. High incidence of superficial and deep medial collateral ligament injuries in 'isolated' anterior cruciate ligament ruptures: a long overlooked injury. Knee Surg Sports Traumatol Arthrosc 2022;30(1):167–75.

42. Svantesson E, Piussi R, Beischer S, et al. Only 10% of Patients With a Concomitant MCL Injury Return to Their Preinjury Level of Sport 1 Year After ACL Reconstruction: A Matched Comparison With Isolated ACL Reconstruction. Sports Health 2023. 19417381231157746.
43. Holuba K, Vermeijden HD, Yang XA, et al. Treating Combined Anterior Cruciate Ligament and Medial Collateral Ligament Injuries Operatively in the Acute Setting Is Potentially Advantageous. Arthroscopy 2023;39(4):1099–107.

Nonoperative Anterior Cruciate Ligament Injury Treatment

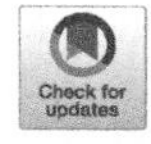

Berte Bøe, MD, PhD

KEYWORDS

• Nonsurgical treatment • Nonoperative treatment • Anterior cruciate ligament
• Exercise therapy • Rehabilitation • Strength exercises

KEY POINTS

- Following trauma where an anterior cruciate ligament (ACL) injury is confirmed, the athlete and physician should advise a schedule that addresses rehabilitation, appropriateness of ACL reconstruction and return to sport.
- An athlete must not be sent back to contact or pivoting sports without being physically and mentally prepared to return.
- The patient's knee strength, balance, and function should be tested and compared with the contralateral healthy side before declaring the patient fully rehabilitated.

INTRODUCTION

After an acute anterior cruciate ligament (ACL) injury, there are 2 possibilities for treatment: either surgical reconstruction of the ligament or nonoperative treatment with training, and both these treatments require intensive rehabilitation. Patients who chose nonoperative treatment will always have the opportunity to choose surgical treatment at a later stage if the instability symptoms persist. Some patients have concomitant injuries that will be an indication for early surgical intervention, such as meniscal and osteochondral injuries. For isolated ACL injuries, there is no high-level evidence to guide clinicians in what treatment to recommend after an acute anterior cruciate injury when it comes to surgical or exercise treatment. In fact, the results in literature reviews report similar outcomes when it comes to patient-reported outcomes, knee function, quality of life, and activity levels between ACL-deficient knees and ACL-reconstructed knees (ACLR).[1–3] For radiologic results, there is even a tendency to inferior results for the ACLR compared with the ACL-deficient knees.[2] There are traditions in choice of treatment and statistics on risk of reinjury and the physicians

Division of Orthopaedics, Oslo University Hospital, Ullevål Sykehus, Postboks 4956, Nydalen, Oslo 0424
E-mail address: berte2@mac.com

Clin Sports Med 43 (2024) 343–354
https://doi.org/10.1016/j.csm.2023.08.003

will inform the patient about this before the patients can be offered shared treatment decision. The shared decision requires knowledge on which criteria predict better outcome. Previously identified predictors in surgically treated patients include activity level, educational level, age, concomitant cartilage, and meniscal injuries. Measurement of knee function including quadriceps muscle strength, single-leg hop test, and patient-reported outcome measurements (PROMs) predicts outcomes in both surgically and nonsurgically treated patients.[4,5] Clinicians and patients can be more confident in a nonsurgical treatment choice in athletes who are female, older in age, and have good knee function, as measured by single-leg hop tests and PROMs, early after an ACL injury. Prediction models that include measures of knee function, assessed either before or after rehabilitation, can estimate 2-year prognoses for nonsurgical treatment, thereby assist shared treatment decision-making.[6] Programs are developed with artificial intelligence (AI) to calculate the risk of additional injuries if the ACL is not surgically reconstructed. The tendency is to recommend surgery to young patients performing pivoting sport. For approximately half of the patients experiencing an ACL injury exercise therapy will lead to a stable knee and these patients can avoid surgical treatment with the possible complications related to an operation. Programs using AI can calculate prognosis and guide clinicians in treatment; however, we still believe in clinical experience when it comes to decisions for the individual patients. To combine what is available in the literature with clinical experience and expert opinions, several consensus reports have been published and become popular, including algorithms for ACL injury treatment.[7–9]

TREATING ACUTE INJURIES

An ACL injury frequently occurs with the knee in valgus with slight flexion when landing or changing direction in contact sport. Most significant acute injuries, whether they affect the muscles, ligaments, tendons, or bone, are characterized by bleeding immediately after the injury. A muscular hematoma can occur as early as 30 seconds after a muscle injury. When the patient sustains an intra-articular ligament rupture and remains untreated, a significant hemarthrosis will be visible within a few minutes in most cases. It is essential that treatment begins as soon as possible after the injury. After a preliminary examination to identify the nature of the injury, and rule out major dislocations or fractures, treatment to limit the extent of damage should begin. The Ottawa Knee Rule (OKR) can be used to decide if the examiner can rule out fracture as a differential diagnosis. OKR is designed to accurately exclude knee fractures and has high sensitivity (98.5%); however, it is not sufficient to rule a fracture in (specificity 48.6%).[10] Patients aged older than 55 years, patients not able to weight-bear for 4 steps, patients not able to flex greater than 90° and patients with tenderness of the patella and/or fibular head should be considered for x-ray imaging. ACL injuries often come with concomitant injuries such as meniscal tears, cartilage injuries, sprains of other ligaments, most frequently the medial collateral ligament (MCL). Adolescents could also have a patellar dislocation or subluxation that will result in tenderness on the medial side of the patella. In experienced hands, a Lachman test is usually sufficient to diagnose an ACL injury in the acute setting. Often the first clinical examinations are performed by less-experienced assessors, and to avoid misdiagnosis, an MRI or repeated examination might be necessary.

ACUTE PHASE

The principles of POLICE include protection, optimal loading, ice, compression, and elevation. Initially, a few hours with brief or total immobilization and unloading are necessary. After the initial examination, to exclude fractures and dislocations, the POLICE principles should be applied as fast as possible. To limit swelling, the POLICE principles emphasize on cooling and good compression after an ACL injury. Bleeding and effusion will continue for 48 hours, and the POLICE treatment should be continued for the whole period.

During this initial stage, in the cases where the athlete is limited by inflammation or pain, the use of nonsteroidal anti-inflammatory drugs or other anti-inflammatory therapy may be called for. Crutches are used until the swelling is minimal and the patient can walk without extension deficit. The anterior cruciate ligament is intra-articular. Following total rupture of an intra-articular ligament, healing will not take place, whereas the capsular ligaments have excellent healing potential.

PRINCIPLES FOR REHABILITATION OF SPORTS INJURIES

All rehabilitation after sports injuries is divided in phases where progression to the next level is decided by pain and swelling (**Table 1**). How fast the athlete can move forward will vary from athlete to athlete, no matter how well trained they are at the time of injury. Based on experience, we can estimate how many weeks each phase normally last and can inform the athlete of their prognosis. However, sometimes additional injuries or unexplained swelling delay the expected progression. In other cases, the athlete wants to speed up the rehabilitation because they feel very little pain or swelling. An important task for the health-care professional is to inform the athlete about the negative sides of training with swelling or to increase the load too fast.

REHABILITATION PHASE

All patients suffering from an ACL injury should be advised to start a rehabilitation program as fast as pain and swelling allows. Guidance from a rehabilitation clinician experienced in rehabilitation of ACL injuries is recommended. This does not mean that the patient needs to do all the exercises under supervision; however, an experienced rehabilitation clinician will ensure adequate progress and recognize complications. The cooperation with a clinician will, in most cases, give access to facilities where the athlete can perform the exercises 2 to 4 times a week. Preoperative quadriceps weakness is a predictor of poorer quadriceps strength after the ACL reconstruction and extension deficit before the operation is a main risk factor for extension deficit after the ACL reconstruction.[11] The only exceptions when it comes to early rehabilitation

Table 1
Phases in nonoperative treatment of anterior crucial ligament injuries

Rehabilitation Phase	Time Frame Non Operative Treatment	Physical Focus
Acute	1–4 wk (2–6 wk postoperative)	Reduce swelling and pain Increase range of movement Initial activation of muscles Minimal load
Active rehabilitation	1–4 mo (2–8 mo postoperative)	Full range of motion Patient can walk normally without pain Strength, stability, and coordination
Intensive training and return to sport	3–9 mo (Gradually from 6 to 12 mo postoperative)	Sport specific exercises High-loading and plyometric exercises

after an ACL injury are those who have additional injuries, such as a bucket handle meniscal injury, a distal MCL rupture, or a significant osteochondral injury that should be treated surgically if diagnosed in the acute phase. In addition, a major injury of the lateral or posterolateral side of the knee is much easier to repair or reconstruct during the first 2 weeks following the injury.

Even if they are young athletes that will be scheduled for early surgery because of their activity level, the recommendation is to start movements of the knee joint to avoid stiffness and lack of extension before the operation. The main tool to determine how much and what kind of training to perform during rehabilitation is to monitor pain and swelling. Rehabilitation protocols have moved from time-based to criterion-based progression to be more individualized. This approach ensures that the athletes do not surpass the capacity of the knee and/or are delayed by time limits. To experience progress, it might be necessary to tolerate some pain, at least as long as pain or swelling does not worsen from one training session to the next. Reduced loading or alternative forms of exercise may be necessary for some patients if they experience increased pain or swelling over time.

To achieve full range of motion, the athlete must be advised to perform active stretching exercises. Especially full extension might be challenging, and after a knee injury, it is comfortable to rest the knee on a pillow. To place the pillow under the ankle while resting the athlete will get some help from gravity in stretching the posterior knee capsule. Lying prone on a bench and letting the weight of the foot stretch the knee is also useful. Knee extension to zero degrees is essential to achieve normal gait pattern.

OUTLINES OF A REHABILITATION PROGRAM

The warmup in the rehabilitation phase would typically be walking on a treadmill, elliptical walker, or cycling on a stationary bicycle (**Fig. 1**). Rehabilitation typically begins with a higher number of repetitions (eg, 4 series of 20–30 repetitions) and lighter loads and should then gradually progress to heavier loads and fewer repetitions (eg, 3 series of 6–8 repetitions).

The exercises in the rehabilitation phase are guided by a dose-respond framework, where the aim for the athlete is to maintain 6 to 8 repetitions in 3 to 4 sets. When they get stronger and can continue doing 10 repetitions in the last set, it is time to increase the load.

Athletes can switch between doing exercises for both legs and for the injured leg. In the beginning, the athletes do not trust the injured leg, and it is natural to start squats on both legs (**Fig. 2**). The flexion angle in the knees can be adjusted and increase with experience. Some patients are familiar with strengthening exercises from injury prevention programs. Other patients might not have performed structured strength training before. Further challenge in squats with both legs will be adding weights on the athlete's shoulders (**Fig. 3**A and B). Mandatory exercises for the injured leg are leg press, knee extension, and leg curl, and most training facilities will have equipment for these exercises. Single leg squats are a neuromuscular challenge increasing both balance and proprioception. Taking it even further is performing the exercise on a balance pad (**Fig. 4**). This is easily available equipment, and the exercise might be performed everywhere, including at home.

Including hamstring in the program can be done when lying supine with flexion in the knee. Lifting the pelvis from the ground will load the hamstring. Initially the athlete will need to start from the floor. Further load and stability training comes with placing the loaded leg on a fitball (**Fig. 5**). Hamstring on fitball including movements is a further challenge (**Fig. 6**A and B).

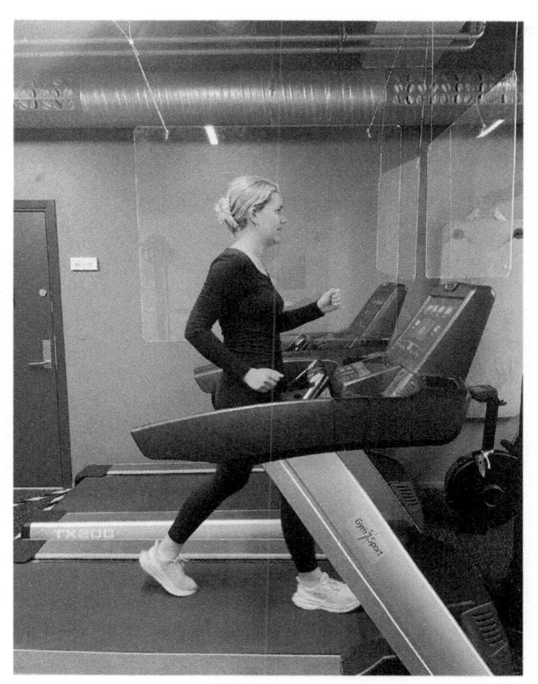

Fig. 1. Warm up before exercise training can be done walking on a treadmill, ellipse walker, or a stationary bike.

Quadriceps strength has been proven to be essential in rehabilitation of ACL-deficient knees. To regain quadriceps muscle strength, open chain exercises should be included as well as closed kinetic chain. Open kinetic chain exercises have been shown to be of importance to increase quadriceps strength.[12]

Plyometric exercises are explosive exercises that require the athlete to generate a large amount of force in a short period. Individuals preparing for return to sport will have to include plyos in their program because different sport activities are heavy on explosive moments. Plyos are the most challenging type of strengthening exercises and will be introduced in a late phase preparing for returning to sport to enhance neuromuscular performance and strength. Plyometrics involves both eccentric and concentric muscle contractions and are all about generating power fast.

In ACL-injured patients, plyometric exercises include single-leg jumps focusing on maintaining knee-over-toe position in landing to avoid injurious dynamic load.[13] Exercise with skating involves jumping from side to side, landing on the single leg (**Fig. 7**A and B).

Supervision

The first weeks after an ACL injury, the athlete might be depressed by the thought of the long way they have to walk before they can return to their favorite activities. It is important to have support both mentally and physically. The exercises should be supervised by a physiotherapist to assure that the exercises are performed at the correct level of difficulty and to ensure compliance. The athlete should meet their therapist at least every other week and replacement of exercises is mandatory to keep the motivation. Replacement of exercises is also important for neuromuscular stimulation and

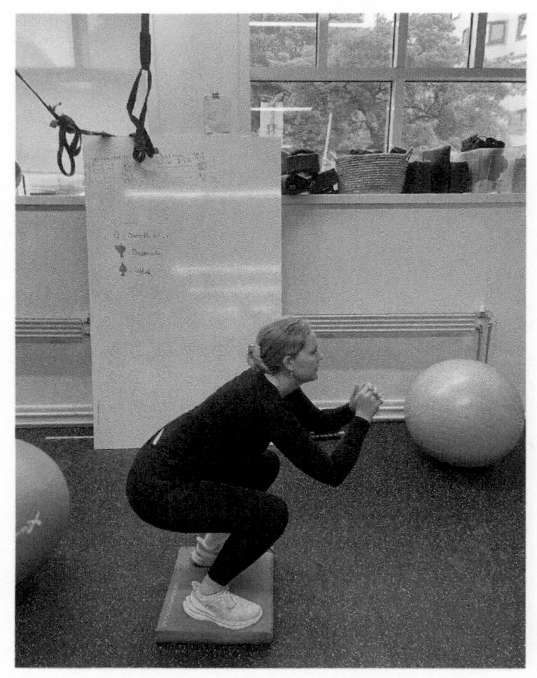

Fig. 2. Simple squats on both legs. First level will limit the angle of knee flexion. Exercise can be more challenging standing on a pillow.

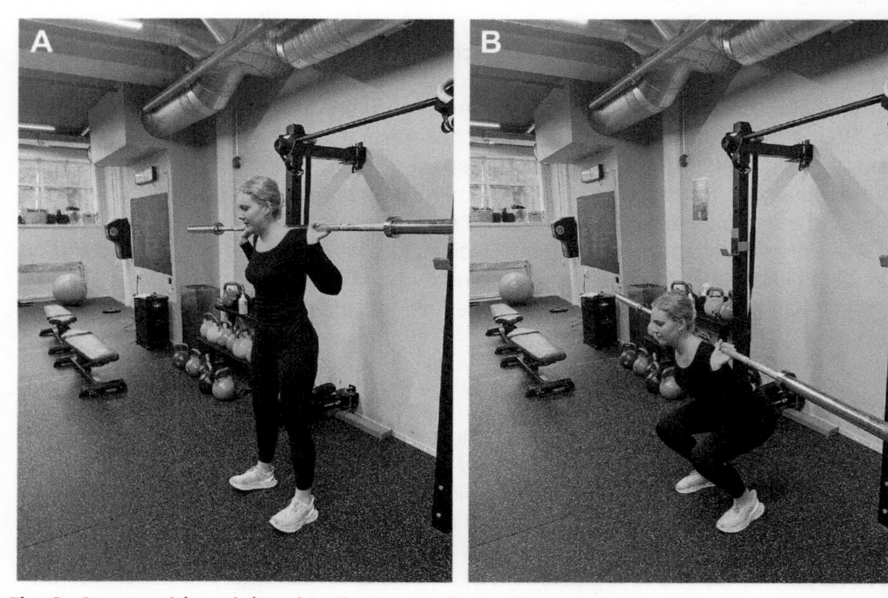

Fig. 3. Squats with weights. (*A, B*) Focus on knee above toe.

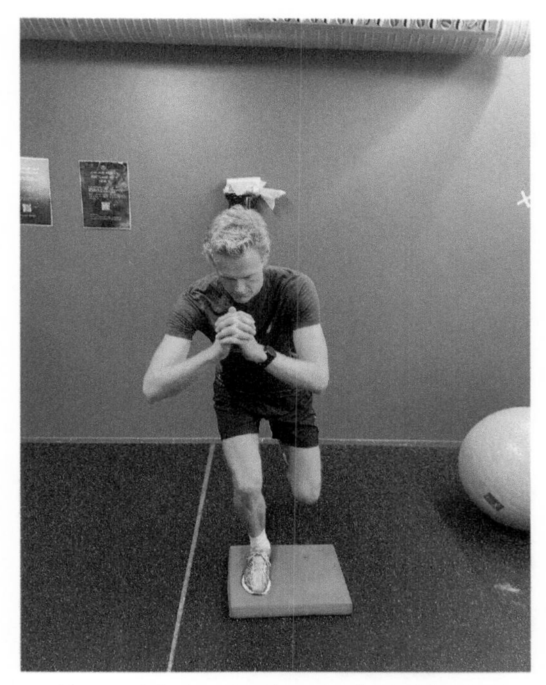

Fig. 4. One leg squat. Non–weight-bearing leg can be held anterior or posterior. Pillow makes it more difficult to maintain balance.

progress. A commonly accepted recommendation is to change only one exercise at a time. This allows the therapist to accurately determine which type of exercise or movement or amount of loading that may be provoking the symptoms. Patients should be reminded to generously apply ice to the joint after exercising.

Postrehabilitation Testing

After completion of the rehabilitation, the athlete should go through testing to assess if they are copers or noncopers to make the final decision whether the athlete needs an ACL reconstruction. Some patients can functionally stabilize the instability caused by the ACL rupture, and these are called "copers."[14] Athletes who do not return to their previous level of activity and experience giving way symptoms are noncopers. Giving way symptoms and/or new injuries affecting the cartilage or meniscus in an ACL-deficient knee is a sign of failure of nonoperative treatment and should be an indication for ACL reconstruction. Some patients might prefer surgery, even if they are copers because of their activity level and desire to return to pivoting sport. Patients who are not referred to surgery will move on to phase 3 in rehabilitation with training.

TRAINING PHASE

An athlete must be highly disciplined, and strong motivation is often required from the athlete, as well as the physician, and physical therapists to achieve the desired result. It is crucial for the athlete to be continuously instructed and, if necessary, to keep a training and pain diary, to record and monitor response to training.

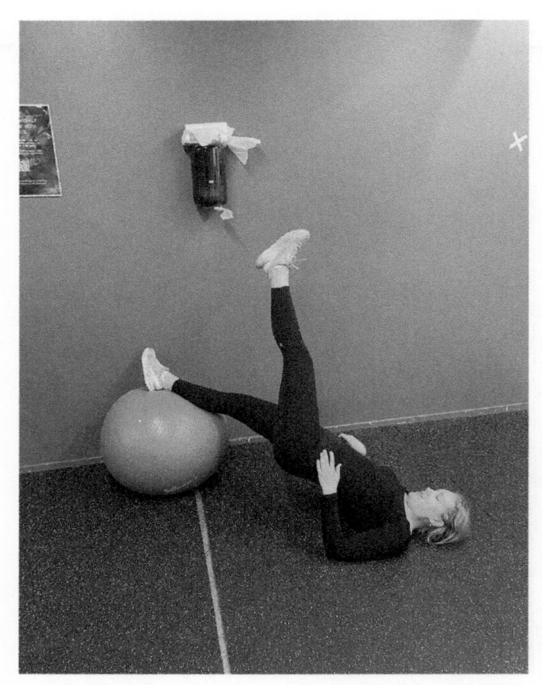

Fig. 5. Hamstring on fitball. One foot on top of the ball. Lift back and pelvis up and maintain a steady position.

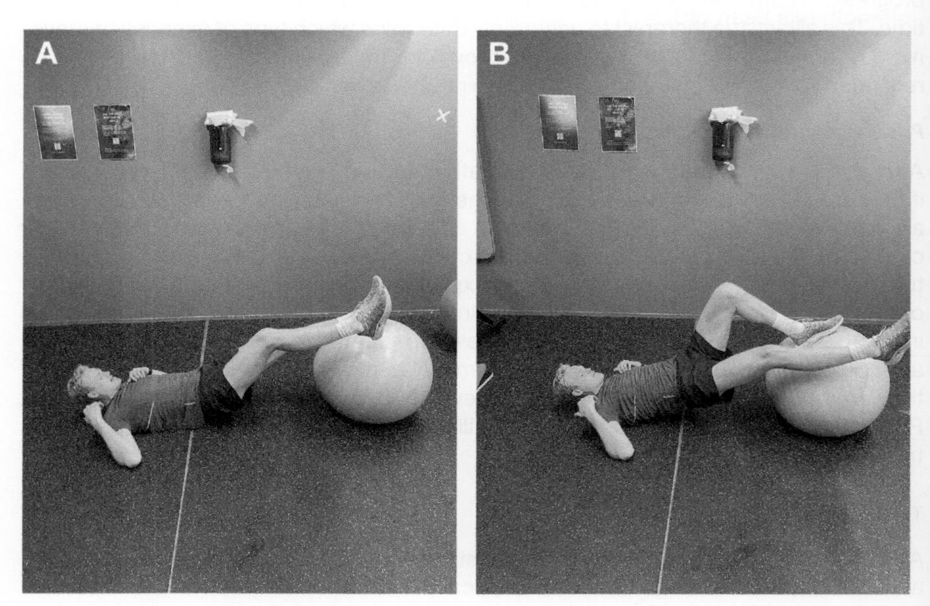

Fig. 6. Hamstring on fitball with movements. (*A, B*) One foot on the ball. Lift back and pelvis and pull the ball toward the pelvis.

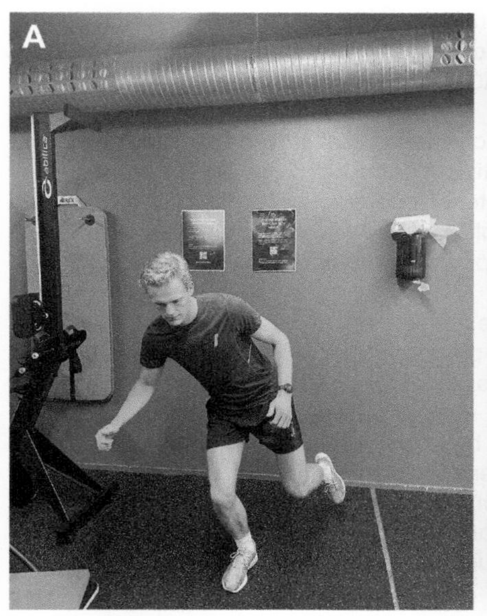
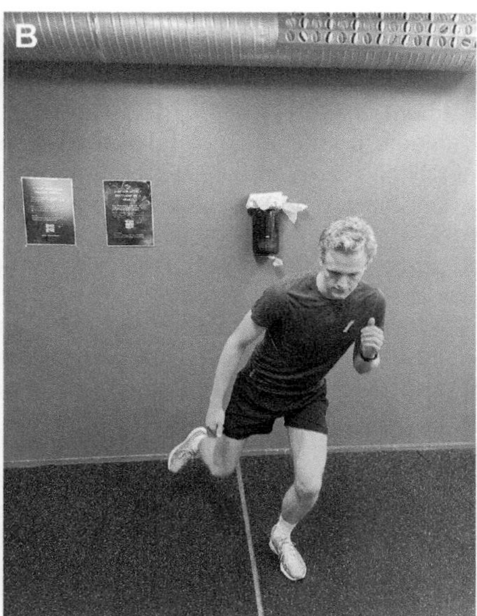

Fig. 7. Skating. (*A, B*) Start on one leg, hop sideways, and aim for a soft, deep, and steady landing on the other leg.

With injuries that require a prolonged rehabilitation period, health-care personnel can be considered more like coaches than caregivers.

During the training phase, the athlete is expected to achieve normal strength in the quadriceps and hamstring group compared with the healthy side. Quadriceps strength has been proven to be the single most important predictor to knee function 2 years after ACL reconstruction.[4] Another aim is normal sensory motor function. Knee injuries may reduce neuromuscular function and a slow reaction to changes of position makes the athlete vulnerable to new injuries caused by cutting and landing. The uninjured leg is often used to compare the standard both when examining an injury and when measuring results of training. For ACL patients, this might lead to a misinterpretation in individuals because of bilateral neuromuscular changes after injury.[13]

Eventually, controlled sport-specific training must be incorporated to reduce the risk of reinjury. The athlete should be fully recovered physically and mentally before resuming competitive activity.

RETURN TO SPORT

A gradual return to sport and activities are integrated in rehabilitation protocols for nonoperative treatment of ACL injuries as the same for rehabilitation after ACL reconstruction. If the patient has an ACL injury, it is common to plan on 6 to 9 months of rehabilitation and recovery time before the athlete can return to sports that involve hard stops and sudden turns. Those patients who are characterized of achieving good knee stability are copers and those who do not achieve satisfactory stability are noncopers. Patients with ACL injury may experience a significant functional improvement after rehabilitation.[15] There are no randomized studies available in the literature that investigate the outcome of patients who are divided into copers and noncopers based on functional criteria. There is one RCT where patients could be randomized into a treatment group of optional delayed ACL reconstruction. Of the 59 patients in this group, 30 patients required ACL reconstruction after initial nonsurgical treatment.[16]

Athletes participating in less pivoting activities, such as running, bicycling, and weightlifting are amenable to nonoperative treatment. Such activities are less demanding on the knee stabilizers and anterior-posterior instability can to a certain degree be maintained by muscular control.[17] In less pivoting activities, the athlete can achieve an earlier return to sport compared with athletes going through an ACL reconstruction.[18]

There are some criteria to fulfill before the athlete can return to sport at a high level. The athlete has to be fully rehabilitated and physically ready. Physically readiness can be measured by certain criteria, such as isokinetic quadriceps strength testing. Equally important is it that the athlete is mentally ready to perform their activity. Assessing psychological readiness might be more challenging. The physician can use patient-reported tools such as the anterior cruciate ligament return to sport after injury scale.[19] Even though the rehabilitation protocols have moved from time-based to criteria-based, depending on the situation and type of injury, biology requires sufficient time for the tissues to heal. Early return to pivoting sports has been associated with a high rate of knee reinjuries.[20]

CLINICS CARE POINTS

- An ACL injury can be treated either nonoperatively with training or operatively with ACL reconstruction. Both treatments require intensive rehabilitation.
- Nonoperative treatment is divided in phases based on physical criteria. The patient has to fulfill physical criteria and be mentally ready before returning to sport.
- After nonoperative treatment, the patient and the treatment team should evaluate the result of the treatment and decide whether to proceed to surgical treatment in a shared decision.
- Measurement of knee function including quadriceps muscle strength, single-leg hop test, and PROMs predict outcomes in both surgically and nonsurgically treated patients.

SUMMARY

Following trauma where an ACL injury is confirmed, the athlete and physician should advise a schedule that addresses rehabilitation, appropriateness of ACL reconstruction, and return to sport. A policy of shared decision-making, after nonoperative treatment, the patient and surgical team should decide whether to proceed with ACL reconstruction surgery to address continued symptoms or instability.

An athlete must not be sent back to contact or pivoting sports without being physically and mentally prepared to return. The patient's knee strength, balance, and function should be tested and compared with the contralateral healthy side before declaring the patient fully rehabilitated.

A clear consensus does not exist for selection of exercises and how many sessions every week in the early phase after an ACL injury. The strength training should be based on regiments for heavy resistant strength training with few repetitions in each series to increase muscle volume and promote neuromuscular adaption.

Future studies, including randomized controlled trials with groups that perform different exercise therapy programs, are needed to verify the potential effectiveness of different programs.

DISCLOSURES

The author, her immediate family, and any research foundations with which she is affiliated have not received any financial payments or other benefits from any commercial entity related to the subject of this article.

REFERENCES

1. Filbay SR, Culvenor AG, Ackerman IN, et al. Quality of life in anterior cruciate ligament-deficient individuals: a systematic review and meta-analysis. Br J Sports Med 2015;49(16):1033–41.
2. Smith TO, Postle K, Penny F, et al. Is reconstruction the best management strategy for anterior cruciate ligament rupture? A systematic review and meta-analysis comparing anterior cruciate ligament reconstruction versus non-operative treatment. Knee 2014;21(2):462–70.
3. Monk AP, Davies LJ, Hopewell S, et al. Surgical versus conservative interventions for treating anterior cruciate ligament injuries. Cochrane Database Syst Rev 2016; 4(4):Cd011166.
4. Eitzen I, Holm I, Risberg MA. Preoperative quadriceps strength is a significant predictor of knee function two years after anterior cruciate ligament reconstruction. Br J Sports Med 2009;43(5):371–6.
5. Logerstedt D, Lynch A, Axe MJ, et al. Pre-operative quadriceps strength predicts IKDC2000 scores 6 months after anterior cruciate ligament reconstruction. Knee 2013;20(3):208–12.
6. Grindem H, Wellsandt E, Failla M, et al. Anterior cruciate ligament injury-who succeeds without reconstructive surgery? the delaware-oslo ACL cohort study. Orthopaedic Journal of Sports Medicine 2018;6(5). 2325967118774255.
7. Petersen W, Guenther D, Imhoff AB, et al. Management after acute rupture of the anterior cruciate ligament (ACL). Part 1: ACL reconstruction has a protective effect on secondary meniscus and cartilage lesions. Knee Surg Sports Traumatol Arthrosc 2023;31(5):1665–74.
8. Petersen W, Häner M, Guenther D, et al. Management after acute injury of the anterior cruciate ligament (ACL), part 2: management of the ACL-injured patient. Knee Surg Sports Traumatol Arthrosc 2023;31(5):1675–89.
9. Diermeier T, Rothrauff BB, Engebretsen L, et al, Panther Symposium ACL Treatment Consensus Group. Treatment after anterior cruciate ligament injury: Panther Symposium ACL Treatment Consensus Group. Knee Surg Sports Traumatol Arthrosc 2020;28(8):2390–402.
10. Bachmann LM, Haberzeth S, Steurer J, et al. The accuracy of the Ottawa knee rule to rule out knee fractures: a systematic review. Ann Intern Med 2004; 140(2):121–4.
11. Carter HM, Littlewood C, Webster KE, et al. The effectiveness of preoperative rehabilitation programmes on postoperative outcomes following anterior cruciate ligament (ACL) reconstruction: a systematic review. BMC Muscoskel Disord 2020;21(1):647.
12. Lepley LK, Wojtys EM, Palmieri-Smith RM. Combination of eccentric exercise and neuromuscular electrical stimulation to improve quadriceps function post-ACL reconstruction. Knee 2015;22(3):270–7.

13. Palmieri-Smith RM, Thomas AC. A neuromuscular mechanism of posttraumatic osteoarthritis associated with ACL injury. Exerc Sport Sci Rev 2009;37(3):147–53.
14. Thoma LM, Grindem H, Logerstedt D, et al. Coper classification early after anterior cruciate ligament rupture changes with progressive neuromuscular and strength training and is associated with 2-year success: the delaware-oslo ACL Cohort Study. Am J Sports Med 2019;47(4):807–14.
15. Moksnes H, Snyder-Mackler L, Risberg MA. Individuals with an anterior cruciate ligament-deficient knee classified as noncopers may be candidates for nonsurgical rehabilitation. J Orthop Sports Phys Ther 2008;38(10):586–95.
16. Frobell RB, Roos HP, Roos EM, et al. Treatment for acute anterior cruciate ligament tear: five year outcome of randomised trial. BMJ 2013;346:f232.
17. Waite JC, Beard DJ, Dodd CA, et al. In vivo kinematics of the ACL-deficient limb during running and cutting. Knee Surg Sports Traumatol Arthrosc 2005;13(5):377–84.
18. Grindem H, Eitzen I, Moksnes H, et al. A pair-matched comparison of return to pivoting sports at 1 year in anterior cruciate ligament-injured patients after a nonoperative versus an operative treatment course. Am J Sports Med 2012;40(11):2509–16.
19. Webster KE, Feller JA, Lambros C. Development and preliminary validation of a scale to measure the psychological impact of returning to sport following anterior cruciate ligament reconstruction surgery. Phys Ther Sport 2008;9(1):9–15.
20. Grindem H, Snyder-Mackler L, Moksnes H, et al. Simple decision rules can reduce reinjury risk by 84% after acl reconstruction: the delaware-oslo ACL cohort study. Br J Sports Med 2016;50(13):804–8.

Perioperative

Value-Based, Environmentally Sustainable Anterior Cruciate Ligament Surgery

Ian D. Engler, MD[a,b,*], Frances L. Koback, BS[c],
Andrew J. Curley, MD[b,d]

KEYWORDS

- ACL reconstruction • Cost • Value • Environmental • Sustainability
- Operating room • Waste

KEY POINTS

- Although clinical factors remain most important, surgeons should consider broader societal impacts of their decisions surrounding anterior cruciate ligament (ACL) reconstruction.
- Value-based ACL reconstruction, in which cost is reduced over the long term, includes operating in outpatient/ambulatory surgery centers, using autograft, choosing meniscus repair over meniscectomy when indicated, and using less costly implants such as metal screws and staples.
- Environmentally sustainable ACL reconstruction, in which greenhouse gas emissions and waste are reduced, includes minimizing waste in the operating room, using surgical packs and trays that only include the needed equipment, and avoiding use of the inhaled anesthetic gas desflurane.

INTRODUCTION

Anterior cruciate ligament (ACL) reconstruction has many technical aspects that surgeons consider with clinical outcomes in mind, but orthopedic surgeons are increasingly recognizing the additional broader societal impacts of their surgical decisions. Of note, cost is an unavoidable factor in patient management decisions given that health care systems at all levels must function financially. Value, herein referring to financial value or maximizing cost-effectiveness, has been an integral part of modern orthopedic surgery literature as US health care costs continue to rise and as individual institutions strive for financial stability.[1]

[a] Central Maine Healthcare Orthopedics, Central Maine Medical Center, 690 Minot Avenue #1, Auburn, ME 04210, USA; [b] UPMC Freddie Fu Sports Medicine Center, University of Pittsburgh, 3200 South Water Street, Pittsbrugh, PA, USA; [c] Geisel School of Medicine at Dartmouth, Dartmouth College, 1 Rope Ferry Road, Hanover, NH 03755, USA; [d] TidalHealth Nanticoke, 801 Middleford Road, Seaford, DE 19973, USA
* Corresponding author. 690 Minot Ave #1, Auburn, ME, 04210.
E-mail address: ianenglermd@gmail.com

Clin Sports Med 43 (2024) 355–365
https://doi.org/10.1016/j.csm.2023.08.004
0278-5919/24/

More recently, environmental sustainability has been recognized as a relevant entity to orthopedics.[2] Environmental sustainability means conducting actions in a manner that reduces harm to the planet and environment while maintaining the desired quality of outcomes from those actions. Although impact on the planet occurs in many ways, the most common are through greenhouse gas emissions—for example, via energy use or material production—which contribute to global warming and through production of waste or trash. The health care sector is one of the biggest contributors to greenhouse gases in the United States, with the operating room having a particularly large impact.[3] Orthopedic surgery is one of the highest volume surgical specialties, so it is an important player in the discussion around environmental sustainability in medicine.[4]

ACL reconstruction is a frequent procedure within sports medicine, with the use of implants and appreciable operating time, so considering both its value and environmental impact is prudent. Cost and sustainability are symbiotic, with less material use leading to both lower cost and generally a lower environmental impact. Therefore, considering these issues together can be helpful. If surgeons wish to fully understand the outcomes of their decisions surrounding ACL reconstruction, they may reflect on both cost and environmental impact.

DISCUSSION: VALUE-BASED ANTERIOR CRUCIATE LIGAMENT SURGERY

As costs in the US health care system rise to likely unsustainable levels, it has become increasingly important for physicians to consider the cost-effectiveness of patient management options.[1] This certainly holds true for patients with ACL injuries. The cost of care is affected by each of the many decisions within ACL injury management, though here the most well-researched decision points will be discussed.

Of note, in many of the following sections, cost-effectiveness analyses results are reported in cost per quality-adjusted life year (QALY). Here, QALY will be defined as "the equivalent of a completely well year of life, or a year of life free of any symptoms, problems, or health-related disabilities,"[5] where quality of life is measured by the Quality of Well-Being scale.[5,6] In addition, costs in the following sections are reported as 2023 currency adjusted for inflation.

Operative Versus Nonoperative Management

The most fundamental question in the management of ACL injuries is in selecting operative versus nonoperative management. Given the impact of this decision on the patient, cost may not play a central role. Nevertheless, research on the cost-effectiveness of ACL reconstruction surgery versus nonoperative management has been performed, with mixed results.

Most literature shows that ACL reconstruction is a cost-effective option for most patients. Literature has defined "very cost-effective procedures" as those having a cost per QALY of less than $41,431 ($29,300 in 2009)[6,7] and concluded that ACL reconstruction was a cost-effective option for patients, at a cost per QALY of $14,601 for ACL reconstruction ($10,326 in 2009) versus, for comparison, $8177 for knee arthroscopy ($5783 in 2009).[6]

Further research on the cost-effectiveness of ACL reconstruction led to similar findings, calculating an average cost of $10,318 ($5857 in 2000) per QALY for ACL reconstruction surgery.[8] The investigators concluded that ACL reconstruction surgery was a cost-effective procedure for many patients, especially for young adults who value a knee capable of participation in sports and other activities of daily living.

Some studies suggest that ACL reconstruction may not be cost-effective when compared with nonoperative management. A 2021 study reported that early ACL reconstruction leads to a slight improvement (0.04) in QALY compared with nonoperative rehabilitation.[9] Yet, the costs associated with ACL reconstruction, which ranged from €55,984/QALY (health care perspective; €48,460 in 2021) to €90,317/QALY (societal perspective; €78,179 in 2021), led the authors to conclude that ACL reconstruction was not a cost-effective option for the standard population, given a maximum willingness-to-pay of €23,105/QALY (€20,000 in 2021).[9] A second study similarly concluded that the additional 0.13 QALY is not worth the €6010 additional cost (€4695 in 2016) for most patients when choosing to undergo early ACL reconstruction as opposed to nonsurgical management.[10]

These cost-effectiveness studies depend greatly on the benefit derived from ACL reconstruction. This benefit has more consistently been demonstrated in the United States than European literature, contributing to the question of cost-effectiveness of reconstruction in European literature above.[6,8–10] Of note, data even out of Europe are increasingly clear on the merits of early ACL reconstruction.[11–13] Therefore, arguments for the cost–benefit of ACL reconstruction continue to strengthen.

Hospital Versus Outpatient Surgical Center Setting

ACL reconstruction may be performed in either a hospital setting or in an outpatient surgical center. Several studies indicate that ACL reconstructions performed in outpatient surgical centers are associated with lower costs and similar patient outcomes.[14–16]

A 2017 analysis found that when compared with ACL reconstruction performed in a hospital setting, outpatient ACL reconstruction resulted in cost savings ranging from $1697 to $9146 ($1371 to $7390 in 2017[14]). Similarly, an older study found that the average cost for an inpatient procedure was $18,353 ($9220 in 1995), whereas the average cost for an outpatient procedure was $7773 ($3905 in 1995)—a cost savings of 58%.[15]

Perhaps most convincingly, a 2023 study found that performing primary ACL reconstruction in ambulatory surgical centers had the largest effect of all measured variables on reducing total health care utilization—including preoperative and postoperative care—associated with ACL reconstruction.[16] ACL reconstructions performed in outpatient hospitals were associated with a $6,789, or 39%, increase in cost when compared with those performed in ambulatory surgical centers.

Anesthesia

Anesthesia and pain management options are associated with variable costs in the perioperative period around ACL reconstruction. Traditionally, general anesthesia alone has been standard during ACL reconstruction.[17] More recent studies have explored regional anesthesia with nerve blocks as an addition or alternative to general anesthesia. Cost analysis of regional anesthesia considers the added expense of the anesthesia provider's time and expertise alongside the potential benefits of improved pain control and therefore facilitation of stable discharge.

A 2016 analysis found that nerve blocks in addition to general anesthesia facilitated reliable same-day surgery discharge and significantly reduced unanticipated hospital admissions in pediatric patients undergoing ACL reconstruction, thereby reducing costs.[18] In addition to the cost benefits, adding regional anesthesia was also associated with improved postoperative comfort, decreased postoperative nausea and vomiting, and reduced recovery time. Nerve blocks similarly contribute to reliable same-day discharge and post-anesthesia care unit bypass in a general ACL reconstruction population.

Regional anesthesia alone may not provide effective pain control—especially because of concerns that a more comprehensive femoral nerve block affects the quadriceps, which many surgeons wish to spare, and the quadriceps-sparing adductor canal block may not provide as much regional pain coverage.[19,20] In addition, there is the concern for nerve injury with nerve blocks. Nevertheless, if the management team is comfortable and efficient with blocks, hospitals and outpatient surgical centers may have the potential to create cost savings by adding regional anesthesia to general anesthesia.

Graft Type

The selection of graft type in ACL reconstruction is one of the most debated and researched variables in sports medicine, and there have been cost analyses in addition to the myriad outcome-related studies. The literature suggests that although autografts require increased operative time and may lead to slightly increased recovery room costs due to pain associated with donor site morbidity, the overall cost of autografts is significantly less than that of allografts.[1,17,21–23] Studies consistently showing higher allograft failure rates in high-risk populations also imply greater lifetime cost of care with allografts.[24,25]

Numerous studies have evaluated the clinical outcomes of bone–patellar tendon–bone (BTB) versus hamstring versus quadriceps autograft. The frequent conflicting results of failure rate by graft make cost-effectiveness analyses challenging because those analyses depend on what failure rate or outcomes are input and those outcomes are variable in the literature. One study on the topic compared BTB autograft, hamstring autograft, and allograft and determined that the hamstring autograft was the most cost-effective for patients.[1] However, the cost savings associated with hamstring autograft were modest—$265 ($207 in 2015) when compared with BTB autograft. Therefore, the investigators concluded that the lower failure rate and increased stability associated with BTB autograft may override a slightly increased cost to make BTB autograft the most cost-effective option for patients.[1]

Meniscus Management

Intraoperative management of meniscus pathology during ACL reconstruction has evolved over time, with more surgeons and literature preferring meniscus preservation via repair when possible to save the meniscus.[26,27] Similar to the decision over operative versus nonoperative management of ACL injury, which is important enough that it may warrant purely clinical evaluation over a cost-based evaluation, this decision may factor in cost less heavily than other variables associated with ACL reconstruction.

Nevertheless, cost-effectiveness analyses also favor meniscus repair. Meniscus repair does have higher initial cost ($8315) than meniscectomy ($6356) ($7094 vs $5423 in 2020).[28] However, given meniscal preservation improving quality of life and prolonging the longevity of the knee, most studies report that meniscus repair is more cost-effective longer term than meniscectomy in the setting of concomitant ACL reconstruction.[29,30] Long-term cost savings of repair are up to $8300 ($6870 in 2018).[29] Considering clinical and cost perspectives, meniscus repair should be the first-line treatment option for patients with concomitant ACL and meniscus injuries in the setting of a reparable meniscus tear.

Implants and Devices

Implants are ubiquitous in ACL reconstruction. Definitive implant costs are generally not available or consistent because they vary based on negotiations between hospitals and device companies. However, several studies have investigated the costs of implants associated with ACL reconstruction, though some report charges and others report cost (**Tables 1** and **2**).[31,32]

Beyond costs of specific implants, evaluation of costs across somewhat comparable categories of implants—such as metal versus bioabsorbable interference screws—can be useful. Newer bioabsorbable interference screws are designed to promote osseous integration and are often more expensive than metal implants. Given limited US studies on the topic, a Brazilian study showed a cost of R$1377 for metal versus R$1972 for bioabsorbable (R refers to Brazilian Real; R$984.00 vs R$1409.00 in 2016).[33] Clinical studies comparing bioabsorbable screws to metal screws are limited; however, most report similar patient outcomes.[33] More research is necessary to better understand the cost-effectiveness of various types of interference screws in the context of patient outcomes.

Cost to Patients

Patient expenses are a consideration in the value-based approach to ACL reconstruction as the health care system should strive to minimize financial burden on patients. Carbone and colleagues analyzed 37,763 patients who underwent primary ACL reconstruction between 2013 and 2017 and reported a 36% increase in patient out-of-pocket expenses alongside a 4.3% decrease in day-of-surgery reimbursement during those years.[4] Therefore, although out-of-pocket expenses continue to rise for patients undergoing primary ACL reconstruction, reimbursement rates have fallen among both commercial insurers and Medicare.[4]

When considering value in health care, one must consider patient willingness-to-pay and the personal importance a patient places on a stable functional knee. Many studies have shown that patients are willing to pay higher out-of-pocket expenses for early ACL reconstruction[34] and are willing to pay much more for ACL reconstruction than traditional payors, including insurance companies and government programs.[35] This suggests that patients value ACL reconstruction more than traditional payors recognize.

Price transparency is an issue for patients and even for researchers. A prospective study attempted to obtain price estimates for ACL reconstruction from 102 hospitals in 2020.[36] Only 30% of hospitals were able to provide a complete price estimate, whereas 52% were unable to provide any price information.

As the US health care system moves toward a value-based approach to care, it is crucial for the field to adopt a more transparent approach to pricing and reimbursement. This will enable accurate evaluation of the correlation between cost and patient outcomes and facilitate identification of the most value-based approaches to ACL reconstruction.

DISCUSSION: ENVIRONMENTALLY SUSTAINABLE ANTERIOR CRUCIATE LIGAMENT SURGERY

Beyond cost, another important societal consideration in precision ACL reconstruction is the environmental impact of the procedure.[37] Climate change is an increasingly

Table 1
Charges of common implants associated with anterior cruciate ligament reconstruction (limited by companies with available data in the referenced study)[31]

Implant Type	Charge (2023 US Dollars)
EndoButton (Smith & Nephew)	2720
Fast-Fix 360 Meniscus Repair (Smith & Nephew)	2559
Bioabsorbable Biointrafix Flexisheath (DePuy Mitek)	1721
EndoButton Closed Loop (Smith & Nephew)	1602
Bioabsorbable Tibial Screw (DePuy Mitek)	1565
Interference Screw (Smith & Nephew)	1510

Table 2
Cost of common anterior cruciate ligament reconstruction femoral and tibial fixation implants[32]

Femoral Implant Device	Cost (2023 Euros)
Rigidfix	360
Endobutton (Smith & Nephew)	235
Metal interference screw	138
Staple	28
Tibial Implant Device	**Cost (2023 Euros)**
Bio-Intrafix (DePuy Mitek; expansion sheath and tapered screw)	450
Rigidfix	360
Metal interference screw	138
AO screw and washer	55
Staple	28

recognized and impactful force facing society, and health care plays a large role in it through the carbon emissions and waste involved in the sector.[38] Although a large environmental impact is to be expected in such a large and complex sector, there is much work that can be done readily to reduce the environmental impact from health care and orthopedic surgery.[39,40] ACL reconstruction presents a useful case study in that regard, and surgeons can consider several variables to reduce the carbon footprint of the procedure without compromising patient care. This has been termed "Greening the OR."

Waste

ACL reconstruction, similar to other surgical procedures,[41,42] produces large volumes of waste. Many facilities use disposable gowns, drapes, towels, and other components of the procedure. Single-use items are convenient because they do not require sterilization or reprocessing to guarantee sterility. Replacing disposable items with reusable ones in the operating room generally leads to a smaller environmental impact, shown most conclusively with gowns and drapes though with less data on surgical instruments.[43] Easily reusable items include cotton towels, basins, sterile tray coverings, tourniquets, sequential compression devices, and gel pads. Even making incremental changes by consistently replacing a few disposable items with reusable ones can have an impact when considering the summation of a year's worth of cases.

When reusing equipment is difficult or unsafe, even disposable equipment can play a role in reducing greenhouse gas emissions. In the operating room, the two primary trash systems are biohazard trash—often in a red bag—and non-contaminated trash—often in a clear bag. Biohazard trash is much more energy-intensive to process as it is generally incinerated instead of simply stored in a waste facility.[44] Therefore, minimizing biohazard trash by properly separating trash types makes a difference.[41]

One strategy to decrease mental burden on operating room staff is to only have non-biohazard trash bags open before the case, or before contamination is possible. Once the case starts, the biohazard bag is opened. Thereafter, the staff should think about in which bag to place a given piece of trash, only placing contaminated items in the biohazard bags.

Surgical Packs and Trays

Streamlining surgical packs and trays involves only including the necessary equipment for the case at hand, leading to a "Smart OR." Naturally surgeons want to be ready for the unexpected, so some items in trays may not be used consistently. Yet if packs and trays are redesigned to only include the most commonly used equipment—for example, those that are used every fifth case or more often—then there will be less disposable items wasted and fewer sterilized instruments that do not need to undergo energy-intensive sterilization.[45]

The easiest version of this is surgeons reevaluating their pick cards, or the items opened for a given surgical procedure. Surgeons should ensure that each item on the card is worth opening. Other intermittently needed items can be kept ”on hold“ in the room, such that they are not wasted if not needed but can be opened quickly in the event that the surgeon wants it.[46]

Surgical packs are difficult to redesign because they are often purchased preassembled from companies. Therefore, basic packs can be ordered instead and supplemented with the surgeon's preferred drapes and other such equipment.

Implants and Devices

The environmental impact of implants and devices is challenging to assess given the proprietary nature of the technology. Although lower volume of disposable implants would seem to have a smaller impact, the energy intensity of production of each implant matters greatly in that calculation and that production is generally not shared with the public. Devices that have reusable inserters, such as reusable taps and punches for anchors or reusable tensioners for graft or suture tension, avoid waste and the carbon emissions associated with the upstream production of the product. However, the energy and materials used to make the reusable taps and punches should also be considered when comparing to single-use materials, requiring further investigation to determine the most environmentally friendly approach. Of note, the clinical implications of implant usage are likely more important to the surgeon and patient than the environmental implications. The environmental implications factor in most in the setting of clinically equivalent implants or techniques.

Anesthesia

Anesthesia has helped lead the way in the study of the environmental impact of the operating room, and their literature shows carbon-reduction strategies.[47,48] The most impactful is cessation of the use of desflurane, an inhaled anesthetic gas.[49] Anesthetic gases are minimally metabolized, and the vast majority of the administered gas is released into the hospital room and ultimately the atmosphere. Desflurane is an incredibly potent greenhouse gas, with a global warming potential of 20 times that of the alternative sevoflurane.[49] Sevoflurane is an easy substitute that the surgeon could request from the anesthesiologist. Regional anesthesia may reduce inhaled gas use, and propofol-only anesthesia avoids all gas use, reducing emissions further.[50]

SUMMARY

Surgeons play a prominent role in society in bringing people back to health, but they also play a prominent role in health care by contributing cost and environmental impact through their work. Therefore, consideration of cost and environmental impacts is prudent. ACL reconstruction presents a prime opportunity for sports medicine surgeons to take value and environmental sustainability into consideration in some of the many variables they face. Certainly, clinical care and outcomes remain the most important factor in each of the decisions. Yet, in the face of clinical equivalency, society could benefit from surgeons preferring value and decreased environmental impact in their ACL reconstructions.

CLINICS CARE POINTS

- Within decisions surrounding anterior cruciate ligament (ACL) reconstruction, surgeons should consider the broader societal impacts of cost and environmental impact in the setting of clinical equivalency.
- Long-term value-based ACL reconstruction includes operating in outpatient surgery centers over hospitals, using autograft over allograft, choosing meniscus repair over meniscectomy when indicated, and using less expensive fixation devices such as metal screws and staples.
- Environmentally sustainable ACL reconstruction, which reduces waste and greenhouse gas emissions, includes refining surgical packs and trays to only the needed equipment, avoiding use of the inhaled anesthetic gas desflurane or gases altogether, and minimizing operating room waste.

DISCLOSURE

The authors have no commercial or financial conflicts of interest pertaining to this article, and there were no funding sources for this article.

REFERENCES

1. Saltzman BM, Cvetanovich GL, Nwachukwu BU, et al. Economic Analyses in Anterior Cruciate Ligament Reconstruction: A Qualitative and Systematic Review. Am J Sports Med 2016;44(5):1329–35.
2. Engler ID, Curley AJ, Fu FH, et al. Environmental Sustainability in Orthopaedic Surgery. J Am Acad Orthop Surg 2022;30(11):504–11.
3. Wu S, Cerceo E. Sustainability Initiatives in the Operating Room. Jt Comm J Qual Patient Saf 2021;47(10):663–72.
4. Carbone AD, Wang K, Tiao J, et al. Trends in Health Care Expenditures and Patient Out-of-Pocket Expenses in Primary Anterior Cruciate Ligament Reconstruction. Am J Sports Med 2022;50(10):2680–7.
5. Seiber WJ, Groessl EJ, David KM, et al. Quality of Well Being Self-Administered (QWB-SA) Scale. 2008. Available at: https://hoap.ucsd.edu/qwb-info/qwb-manual.pdf.
6. Lubowitz JH, Appleby D. Cost-Effectiveness Analysis of the Most Common Orthopaedic Surgery Procedures: Knee Arthroscopy and Knee Anterior Cruciate Ligament Reconstruction. Arthrosc J Arthrosc Relat Surg 2011;27(10):1317–22.
7. Laupacis A, Feeny D, Detsky AS, et al. How attractive does a new technology have to be to warrant adoption and utilization? Tentative guidelines for using clinical and economic evaluations. CMAJ Can Med Assoc J 1992;146(4):473–81.
8. Gottlob CA, Baker CL. Anterior cruciate ligament reconstruction: socioeconomic issues and cost effectiveness. Am J Orthop Belle Mead NJ 2000;29(6):472–6.
9. Eggerding V, Reijman M, Meuffels DE, et al. ACL reconstruction for all is not cost-effective after acute ACL rupture. Br J Sports Med 2022;56(1):24–8.

10. Kiadaliri AA, Englund M, Lohmander LS, et al. No economic benefit of early knee reconstruction over optional delayed reconstruction for ACL tears: registry enriched randomised controlled trial data. Br J Sports Med 2016;50(9):558–63.
11. Beard DJ, Davies L, Cook JA, et al. Rehabilitation versus surgical reconstruction for non-acute anterior cruciate ligament injury (ACL SNNAP): a pragmatic randomised controlled trial. Lancet Lond Engl 2022;400(10352):605–15.
12. Persson K, Bergerson E, Svantesson E, et al. Greater proportion of patients report an acceptable symptom state after ACL reconstruction compared with non-surgical treatment: a 10-year follow-up from the Swedish National Knee Ligament Registry. Br J Sports Med 2022;56(15):862–9.
13. Bergerson E, Persson K, Svantesson E, et al. Superior Outcome of Early ACL Reconstruction versus Initial Non-reconstructive Treatment With Late Crossover to Surgery: A Study From the Swedish National Knee Ligament Registry. Am J Sports Med 2022;50(4):896–903.
14. Ferrari D, Lopes TJA, França PFA, et al. Outpatient versus inpatient anterior cruciate ligament reconstruction: A systematic review with meta-analysis. Knee 2017;24(2):197–206.
15. Kao JT, Giangarra CE, Singer G, et al. A comparison of outpatient and inpatient anterior cruciate ligament reconstruction surgery. Arthrosc J Arthrosc Relat Surg 1995;11(2):151–6.
16. Tiao J, Wang K, Carbone AD, et al. Ambulatory Surgery Centers Significantly Decrease Total Health Care Expenditures in Primary Anterior Cruciate Ligament Reconstruction. Am J Sports Med 2023;51(1):97–106.
17. Foster BD, Terrell R, Montgomery SR, et al. Hospital Charges and Practice Patterns for General and Regional Anesthesia in Arthroscopic Anterior Cruciate Ligament Repair. Orthop J Sports Med 2013;1(5). 2325967113505270.
18. Hall-Burton DM, Hudson ME, Grudziak JS, et al. Regional Anesthesia Is Cost-Effective in Preventing Unanticipated Hospital Admission in Pediatric Patients Having Anterior Cruciate Ligament Reconstruction. Reg Anesth Pain Med 2016;41(4):527–31.
19. Runner RP, Boden SA, Godfrey WS, et al. Quadriceps Strength Deficits After a Femoral Nerve Block Versus Adductor Canal Block for Anterior Cruciate Ligament Reconstruction: A Prospective, Single-Blinded, Randomized Trial. Orthop J Sports Med 2018;6(9). 2325967118797990.
20. Williams BA, Kentor ML, Vogt MT, et al. Economics of nerve block pain management after anterior cruciate ligament reconstruction: potential hospital cost savings via associated postanesthesia care unit bypass and same-day discharge. Anesthesiology 2004;100(3):697–706.
21. Mistry H, Metcalfe A, Colquitt J, et al. Autograft or allograft for reconstruction of anterior cruciate ligament: a health economics perspective. Knee Surg Sports Traumatol Arthrosc 2019;27(6):1782–90.
22. Oro FB, Sikka RS, Wolters B, et al. Autograft Versus Allograft: An Economic Cost Comparison of Anterior Cruciate Ligament Reconstruction. Arthrosc J Arthrosc Relat Surg 2011;27(9):1219–25.
23. Nagda SH, Altobelli GG, Bowdry KA, et al. Cost Analysis of Outpatient Anterior Cruciate Ligament Reconstruction: Autograft versus Allograft. Clin Orthop 2010;468(5):1418–22.
24. Kaeding CC, Aros B, Pedroza A, et al. Allograft Versus Autograft Anterior Cruciate Ligament Reconstruction: Predictors of Failure From a MOON Prospective Longitudinal Cohort. Sports Health 2011;3(1):73–81.

25. Bottoni CR, Smith EL, Shaha J, et al. Autograft Versus Allograft Anterior Cruciate Ligament Reconstruction: A Prospective, Randomized Clinical Study With a Minimum 10-Year Follow-up. Am J Sports Med 2015;43(10):2501–9.
26. Biedert RM. Treatment of intrasubstance meniscal lesions: a randomized prospective study of four different methods. Knee Surg Sports Traumatol Arthrosc 2000;8(2):104–8.
27. Wen Qiang Lee, Jonathan Zhi-Wei Gan, Denny Tjiauw Tjoen Lie. Save the meniscus – Clinical outcomes of meniscectomy versus meniscal repair. J Orthop Surg 2019. https://doi.org/10.1177/2309499019849813.
28. Sochacki KR, Varshneya K, Calcei JG, et al. Comparing Meniscectomy and Meniscal Repair: A Matched Cohort Analysis Utilizing a National Insurance Database. Am J Sports Med 2020;48(10):2353–9.
29. Lester JD, Gorbaty JD, Odum SM, et al. The Cost-Effectiveness of Meniscal Repair Versus Partial Meniscectomy in the Setting of Anterior Cruciate Ligament Reconstruction. Arthrosc J Arthrosc Relat Surg 2018;34(9):2614–20.
30. Herzog MM, Marshall SW, Lund JL, et al. Cost of Outpatient Arthroscopic Anterior Cruciate Ligament Reconstruction Among Commercially Insured Patients in the United States, 2005-2013. Orthop J Sports Med 2017;5(1). 2325967116684776.
31. Pan T, Gottshall J, King TS, et al. Meniscus Work and Implant Selection Are Major Cost Drivers of Anterior Cruciate Ligament Reconstruction. Cureus 2023;15(2). e34647.
32. Forssblad M, Valentin A, Engström B, et al. ACL reconstruction: patellar tendon versus hamstring grafts—economical aspects. Knee Surg Sports Traumatol Arthrosc 2006;14(6):536–41.
33. Debieux P, Franciozi CE, Lenza M, et al. Bioabsorbable versus metallic interference screws for graft fixation in anterior cruciate ligament reconstruction. Cochrane Database Syst Rev 2016;2016(7):CD009772.
34. Memon M, Ginsberg L, de SA D, et al. Patient perceptions regarding physician reimbursements, wait times, and out-of-pocket payments for anterior cruciate ligament reconstruction in Ontario. J Exp Orthop 2017;4:1.
35. Hall MP, Chiang-Colvin AS, Bosco JA. Willingness to pay for anterior cruciate ligament reconstruction. Bull Hosp Jt Dis 2013;71(3):218–21.
36. Lee J, Guzek RH, Shah NS, et al. How Much Will My Child's ACL Reconstruction Cost? Availability and Variability of Price Estimates for Anterior Cruciate Ligament Reconstruction in the United States. J Pediatr Orthop 2022;42(10):614–20.
37. Engler ID, Curley AJ. Environmental Sustainability in Orthopaedic Surgery – Where We Are and Where We Are Going. Oper Tech Orthop 2022;32(4). 100995.
38. Sherman JD, MacNeill A, Thiel C. Reducing Pollution From the Health Care Industry. JAMA 2019;322(11):1043–4.
39. Smith JT, Boakye LAT, Ferrone ML, et al. Environmental Sustainability in the Orthopaedic Operating Room. JAAOS - J Am Acad Orthop Surg. 2022;30(21):1039.
40. Saleh JR, Mitchell A, Kha ST, et al. The Environmental Impact of Orthopaedic Surgery. JBJS 2023;105(1):74.
41. de Sa D, Stephens K, Kuang M, et al. The direct environmental impact of hip arthroscopy for femoroacetabular impingement: a surgical waste audit of five cases. J Hip Preserv Surg 2016;3(2):132–7.
42. Stall NM, Kagoma YK, Bondy JN, et al. Surgical waste audit of 5 total knee arthroplasties. Can J Surg J Can Chir 2013;56(2):97–102.
43. Drew J, Christie SD, Tyedmers P, et al. Operating in a Climate Crisis: A State-of-the-Science Review of Life Cycle Assessment within Surgical and Anesthetic Care. Environ Health Perspect 2021;129(7):076001.

44. Kagoma Y, Stall N, Rubinstein E, et al. People, planet and profits: the case for greening operating rooms. CMAJ Can Med Assoc J 2012;184(17):1905–11.
45. Van Demark RE, Smith VJS, Fiegen A. Lean and Green Hand Surgery. J Hand Surg 2018;43(2):179–81.
46. Thiel CL, Fiorin Carvalho R, Hess L, et al. Minimal Custom Pack Design and Wide-Awake Hand Surgery: Reducing Waste and Spending in the Orthopedic Operating Room. Hand N Y N 2019;14(2):271–6.
47. Thiel CL, Eckelman M, Guido R, et al. Environmental Impacts of Surgical Procedures: Life Cycle Assessment of Hysterectomy in the United States. Environ Sci Technol 2015;49(3):1779–86.
48. MacNeill AJ, Lillywhite R, Brown CJ. The impact of surgery on global climate: a carbon footprinting study of operating theatres in three health systems. Lancet Planet Health 2017;1(9):e381–8.
49. Sherman J, Le C, Lamers V, et al. Life Cycle Greenhouse Gas Emissions of Anesthetic Drugs. Anesth Analg 2012;114(5):1086.
50. Herr MM, Outterson RE, Aggarwal S. Lost in the Ether: The Environmental Impact of Anesthesia. Oper Tech Orthop 2022;32(4):100997.

Avoiding Graft Failure

Lessons Learned from the Stability Trial

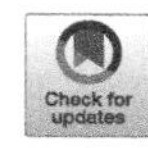

Alan M.J. Getgood, MPhil, MD, FRCS(Tr&Orth)

KEYWORDS

- Lateral extra-articular tenodesis • Stability study
- Anterior cruciate ligament reconstruction

KEY POINTS

- Adequately powered study investigating an important primary outcome in a high-risk population.
- The addition of lateral extra-articular tenodesis (LET) to hamstring tendon autograft anterior cruciate ligament reconstruction reduces graft failure and persistent rotatory laxity at 2 years postoperative.
- No differences demonstrated in patient-reported outcomes, return to sport, or adverse events.
- LET causes slight increase in pain and quadriceps weakness up to 6 months postoperative but equals out by 12 months postoperative.
- LET is a cost-effective procedure.

INTRODUCTION/BACKGROUND

Over the past number of decades, we have witnessed the evolution of surgical techniques to address anterior cruciate ligament (ACL) deficiency.[1] The early days of ACL repair in the first part of the twentieth century were replaced by extra-articular procedures in the 1950s with limited success. ACL repair would again take center stage with promising early results in the 1980s, only to be found to be deficient at longer term follow-up, with high rates of recurrent instability, knee dysfunction, and ultimately failure.[2] Open ACL reconstruction (ACLR) became the gold standard, with the ACL being replaced by a variety of materials including autologous grafts and later synthetics. Satisfactory results were encountered with the former, but synthetics fell out of favor due to high rates of synovitis and fatigue failure. The introduction of arthroscopy led to a new era of minimally invasive surgical techniques, with industry developing a myriad of tools and devices to preferentially fix graft material in "so called" optimal graft

Western University, Fowler Kennedy Sport Medicine Clinic, 3M Centre, London, Ontario N6A 3K7, Canada
E-mail address: alan.getgood@uwo.ca
Twitter: @FKSMC_Getgood (A.M.J.G.)

Clin Sports Med 43 (2024) 367–381
https://doi.org/10.1016/j.csm.2023.08.005
0278-5919/24/

positions. The early days witnessed transtibial tunnel drilling with a focus on isometric graft position, evolving to medial portal drilling, allowing for a more "anatomic" graft placement and improved replication of knee kinematics. This paved the way for the introduction of double-bundle techniques, again aiming for better control of knee stability. However, even these techniques would ultimately fail to last the test of time as clinical results, and more specifically, failure rates were not improved. Throughout this time was the consistent discussion of optimal graft material, in terms of strength, donor site morbidity, and availability.

But what was the point of this evolution in technique? Putting aside the obvious role of industry in driving commercialism of surgical tools and consumables, clinicians ultimately hoped for improved outcomes for their patients. As ACL injuries primarily occurred in young, active individuals and athletes, it was disheartening to see them unable to return to their preinjury level of activity, and worse still, develop significant complications in later life such as post-traumatic osteoarthritis (PTOA).[3]

The introduction of evidence-based medicine into orthopedics led to a change in focus on outcomes. Traditional laxity measurements in small case series evolved to comparisons of patient-reported outcomes (PROs) in prospective cohorts and randomized studies, focusing on graft type and technique options. Unfortunately, these studies often involved small populations of patients and were often dogged with being underpowered for the primary outcome of choice. Systematic reviews and meta-analytic techniques followed, ultimately showing little difference between techniques and graft options that either killed the development of technique or determined potentially incorrectly that there was no difference in technique and therefore the procedure would be abandoned.

A great example of this is the study by O'Brien and colleagues, in which a retrospective analysis of two surgical techniques was performed, comparing ACLR with bone-tendon-bone (BTB) autograft with or without an extra-articular procedure.[4] With 40 patients in each group, the investigators found that there were no differences in PROs or graft failure between groups and therefore they concluded that extra-articular reconstruction was not required as an augmentation to ACLR. This study was a key reason as to why extra-articular reconstruction was abandoned in North America.

Another key example of this is the age-old argument around graft choice. Multiple systematic reviews have ultimately led to the same conclusion that there is no difference between hamstring tendon (HT) autograft or BTB autograft for primary ACLR.[5] Most of the systematic reviews have pooled data that include patients of all ages and activity levels and have shown no difference in PRO scores, with only small differences in graft failure between groups observed.[6] Even though a subjective assessment of anterolateral rotatory laxity (the pivot shift test) would favor the use of BTB autograft.

Here lies the problem with data from earlier studies. The primary outcome of choice often focused on PROs that potentially are not sensitive enough to pick up important differences in surgical techniques specific to ACL injury or have significant ceiling effects when dealing with a young active population.[7] Second, they tend to include a wide spectrum of patients of all ages with differing demands and goals regarding return to sport and activity. The Multicenter Orthopedic Outcomes Network (MOON) group clearly demonstrated that younger patients experience a higher rate of ACL graft failure than older patients,[8] which is probably a surrogate measure of activity level, that is, younger patients are generally involved in higher risk activities such as cutting and pivoting sports.

What Does Your Patient Want Following Anterior Cruciate Ligament Reconstruction?

We asked our patients what their goal was following ACLR surgery.[9] Most were interested in an injury-free return to their preinjury activity level in a short a time as possible. This was in contrast to surgeons' point of view who were more interested in longer term outcomes such as being free from PTOA.

It is this notion that younger patients want a reduction in graft failure, coupled with our recognition that contemporary ACLR techniques did not provide optimal knee stability that was the impetus of designing the Stability Study. In Canada and Europe, the most common ACLR being performed in 2010 was a medial portal drilling technique with an HT autograft. We recognized that there was great variability in outcome, in terms of stability and failure rates, and that this was particularly an issue in the younger more active population. For example, studies from Australia had demonstrated up to 20% failure in young active individuals with a further 10% risk of contralateral ACL injury, indicating up to 30% of patients were at risk of having another ACL injury within 2 years from index surgery—a devastating issue for any young aspiring athlete.[10] Added to this was the poor rates of return to sport. Systematic reviews have suggested only 63% of patients would return to their pre-injury level.[11]

Claes and colleagues published their anatomic study on the anterolateral ligament (ALL), suggesting that this structure within the anterolateral capsule of the knee was the key to controlling anterolateral rotatory laxity.[12] Multiple anatomic and biomechanical studies ensued demonstrating that several structures, collectively named the anterolateral complex, played a significant role in controlling the pivot shift and that an extra-articular procedure, such as an iliotibial band lateral extra-articular tenodesis (LET) or ALL reconstruction, could play a role in reducing rotatory laxity and graft failure.[13]

As discussed previously, LET was not a new concept. In fact, it had continued use in many parts of Europe, particularly in high-level athletes playing pivoting sports. Several systematic reviews of historic comparative studies clearly showed that a reduction in the pivot shift was observed when an anterolateral procedure was combined with contemporary intra-articular ACLR.[14–16] However, for this "older" technique to be reintroduced back into current treatment paradigms, we recognized that an adequately powered randomized clinical trial was required to determine if the addition of an LET to HT autograft ACLR could reduce anterolateral rotatory laxity and ACL graft failure in a specific at-risk population.

THE STABILITY RANDOMIZED CLINICAL TRIAL

In 2014, we commenced recruitment of the Stability Study.[17] The International Society of Arthroscopic Knee Surgery and Orthopedic Sports Medicine sponsored Stability Study was designed as a multicenter, multi-continent pragmatic parallel groups randomized clinical trial comparing contemporary HT autograft ACLR with or with a modified Lemaire LET in young patients at high risk of graft failure. The latter aspect of this was particularly important; recognizing that failure rates were higher in younger, more active individuals, we aimed to focus on this high-risk group so that the event rate would be large enough where we could power the study to achieve a clinically reasonable reduction in event rate, if the additional procedure were to be efficacious. As such, the eligibility included patients less than the age of 25 year old with 2 or more of the following criteria making them at higher risk of reinjury.

1. A pivot shift equal or greater than 2
2. Returning to competitive pivoting sport

3. Beighton score equal or greater than 4 OR knee hyperextension equal or greater than 10°

Nine centers across Canada and Europe recruited 618 patients over more than 3 years.

Primary Outcome

The primary outcome of choice was what we described as "clinical failure." This was a composite measure of persistent rotatory laxity and graft failure. The argument behind using this as a primary outcome was that this has been the goal of the majority of ACLR technique evolutions over the last 2 decades—changes in graft material, graft position, tunnel drilling technique, and so forth to improve rotational laxity and reduce failure. If the addition of an LET failed to reduce either of these two measures, then it would not be worth adding the procedure. Of course, the pivot shift test is a subjective measure, the use of which as an outcome of importance has been questioned over the years. To mitigate this issue, an independent blinded observer was used to record the pivot shift at each follow-up time, with the documentation of a positive outcome as the following.

1. Grade 1 asymmetric pivot shift recorded on at least two separate clinic visits
2. Grade 2 pivot shift recorded on at least one clinic visit
3. Graft failure demonstrated on either MRI or at arthroscopy

Based on an event rate of 40%, a total of 600 patients (300 per group) would be required to demonstrate a 40% reduction in clinical failure at 2 years postoperative. Following a group discussion of investigators, we determined that a 40% reduction in failure would be adequate to represent a clinically meaningful difference and thus, if demonstrated, would be enough to change clinical practice.

Interventions

A standardized medial portal HT autograft ACLR was chosen due to its worldwide popularity. In an attempt to mitigate against graft size being an independent risk factor for graft failure,[18] semitendinosus and/or gracilis was tripled to provide a graft diameter of greater than 8 mm when possible. The experimental intervention comparator was the addition of a modified Lemaire LET. A full technique description has previously been described.[19] In brief, a 1-cm wide, 8-cm long strip of the posterior half of the iliotibial band was harvested, freed proximally, and left intact on Gerdy's tubercle distally. It was routed under the fibular collateral ligament then attached on the metaphyseal flare of the lateral femoral condyle with a Richards staple (Smith and Nephew, Inc.; Andover, MA), with minimal tension applied to the graft with the knee at 60° of flexion, neutral tibial rotation.

Rehabilitation

Owing to the pragmatic nature of the study, rehabilitation following the ACLR followed the traditional protocol from participating centers. Return to sport was not recommended until at least 9 months postoperative.

Secondary Outcomes

A range of secondary outcomes were collected over the course of the study period. Patients were seen at 6 weeks and 3, 6, 12, and 24 months postoperative when a range of outcomes were collected as detailed in **Table 1**. Details of adverse events were collected at these time points as well as at any other unscheduled visits if they arose. Cost data were also collected in the event of an adverse event so that a later cost-effective analysis could be performed.

Table 1
Secondary outcomes of the Stability Study

	Baseline	Surgery	6 wk	3 mo	6 mo	12 mo	24 mo	PRN
PROs								
ACL QOL	X		X	X	X	X	X	
KOOS	X		X	X	X	X	X	
IKDC-SKF	X		X	X	X	X	X	
Marx Activity	X		X	X	X	X	X	
EQ5D	X		X	X	X	X	X	
Sport Participation	X							
Return to Sport					X	X	X	
Clinical Assessment	X		X	X	X	X	X	
Plain Radiographs	X						X	
ROM and Muscle Function								
Range of Motion (ROM)	X		X	X	X	X	X	
Strength Testing (select sites)					X	X	X	
Performance Tests (selected sites)								
Hop Test					X	X	X	
Clinician-Rated Drop Vertical Jump					X	X		
As Needed								
Adverse Event								X
Withdrawal Form								X
Cost Forms for failed ACLs			X	X	X	X	X	

Abbreviations: ACL-QOL, anterior cruciate ligament quality of life; IKDC-SKF, International Knee Documentation Committee Subjective Knee Form; KOOS, Knee Osteoarthritis Outcome Score.

PARTICIPANTS

Over the course of 3 years, 618 patients, with a mean age of 19 year old were recruited to the Stability Study. At 2 years postoperative, 298 of 312 patients who received ACLR alone and 291 of 306 patients who received ACLR + LET were reviewed with less than 5% loss to follow up. No difference between groups was observed in terms of the patient demographics. An average of 73% had a noncontact ACL injury with a mean of 9 months between injury and surgery. Most of the patients (>75%) were involved in pivoting sport preinjury. Similar graft sizes and rates of meniscal injury were found between groups.

OUTCOMES

The following is a summary of clinical outcomes found from the Stability Study. Most of these outcomes have been previously published in peer-reviewed journals, the details of which may be found in these specific publications.

Clinical Failure and Graft Rupture

At 2 years postoperative, a 40% reduction in clinical failure [relative risk reduction (RRR) = 0.39 (95%CI 0.22–0.52), $P < .0001$] was observed, representing a clinically and statistically significant reduction in favor of the additional LET.[20] A 66% reduction in graft failure was observed in favor of the additional LET (RRR = 0.66 [95%CI 0.35–

0.81], $P < .001$), a statistical that remained consistent for both the under 20 age group and the 20 to 25 year age group.

Patient-Reported Outcomes

No differences in any of the PROs were observed between the two treatment groups at 12 or 24 months.[20] At 3 and 6 months postoperative, there were statistically significant differences in both the International Knee Documentation Committee (IKDC) and Knee Osteoarthritis Outcome Score (KOOS) scores in favor of the ACL alone group; however, these differences did not reach a minimum clinically important difference. That said, an increase in pain was observed on the P4 questionnaire in the LET group at 3 months with a reduction in Lower Extremity Functional Score (LEFS) in the same group at 6 months, suggesting that the addition of LET may result in more discomfort and a slower recovery in the early time periods.

Quadriceps and Hamstring Strength

A similar trend was observed in the quadriceps and hamstring isokinetic testing.[21] In a subcohort of patients in three of the study centers, a statistically significant reduction in quadriceps peak torque and average power was observed in the LET group; however, the clinical significance of these differences was questionable. When observed in the context of greater pain and reduced LEFS at the 6-month time point, it again points to a slower recovery with the addition of LET, a finding that should be taken into consideration when adding any additional surgical procedures to an ACLR. Of note, no differences in hamstring strength were observed, again suggesting that the LET procedure, with the surgical incision and approach involving the distal insertion of the vastus lateralis was implicated.

Hop Testing

A functional assessment was performed on a subset of patients across three of the centers in the study using hop testing.[21] No difference was observed between groups, with the majority of patients achieving at least 90% limb symmetry index (LSI) at 6 months, with over 95% at 12 months and close to 100% at 24 months. On further analysis, none of the functional metrics of strength or LSI hop tests were predictive of clinical failure or graft failure at the 12 or 24 month time frame, questioning their predictive ability for graft failure.

Drop Vertical Jump

In an unpublished series of patients from the Fowler Kennedy Sport Medicine clinic, drop vertical jump (DVJ) tests were performed on 120 patients at 6, 12, and 24 months post-op. No differences in external knee moments were observed between groups at any time point indicating that LET was at least a safe procedure, with the additional surgery observed to not result in altered knee kinetics during a functional landing task. However, the DVJ has been described as a method of determining risk of reinjury, through assessment of landing patterns such as valgus collapse, and ligament dominant landing patterns. None of these parameters were found to be predictive of graft failure in this Stability subcohort.

Return to Sport

No difference in Marx activity score was noted between groups, nor was there any statistical difference in return to sport time, with both groups returning to sport at a mean of between 11 and 12 months postsurgery.[21] In total, 87% of the study population returned to their preinjury sport by 2 years postoperative, significantly higher than what is reported in the literature. However, this is likely a measure of the fact that most of the patients that were included in the study were young and active and intended on returning to sport postsurgery. The proportion of patients who did not return to sport was similar between the ACLR (11%) and ACLR + LET (14%) groups ($P < .05$).

Similar to what has been previously published, the reasons why patients did not return to sport included adverse events such as graft failure, others had timed out of being eligible for their particular sport due to age or finished school/college (**Table 2**). The most common reason for not returning to sport was fear of reinjury or lack of confidence. This is similar to a study by Webster and colleagues in which they also found fear of reinjury was the most common reason for a postoperative reduction or cessation of sports participation.[11]

In a subsequent study, we analyzed the rate and level of return to sport, along with the predictive factors that may be associated with that return.[22] Classifying patients as either returning to no sport, to low-risk sport (eg, swimming), to high risk/low level of sport (eg, recreational soccer or rugby) and high risk/high level of sport (eg, competitive varsity/elite soccer/rugby/football) we found that there was no difference in rates of return between groups.

Again, hop test LSI was not associated with rate and level of return to sport; however, quadriceps torque symmetry showed a pattern of improved risk and level of sport that was independent of treatment group. Furthermore, a stable knee was associated with two times higher odds of returning to high-risk sports than not returning at all, again independent of treatment group. This latter statistical is somewhat counterintuitive, when the addition of LET was found to be predictive of having a more stable knee in the overall study. However, it is likely that during this latter subgroup analysis that the comparisons were underpowered to determine an effect of the LET.

ADVERSE EVENTS AND COMPLICATIONS

A full analysis of complications and adverse events were recently published.[23] Adverse events were broken down into minor medical (an event that either resolved spontaneously or with minimal medical management), minor surgical (an adverse event such as meniscus tear or stiffness that required surgical intervention but was not a graft rupture), contralateral ACL rupture, and graft rupture. There were no differences in rates of general adverse events (effusion or infection) between groups. There were also no clinically significant differences in range of motion between groups.

Table 2
Reasons for not returning to sport

Did Not Return to Any Sport (n = 76)	ACLR Alone (n = 34)	ACLR + LET (n = 42)
Why?		
Significant reinjury or complication	2	0
Lost interest/too busy	6	9
Lack of confidence/fear of reinjury	15	15
Not yet cleared to play	2	0
Decline in physical fitness	6	9
Out of season	1	1
Aged out/graduated	4	6

Note: Sums to greater than 100% because patients could give more than one reason; does not include patients who were not participating in sports preoperatively.

The ACLR + LET group experienced an increased number of patients complaining of hardware irritation from the LET staple and therefore underwent hardware removal, compared with the ACLR alone group that complained of ACL-related hardware irritation (10 vs 4). Overall, the rate of minor medical adverse events (11.2%), minor surgical adverse events (7.4%), and ipsilateral or contralateral ACL tears (10.3%) at 24 months postoperative were low considering the high-risk patient profile.

Interestingly, when we analyzed the PROs in the overall study groups, no between group differences were observed, even though a significantly higher number of patients experienced an ACL failure in the ACL alone group. This is likely because the overall rate of graft rupture was still small, with only 10.3% of the overall study group experiencing either an ipsilateral or contralateral ACL injury. As such, the effects of these events were likely washed out by the overall good results from the other study participants. When we purely focused on patients that had an adverse event, an increasing severity of adverse events was associated with lower PRO measures (KOOS, IKDC, ACL-QOL) at 24 months postoperative.

MENISCUS REPAIR

As previously stated, there were no differences between groups in terms of meniscus status and subsequent treatment. The MOON group had previously studied the impact of meniscus repair on outcome, finding that PROs can be negatively affected by meniscus repair and that one of the biggest predictors of poor outcome following ACLR was reoperation within the first 2 years postsurgery, with meniscus complications often being the main culprit for repeat surgery.[24]

We analyzed the Stability cohort regarding outcomes associated with medial and lateral meniscus repair.[25] Similar to the MOON study, medial meniscus repair was associated with worse outcomes on the KOOS ($b = -1.32$, 95% CI: -1.57 to -1.10, $P = .003$), IKDC ($b = -1.66$, 95% CI: -1.53 to -1.02, $P = .031$), and ACL-QOL ($b = -1.25$, 95% CI: -1.61–1.02, $P = .087$). However, these associations indicated small, clinically insignificant changes based on reported measures of clinical relevance. Lateral meniscus repair had no impact of outcome scores. There was no significant association between meniscal treatment and graft rupture or rotatory knee laxity ($c^2 = 0.18$, $P = .91$ and $c^2 = 1.36$, $P = .50$, respectively).

Based on the information gained form this study, it would support meniscus repair and preservation as there is no short-term harm from repairing the meniscus, whereas the long-term effects are not indicated for this study. With long-term studies of meniscal resection being associated with the development of PTOA, this would suggest that meniscal preservation should be continued to be supported.

PREDICTORS OF FAILURE/INDICATIONS

In our consensus statement published in 2017, we identified that there was reasonable evidence for the support of an anterolateral procedure to reduce rotatory laxity.[26] However, a high level of evidence that would provide indications for when and in whom to add an LET or equivalent was lacking. Following Stability, we performed a multivariable regression analysis, investigating several predictors of outcome that could be used to determine the risk of graft failure and the subsequent need for LET.[27] A younger age was associated with higher odds of graft rupture, with every 1-year increase in age reducing the odds of rotational laxity by 38%. Preoperative high-grade rotational laxity, as measured by either a grade 2 pivot shift or high Beighton score was associated with 3.27 times higher odds of graft rupture (OR = 3.27, 95%CI: 1.45–7.41). Interestingly, in a separate publication, we determined that knee hyperextension was the predominant factor within the Beighton score that was associated with high grades of pivot shift.[28] This is in keeping with studies by Larson and colleagues[29] and Guimaraes and colleagues,[30] both of whom identified knee hyperextension as being an independent risk factor for ACLR failure. Posterior tibial slope was also identified in our analysis as being a risk factor for failure. This is similar to a multitude of other studies that have found a posterior tibial slope (PTS) of greater than 12° to be a significant risk of ACLR failure.[31,32] In contrast to these studies, we found that for every 1° increase of PTS, the odds of graft rupture increased by 15%. We did not identify a clear cutoff value where an LET would be more helpful in reducing the failure risk. However, when plotting age against PTS, we observed a low risk of failure that would change to a moderate risk of failure at 10° of PTS, indicating that this may be a reasonable value to add LET into the surgery.

All of these risk factors can be assessed at the time of seeing a patient in clinic, during the initial preoperative visit. As such, a decision may be made as to whether an LET should be added based on the presence of these risk factors, with the addition of LET reducing the odds of graft failure by 60%.

Importantly, this only pertains to patients under the age of 25 year old undergoing ACLR with an HT autograft. It is not clear what impact another graft, such as BTB or quadriceps tendon (QT) autograft, would have on the need for LET augmentation. We performed an indirect comparison of the Stability data with that from the MOON group, using their risk calculator.[33] Data from this study suggested that the combination of HT with LET provided equivalent outcomes to BTB autograft alone in young patients returning to sport. However, this primarily highlighted the need for a further randomized controlled trial (RCT) comparing BTB and QT with or without LET in a similar population, which has spurred the idea for the Stability 2 trial, which is currently ongoing.

Postoperatively slowing down rehabilitation and delaying return to sport also have an impact. Every 1 month of delay in returning to sport resulted in a 14% reduction in graft rupture (OR = 0.86, 95%CI: 0.79–0.94). This is in keeping with previous studies by Nagelli and Hewett who have also shown that a delay in return to at risk activities, that is, sport, can have an impact on reducing failure rates.[34]

COST-EFFECTIVENESS

We evaluated the cost-effectiveness of ACLR with LET compared with ACLR alone using three different outcome measures of effectiveness: (1) quality-adjusted life years over 24 months, (2) the Marx Activity Rating Scale at 24 months (controlling for the baseline score), and (3) the number of participants who returned to a level of sport equal or greater than the baseline level at 24 months following surgery. We prospectively documented any reported adverse events at postsurgical follow-up visits with the surgeon, including at 2 and 6 weeks and at 3, 6, 12, and 24 months after ACLR. We recorded costs from the Canadian health care payer perspective, which includes any direct costs associated with health care resources consumed and covered by Ontario's publicly funded health care system. For each of the three outcomes, we calculated either an incremental cost-utility ratio or incremental cost-effectiveness ratios (ICER).

The mean difference in overall costs between the ACLR with LET group and the ACLR alone group was small (mean difference = 145.18 [95% CI, −128.17–418.53]) from a health care payer perspective. Only revision ACLR costs were significantly different between groups, where costs were $223.35 (95%CI, 28.73–417.96) lower in the ACLR with LET group. Primary ACLR costs were also $348 higher for ACLR with LET. The mean difference between groups in QALY over 24 months was negligible and not statistically significant (mean difference = 0.004 [95% CI, −0.01–0.01]). The ACLR with LET group had significantly higher 24-month Marx scores while adjusting for the baseline Marx score (mean difference = 0.72 [95% CI, 0.07–1.37]). Using the Marx Activity Rating Scale as the outcome, the ICER was $201.64 per 1-point increase in Marx at 24 months when using the ACLR with LET procedure. Using net benefit regression, ACLR with LET was cost-effective if an individual was willing to pay $300 or more for a 1-unit improvement in the Marx at 24 months after ACLR.

Although ACLR with LET is likely to be cost-effective when evaluating a 24-month Marx Activity Rating Scale as the outcome, there was uncertainty in interpretation of cost-effectiveness for QALYs and return to sport with negligible differences in effect between groups. Patient selection and individual characteristics should therefore be considered when deciding between the two approaches. Future research should explore predictors of cost-effectiveness and provide clearer guidelines for the indication of lateral augmentation.

LOSS TO FOLLOW-UP

When performing a large RCT, it is important that as many participants as possible are reviewed at the final follow-up to achieve adequate statistical power for the primary outcome of choice. When designing the study, we factored in a 15% loss to follow up rate to give some breathing space for potential participant dropouts. Overall, we were able to achieve an 8% loss to follow up rate allowing us to hit our goal. We performed a subsequent analysis that focused on reasons for loss to follow up that could then help inform future investigators on how to minimize loss of patients in large studies.[35] We found that smoking, part-time employment, and body mass index (BMI) greater than 25 were significant predictors of loss to follow-up (LTF), and part-time employment was significantly associated with early LTF. One of the most significant predictors was the clinical site involved, in terms of personnel and infrastructure available for research studies. Clinical site was significantly associated with missing data at any visit. This speaks to the importance of site assessments, and initiation visits to ensure adequate resources are available.

WHAT ARE THE POTENTIAL DOWNSIDES?

It is clear from the data from Stability that in the short term, the addition of LET to HT autograft ACLR has a significant impact on reducing ACLR failure. However, we are not able to determine the long-term implications of adding an LET to an intra-articular ACLR. Several systematic reviews have been performed specifically looking at the prevalence of osteoarthritis following LET.[36] At long-term follow-up, there is currently no evidence to suggest that a lateral procedure places knees at higher risk of developing PTOA. A more recent study by Castoldi and colleagues looked at the 20-year outcomes following BTB ACLR with a gracilis tendon graft used as an extra-articular tenodesis, placed under the fibular collateral ligament, and attached to the tibia.[37] In a small cohort of the overall study population, a greater amount of lateral osteoarthritis (OA) was identified in those patients treated with the extra-articular procedure than ACLR alone. However, this may have been associated with greater meniscus loss, and the significant loss to follow up is a major confounding variable. Furthermore, the use of a gracilis tendon instead of a strip of the iliotibial band is a more stiff-constraining construct. In any case, this speaks to the need for close surveillance of the Stability population to determine if there are any potential downsides to the addition of the LET.

In a consecutive subgroup of patients at the Fowler Kennedy Sports Medicine Clinic, we performed bilateral 3T MRI at 2-year postsurgery to determine if there were any differences in cartilage health between groups using T1rho and T2 relaxation times. Ninety-five participants (44 ACL, 51 ACL + LET) with a mean age of 18.8 years (59.8% female, 58/97) underwent MRI 2-year postoperative (range = 20–36 months). T1rho relaxation times were significantly elevated for the ACLR + LET group in the anterior aspect of the tibia (ACLR = 34.1 ± 0.8, ACLR + LET = 37.3 ± 0.7, P = .005) and the anterior aspect of the femur (ACLR = 34.7 ± 0.8, ACLR + LET = 37.3 ± 0.7, P = .007) demonstrating moderate effect sizes, whereas T2 relaxation times were significantly elevated for the ACLR + LET group in the anterior tibia (ACLR = 34.7 ± 0.8, ACLR + LET = 37.3 ± 0.7, ES = moderate) and posterior femur (ACLR = 34.7 ± 0.8, ACLR + LET = 37.3 ± 0.7, ES = moderate) demonstrating small effect sizes. These changes, while statistically significant, remain small and the clinical relevance is questionable. Furthermore, MRI articular cartilage relaxation times were not associated with PROs at the 2-year time point. These results however do highlight the need for future surveillance to determine if there are any unwanted side effects to the addition of LET.

FUTURE PERSPECTIVES

It is clear from the Stability Study that LET has a positive impact on reducing persistent rotatory laxity and graft failure following ACLR with HT autograft in young active patients. This benefit must be weighed up against any potential downsides as previously mentioned. As such, long-term follow-up of the full Stability cohort will be completed from 10 years on to investigate if there is an increased risk of PTOA development.

Understanding that there is slightly increased morbidity following the LET procedure, the question of whether LET is required when performing a BTB or QT autograft ACLR also will be investigated through the Stability 2 trial, the recruitment for which is ongoing. Using the same inclusion/exclusion criteria as the original Stability study, we will ultimately be able to compare three autograft options (HT, BTB, QT) with or without LET in 1800 patients all under the age of 25 year old with characteristics that make them at higher risk of reinjury. Like the MOON group, we will be able to generate a risk calculator that will help inform patients and surgeons as to the individual risk of the presenting patient and will be able to recommend a specific procedure on an individual case–by-case basis. This will further allow for individualized risk analysis and ultimately a more precise surgical plan at the individual patient level.

KEY LESSONS LEARNED

- Study design and target population

When designing a study in ACL surgery, it is important to target a specific population that is at risk of the primary outcome of choice. Stability highlighted the need for performing a study with a large number of patients with a primary outcome that had an appropriate event rate, which would determine if the intervention of choice had a clinical impact on the target population. This gave the most chance of changing clinical practice in the advent of a positive outcome.

- PROs in the context of an ACL study

Stability highlighted some of the issues that we face with current PROs. Many questionnaires such as KOOS, which are used throughout the multinational ligament registries, are not sensitive to pick up important changes, have significant ceiling effects, and simply are inadequate to differentiate between surgical techniques.

- LET may not be required for everyone

Although LET can have a major impact of ACLR failure when combined with HT autograft ACLR, it does have some associated morbidity and the long-term implications are not fully determined yet. As such, LET may not be necessary for everyone, particularly if different grafts are chosen for the primary ACLR. Later evidence from Stability 2 should help in determining individual risk of ACLR graft failure and lead to a more precise ACLR surgical plan. It also speaks to the need for long-term follow-up of any surgical intervention in ACLR.

- Cost-effectiveness

Stability has shown LET to be cost-effective based on the use of a cheap metal staple in a public health paying system. With a greater push from industry partners to be using more expensive anchors for LET fixation, we must be careful not to increase the burden of cost on our health systems, particularly in individuals at low risk of reinjury. Further data from Stability 2 will help inform clinicians, patients and payers as to the incremental benefit, or lack thereof, of these interventions.

- Individualized risk assessment and "Precision ACL surgery"

The results from Stability and its subsequent publications highlight the ability to individually assess patients and determine several factors that make them at higher risk of reinjury. Using this information allows for an individualized assessment of risk and a determination of a specific ACLR plan with the aim of reducing ACLR graft failure and providing optimal results. The days of "one size fits all" ACLR with one specific graft of choice are numbered. Future studies such as Stability 2 will provide patients and surgeons with the information required to provide an individualized risk assessment and a patient-specific surgical plan—"Precision ACL Surgery."

DISCLOSURE

The Stability Study was funded through a multicenter grant award by the International Society of Arthroscopic, Knee Surgery and Orthopedic Sports Medicine (ISAKOS).

REFERENCES

1. Schindler OS. Surgery for anterior cruciate ligament deficiency: a historical perspective. Knee Surg Sports Traumatol Arthrosc 2012;20(1):5–47.
2. Feagin JA, Curl WW. Isolated tear of the anterior cruciate ligament: five-year follow-up study. J Orthop Sports Phys Ther 1990;12(6):232–6.
3. Lohmander LS, Englund PM, Dahl LL, et al. The long-term consequence of anterior cruciate ligament and meniscus injuries: osteoarthritis. Am J Sports Med 2007;35(10):1756–69.
4. O'Brien SJ, Warren RF, Wickiewicz TL, et al. The iliotibial band lateral sling procedure and its effect on the results of anterior cruciate ligament reconstruction. Am J Sports Med 1991;19(1):21–4, discussion 24-5.
5. Mohtadi NG, Chan DS, Dainty KN, et al. Patellar tendon versus hamstring tendon autograft for anterior cruciate ligament rupture in adults. Cochrane Database Syst Rev 2011;9:CD005960.
6. Samuelsen BT, Webster KE, Johnson NR, et al. Hamstring autograft versus patellar tendon autograft for ACL reconstruction: is there a difference in graft

failure rate? a meta-analysis of 47,613 patients. Clin Orthop Relat Res 2017; 475(10):2459–68.
7. Marmura H, Tremblay PF, Getgood AMJ, et al. The knee injury and osteoarthritis outcome score does not have adequate structural validity for use with young, active patients with ACL tears. Clin Orthop Relat Res 2022;480(7):1342–50.
8. Kaeding CC, Pedroza AD, Reinke EK, et al. Risk factors and predictors of subsequent ACL injury in either knee after ACL reconstruction: prospective analysis of 2488 primary ACL reconstructions from the MOON cohort. Am J Sports Med 2015;43(7):1583–90.
9. Marmura H, Bryant DM, Birmingham TB, et al. Same knee, different goals: patients and surgeons have different priorities related to ACL reconstruction. Knee Surg Sports Traumatol Arthrosc 2021;29(12):4286–95.
10. Webster KE, Feller JA. Exploring the high reinjury rate in younger patients undergoing anterior cruciate ligament reconstruction. Am J Sports Med 2016;44(11): 2827–32.
11. Ardern CL, Webster KE, Taylor NF, et al. Return to sport following anterior cruciate ligament reconstruction surgery: a systematic review and meta-analysis of the state of play. Br J Sports Med 2011;45(7):596–606.
12. Claes S, Vereecke E, Maes M, et al. Anatomy of the anterolateral ligament of the knee. J Anat 2013;223(4):321–8.
13. Getgood AB C, Lording T, Amis A, et al, ALC Concensus Group. The Anterolateral Complex of the Knee: Results from the International ALC Consensus Group Meeting. Knee Surg Sports Traumatol Arthrosc 2018. Submitted for publication.
14. Devitt BM, Bell SW, Ardern CL, et al. The role of lateral extra-articular tenodesis in primary anterior cruciate ligament reconstruction: a systematic review with meta-analysis and best-evidence synthesis. Orthopaedic Journal of Sports Medicine 2017;5(10). https://doi.org/10.1177/2325967117731767. 2325967117731767.
15. Hewison CE, Tran MN, Kaniki N, et al. Lateral extra-articular tenodesis reduces rotational laxity when combined with anterior cruciate ligament reconstruction: a systematic review of the literature. Arthroscopy 2015;31(10):2022–34.
16. Song GY, Hong L, Zhang H, et al. Clinical outcomes of combined lateral extra-articular tenodesis and intra-articular anterior cruciate ligament reconstruction in addressing high-grade pivot-shift phenomenon. Arthroscopy 2016;32(5): 898–905.
17. Getgood A, Bryant D, Firth A, et al. The Stability study: a protocol for a multicenter randomized clinical trial comparing anterior cruciate ligament reconstruction with and without Lateral Extra-articular Tenodesis in individuals who are at high risk of graft failure. BMC Muscoskel Disord 2019;20(1):216.
18. Magnussen RA, Lawrence JT, West RL, et al. Graft size and patient age are predictors of early revision after anterior cruciate ligament reconstruction with hamstring autograft. Arthroscopy 2012;28(4):526–31.
19. Jesani S, Getgood A. Modified Lemaire Lateral Extra-Articular Tenodesis Augmentation of Anterior Cruciate Ligament Reconstruction. JBJS Essent Surg Tech 2019;9(4). https://doi.org/10.2106/JBJS.ST.19.00017.
20. Getgood AMJ, Bryant DM, Litchfield R, et al. Lateral Extra-articular Tenodesis Reduces Failure of Hamstring Tendon Autograft Anterior Cruciate Ligament Reconstruction: 2-Year Outcomes From the STABILITY Study Randomized Clinical Trial. Am J Sports Med 2020;48(2):285–97.
21. Getgood A, Hewison C, Bryant D, et al. No difference in functional outcomes when lateral extra-articular tenodesis is added to anterior cruciate ligament

reconstruction in young active patients: the stability study. Arthroscopy 2020; 36(6):1690–701.

22. Rezansoff A, Firth AD, Bryant DM, et al. Anterior cruciate ligament reconstruction plus lateral extra-articular tenodesis has a similar return to sports rate as ACLR alone, but lower failure rate. Arthroscopy 2023. https://doi.org/10.1016/j.arthro.2023.05.019.
23. Heard M, Marmura H, Bryant D, et al. No increase in adverse events with lateral extra-articular tenodesis augmentation of anterior cruciate ligament reconstruction - Results from the stability randomized trial. J ISAKOS 2023. https://doi.org/10.1016/j.jisako.2022.12.001.
24. Brophy RH, Huston LJ, Briskin I, et al. Articular Cartilage and Meniscus Predictors of Patient-Reported Outcomes 10 Years After Anterior Cruciate Ligament Reconstruction: A Multicenter Cohort Study. Am J Sports Med 2021;49(11):2878–88.
25. Marmura H, Firth A, Batty L, et al. Meniscal repair at the time of primary ACLR does not negatively influence short term knee stability, graft rupture rates, or patient-reported outcome measures: the STABILITY experience. Knee Surg Sports Traumatol Arthrosc 2022. https://doi.org/10.1007/s00167-022-06962-z.
26. Getgood A, Brown C, Lording T, et al. The anterolateral complex of the knee: results from the International ALC Consensus Group Meeting. Knee Surg Sports Traumatol Arthrosc 2019;27(1):166–76.
27. Firth AD, Bryant DM, Litchfield R, et al. Predictors of graft failure in young active patients undergoing hamstring autograft anterior cruciate ligament reconstruction with or without a lateral extra-articular tenodesis: the stability experience. Am J Sports Med 2022;50(2):384–95.
28. Batty LM, Firth A, Moatshe G, et al. Association of ligamentous laxity, male sex, chronicity, meniscal injury, and posterior tibial slope with a high-grade preoperative pivot shift: a post hoc analysis of the stability study. Orthopaedic Journal of Sports Medicine 2021;9(4). https://doi.org/10.1177/23259671211000038. 23259671211000038.
29. Larson CM, Bedi A, Dietrich ME, et al. Generalized hypermobility, knee hyperextension, and outcomes after anterior cruciate ligament reconstruction: prospective, case-control study with mean 6 years follow-up. Arthroscopy 2017;33(10): 1852–8.
30. Guimaraes TM, Giglio PN, Sobrado MF, et al. Knee hyperextension greater than 5 degrees is a risk factor for failure in ACL Reconstruction using hamstring graft. Orthopaedic Journal of Sports Medicine 2021;9(11). https://doi.org/10.1177/23259671211056325. 23259671211056325.
31. Webb JM, Salmon LJ, Leclerc E, et al. Posterior tibial slope and further anterior cruciate ligament injuries in the anterior cruciate ligament-reconstructed patient. Am J Sports Med 2013;41(12):2800–4.
32. Salmon LJ, Heath E, Akrawi H, et al. 20-year outcomes of anterior cruciate ligament reconstruction with hamstring tendon autograft: the catastrophic effect of age and posterior tibial slope. Am J Sports Med 2018;46(3):531–43.
33. Marmura H, Getgood AMJ, Spindler KP, et al. Validation of a risk calculator to personalize graft choice and reduce rupture rates for anterior cruciate ligament reconstruction. Am J Sports Med 2021;49(7):1777–85.
34. Nagelli CV, Hewett TE. Should return to sport be delayed until 2 years after anterior cruciate ligament reconstruction? biological and functional considerations. Sports Med 2017;47(2):221–32.
35. Andrew D, Firth DMB, Andrew M, Johnson Alan MJ, et al. Getgood, the STABILITY 1 Study Group. Predicting Patient Loss to Follow-up in the STABILITY 1 Study:

A Multicenter, International, Randomized Controlled Trial of Young, Active Patients Undergoing ACL Reconstruction. J Bone Joint Surg 2022;104(7):594.
36. Devitt BM, Bouguennec N, Barfod KW, et al. Combined anterior cruciate ligament reconstruction and lateral extra-articular tenodesis does not result in an increased rate of osteoarthritis: a systematic review and best evidence synthesis. Knee Surg Sports Traumatol Arthrosc 2017;25(4):1149–60.
37. Castoldi M, Magnussen RA, Gunst S, et al. A Randomized Controlled Trial of Bone-Patellar Tendon-Bone Anterior Cruciate Ligament Reconstruction With and Without Lateral Extra-articular Tenodesis: 19-Year Clinical and Radiological Follow-up. Am J Sports Med 2020;48(7):1665–72.

The Role of Osteotomy in Anterior Cruciate Ligament Reconstruction

Zachary J. Herman, MD*, Laura E. Keeling, MD,
Michael A. Fox, MD, Sahil Dadoo, BS, Volker Musahl, MD

KEYWORDS

- ACL reconstruction (ACLR) • Revision • Coronal and sagittal plane malalignment
- Medial opening wedge high tibial osteotomy
- Lateral closing wedge high tibial osteotomy • Anterior closing wedge osteotomy

KEY POINTS

- Coronal and sagittal knee imbalance have been shown to contribute to graft failure after ACLR.
- Medial opening wedge HTO and lateral closing wedge HTO are well-established treatment options in the setting of ACL deficiency with varus alignment.
- Anterior closing wedge HTO can be used in revision ACLR to decrease posterior tibial slope and improve clinical outcomes.

INTRODUCTION

Revision anterior cruciate ligament reconstruction (ACLR) is becoming more common as the age of athletes sustaining ACL injuries decreases.[1] Clinical failure after ACLR can be due to several factors, most commonly loss of motion and graft failure. Graft failure may result from technical errors including tunnel malposition, trauma, or patient-specific factors such as age, participation in high-level pivoting sports, or pre-existing tibiofemoral malalignment.[2]

Biomechanical studies have shown that varus knee deformity results in increased strain on the native ACL,[3] and clinical data have identified that knees with varus deformity may be more likely to fail ACLR if the malalignment is not addressed.[4,5] In the sagittal plane, increased posterior tibial slope (PTS) of more than 12° has also been recognized as a risk factor for failure after ACLR, as increased PTS results in greater anterior tibial translation during weight-bearing, placing higher stress on the ACL and grafts.[6–10]

Department of Orthopaedic Surgery, UPMC Freddie Fu Sports Medicine Center, University of Pittsburgh, 3200 S. Water Street, Pittsburgh, PA 15203, USA
* Corresponding author.
E-mail address: hermanz@upmc.edu

Clin Sports Med 43 (2024) 383–398
https://doi.org/10.1016/j.csm.2023.08.006 sportsmed.theclinics.com
0278-5919/24/

Studies have shown the benefit of high tibial osteotomy (HTO) to address coronal and sagittal malalignment in ACLR.[9,11–14] Osteotomy is most performed in the patient with chronic ACL insufficiency or failed ACLR. The purpose of this article is to further describe the use of osteotomy by reviewing indications, techniques, and outcomes of high tibial osteotomy in the setting of ACLR.

Evaluation of Failed Anterior Cruciate Ligament Reconstruction or Chronic Insufficiency

Clinical evaluation

Evaluation of patients with chronic ACL injury or failed ACLR should begin with a comprehensive history and physical examination. Key factors to consider are the initial mechanism of injury, time since primary reconstruction, postoperative rehabilitation protocol utilized, occurrence of new traumatic injury, and whether knee stability was achieved following the index procedure.[15] The presence of patient-specific risk factors, including level of activity and sport participation, should also be noted.

Physical examination includes a detailed assessment of gait, alignment, range of motion, and ligamentous stability. One should evaluate standing limb alignment and assess for varus/valgus thrust or hyperextension during gait. One should also determine active and passive range of motion and evaluate for muscular atrophy or asymmetry. Attention should be paid to quadriceps function and patellar tracking. A complete ligamentous examination should test the competency of the ACL, including Lachman and pivot shift testing, as well as of the posterior cruciate ligament (PCL), medial collateral ligament (MCL), and lateral collateral ligament (LCL), and the posterolateral corner (PLC) and posteromedial corner (PMC). Finally, prior skin incisions and the presence or absence of effusion should be documented.[15]

Radiographic evaluation

Plain radiographic imaging is critical in the evaluation of ACL failure as well as chronic ACL insufficiency. An initial radiographic series should include standing anteroposterior (AP) radiographs at 0° of flexion, lateral radiographs in full extension, posteroanterior 45° flexion weight-bearing (Rosenberg) views, and patellofemoral axial views.[16] Standing AP and Rosenberg views are useful for assessing bone quality, notch architecture, and degenerative changes, while AP and lateral views enable evaluation of the position and size of prior tunnels and the type of graft fixation used.[17] Full-length standing radiographs of both lower extremities, including the femoral heads and ankle joints, should be performed to evaluate the mechanical axis, particularly if coronal plane malalignment is a concern. Finally, varus-valgus or lateral stress views may be used to objectively evaluate the integrity of the ligamentous structures about the knee.[18]

MRI of the injured knee is useful as it provides information about the primary graft, including the location, orientation, and diameter of existing bone tunnels. MRI also allows for the evaluation of concomitant meniscal, chondral, and ligamentous pathology. Finally, it offers insight into the mechanism of primary graft failure. The presence of osseous edema in the lateral compartment may indicate a traumatic mechanism of injury, while irregular, increased signal and midsubstance thinning are suggestive of graft impingement. Finally, computed tomography can be performed to further assess previous tunnel placement as well as the extent and trajectory of bony deficiency.

Preoperative Planning

Knowledge of lower limb alignment is of utmost importance. The anatomic axes of the femur and tibia are represented by the respective mid-diaphyseal lines. The mechanical axis of the lower limb corresponds with the line drawn from the center of the femoral head to the center of the ankle joint. The horizontal distance between the mechanical lower limb axis and the center of the knee joint, which is measured in the frontal plane, is termed mechanical axis deviation and is used to quantify frontal plane alignment.[19,20] The mechanical femorotibial angle is also used to quantify frontal plane alignment. It is defined as the angle between the mechanical axes of the femur and tibia, which can be determined by connecting the center of the knee joint with the center of the femoral head and ankle, respectively (**Fig. 1**).[19]

Femoral and tibial joint lines are also utilized to evaluate joint orientation angles and the joint line convergence angle. The medial proximal tibial angle and the lateral distal femoral angle are commonly used. They are defined as the angles between the respective joint line and corresponding mechanical axis (**Fig. 2**).[19] Physiologic ranges

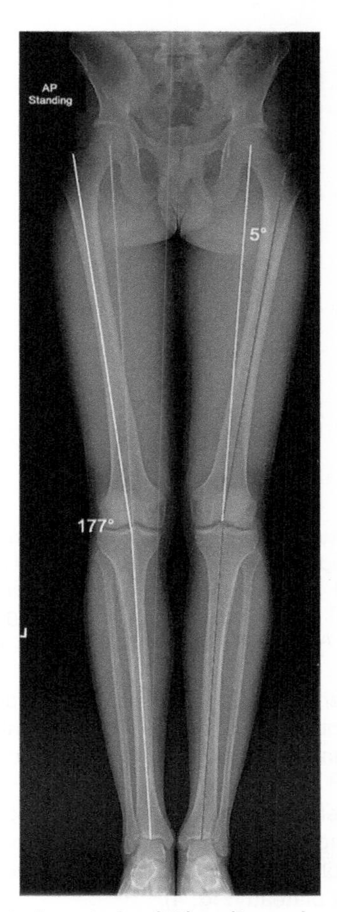

Fig. 1. Standing long leg anterioposterior (AP) radiograph with mechanical (yellow) and anatomic (red) axes of the femur and tibia of the left lower extremity. The anatomic mechanical femoral angle is 5°. The mechanical axis of the left lower extremity is marked with a blue line. The anatomic axis of the femur and tibia of the left leg is marked with a white line and forms a 177° anatomic femorotibial angle. (*Adapted from* Murray R, Winkler PW, Shaikh HS, Musahl V. High Tibial Osteotomy for Varus Deformity of the Knee. J Am Acad Orthop Surg Glob Res Rev. 2021;5(7).)

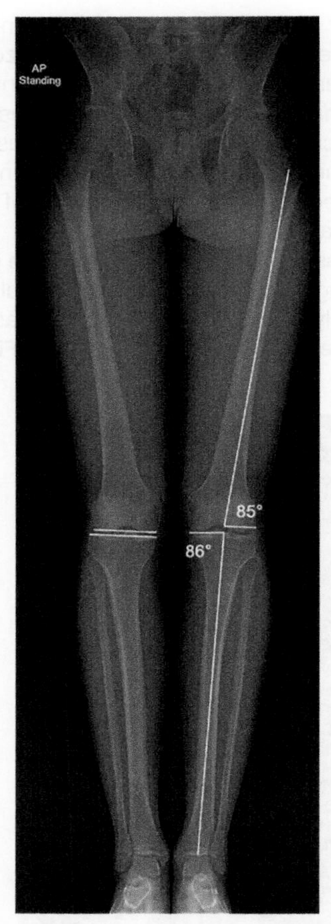

Fig. 2. Full-length standing lower extremity radiograph demonstrating the anatomic medial proximal tibial angle of 86° and anatomic lateral distal femoral angle of 85° of the left lower extremity. Femoral and tibial joint lines are demonstrated on the right lower extremity. (*Adapted from* Murray R, Winkler PW, Shaikh HS, Musahl V. High Tibial Osteotomy for Varus Deformity of the Knee. J Am Acad Orthop Surg Glob Res Rev. 2021;5(7).)

of these parameters are seen in **Table 1**. Specifically, in varus malalignment, the mechanical axis of the lower limb crosses the knee joint medial to its center. This is quantified by an increased medial mechanical axis deviation or a decreased mechanical femorotibial angle (**Fig. 3**).[20]

In the sagittal plane, the senior author's preferred method for measuring PTS utilizes the standard lateral knee radiographs and the "circle 3-point method", in which the PTS is measured as the angle between the longitudinal axis of the tibia and the posterior inclination of the tibial plateau (**Fig. 4**).[21,22]

High Tibial Osteotomy for Varus Malalignment

Varus alignment is frequently observed in the setting of chronic ACL insufficiency or failed ACLR. Progressive varus places heightened forces on the ACL, increasing the likelihood of graft failure.[3,23] These effects are further compounded by the classically described "double" or "triple" varus, which are associated with insufficiency of the

Table 1
Essential parameters and physiologic ranges

Parameter	Physiologically Acceptable Range
mFTA (°)	177–181
mMPTA (°)	85–90
mLDFA (°)	85–90
JLCA (°)	0–3
MAD (mm)	3–17
PTS (°)	0–15

Abbreviations: JLCA, joint line convergence angle (positive values indicate medial convergence); MAD, mechanical axis deviation (positive values indicate medial MAD); mFTA, mechanical femorotibial angle (values > 180° indicate valgus alignment; mLDFA, mechanical lateral distal femoral angle; mMPTA, mechanical medial proximal tibial angle; PTS, posterior tibial slope; values, <180° indicate varus alignment).

Adapted from Murray R, Winkler PW, Shaikh HS, Musahl V. High Tibial Osteotomy for Varus Deformity of the Knee. J Am Acad Orthop Surg Glob Res Rev. 2021;5(7). Physiologic ranges based on Willinger L, Lang JJ, von Deimling C, et al. Varus alignment increases medial meniscus extrusion and peak contact pressure: a biomechanical study. Knee Surg Sports Traumatol Arthrosc. 2020;28(4):1092-1098.

LCL and PCL, respectively.[24] In evaluating the patient with chronic ACL insufficiency or failed ACLR in the setting of varus alignment, it is therefore critical to assess the integrity of the PCL and lateral capsuloligamentous stabilizers of the knee.

HTO is a well-established treatment for medial compartment osteoarthritis (OA)[24] and, increasingly, ACL deficiency in the setting of varus alignment.[23,25] In spite of this, there remains controversy regarding optimal patient selection and surgical planning, including staging and concomitant procedures.

Indications

Indications for valgus-producing HTO in the setting of medial OA are well established and include highly active patients up to 60 years of age with a body mass index (BMI) of less than 30 kg/m^2, mild to moderate medial compartment OA (Kellgren-Lawrence grade II or less), and intact lateral meniscus and cartilage.[20] However, indications for valgus-producing HTO in the ACL-deficient patient are less clear. Studies have reported favorable mid-term outcomes in patients undergoing primary or revision ACLR and lateral closing wedge HTO in the setting of ACL deficiency, mild medial compartment OA, and varus alignment (defined as a hip-knee-ankle angle >180°).[23] Similarly, a 2006 study implicated varus malalignment as a contributing factor to failure of ACLR in 25% of patients,[26] while a more recent study demonstrated a significantly higher incidence of varus alignment more than 5° in patients undergoing revision versus primary ACLR.[27] However, a 2011 study found no difference in functional outcomes in patients undergoing ACLR with differing degrees of primary varus, although the authors excluded patients with double or triple varus from their study. Thus, the precise degree of varus as well as the number of ACL failures that mandate a corrective osteotomy remain poorly defined.[4]

Nevertheless, the literature does support the use of valgus-producing HTO in patients with combined instability and early unicompartmental OA,[28] as well as in those with insufficiency of the lateral or posterolateral knee stabilizers.[24,29] HTO should therefore be considered in patients of the appropriate age, activity level, and BMI who present with ACL insufficiency with concomitant double or triple varus, medial compartment OA, and/or meniscal deficiency requiring meniscal allograft transplantation.[30] Relative

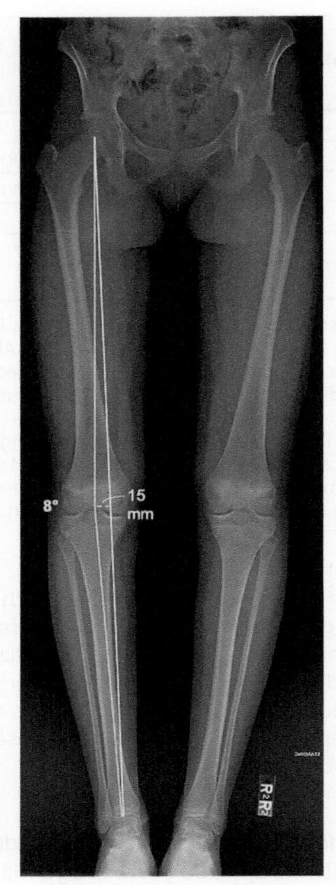

Fig. 3. Standing long leg AP radiograph demonstrating varus alignment of the right lower extremity. The femorotibial angle is 8° varus (yellow). The mechanical axis of the right lower extremity (white) is 15 mm medial to the center of the knee joint. (*Adapted from* Murray R, Winkler PW, Shaikh HS, Musahl V. High Tibial Osteotomy for Varus Deformity of the Knee. J Am Acad Orthop Surg Glob Res Rev. 2021;5(7).)

contraindications to valgus-producing HTO include patellofemoral or tricompartmental arthritis, severe medial compartment OA (Kellgren-Lawrence grade IV), decreased knee range of motion including a flexion contracture more than 10° or total arc of motion less than 120°, inflammatory arthritis, and nicotine use.[31]

Surgical techniques

High tibial osteotomy may be performed via a medial opening wedge (MOW) or a lateral closing wedge (LCW) technique. While each has unique advantages and disadvantages, both techniques have demonstrated efficacy in unloading the medial compartment via lateral translation of the lower limb mechanical axis.[32]

LCW osteotomy is performed via a lateral approach to the proximal tibia and requires identification and protection of the common peroneal nerve. Proximal tibial and fibular osteotomies are performed, maintaining a medial cortical hinge on the tibia to prevent loss of correction due to inadequate fixation. The LCW necessitates careful

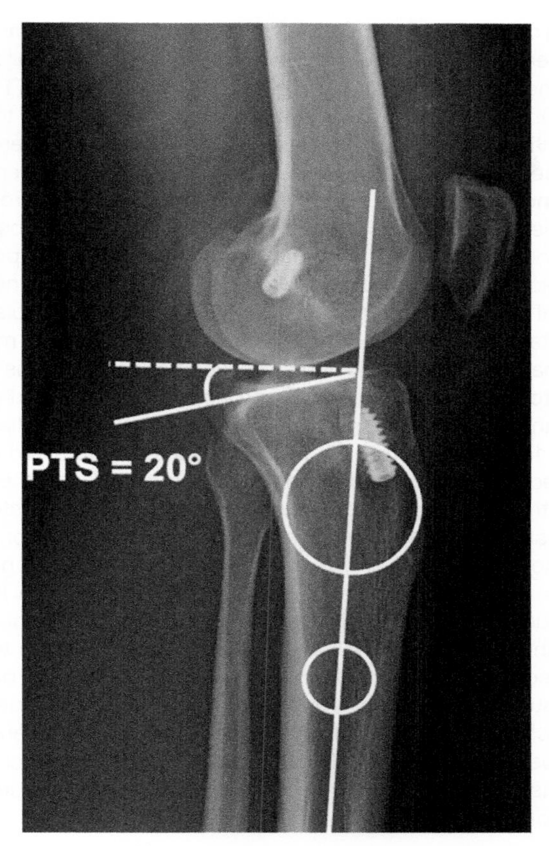

Fig. 4. "Circle 3-point method"[22] to illustrate measurement of the PTS. (*Adapted from* Nazzal EM, Zsidai B, Pujol O, Kaarre J, Curley AJ, Musahl V. Considerations of the Posterior Tibial Slope in Anterior Cruciate Ligament Reconstruction: a Scoping Review. Current Reviews in Musculoskeletal Medicine. 2022;15(4):291-299.)

preoperative planning to ensure resection of an appropriate-sized tibial wedge based on the degree of desired correction. Following tibial and fibular osteotomies, the tibial gap is slowly closed and fixed using a locking plate or staples.[33] Benefits of the LCW osteotomy include direct bone-to-bone contact, which has been theorized to enhance construct stability and healing, although this has been disputed in randomized comparative studies.[34] A further benefit specific to the ACL-deficient patient is the association of LCW-HTO with a slight decrease in PTS compared to MOW, which may produce a slight increase in PTS.[35] However, it is important to note that with meticulous technique, the surgeon may avoid a change in tibial slope with either technique, and even effect a decrease in PTS using the MOW with posterior releases and deliberate plate placement.

The authors' preferred technique is the MOW osteotomy. The patient is positioned supine with a tourniquet on the proximal thigh. The tourniquet is inflated for arthroscopic confirmation of the status of the cartilage and menisci, as well as preparation for concomitant ACLR. Meniscal work is performed as necessary, and the lateral femoral notch is debrided of all soft tissue. ACLR may be performed via anteromedial

(AM) portal drilling of the femoral tunnel, or an over-the-top (OTT) technique, according to surgeon preference.[23] In the revision setting with an anatomic or nearly anatomic femoral tunnel, the authors prefer a single-stage ACLR with OTT technique and concomitant HTO. Following femoral preparation and/or drilling, the tourniquet is deflated and attention is turned to the osteotomy. An 8 to 10 cm anteromedial incision is made midway between the tibial tubercle and posteromedial border of the tibia. The sartorial fascia is incised and the superficial MCL is bluntly elevated from the tibia while preserving the insertion of the pes anserine. The planned biplanar osteotomy is then marked under fluoroscopy with 2 Kirschner wires, aiming from approximately 5 cm distal to the medial joint line toward the tip of the fibular head, and parallel to the PTS in the sagittal plane. Retractors are placed posterior to the tibia and anteriorly, protecting the patellar tendon. The planned depth of osteotomy is measured via the guidewires and marked on an oscillating saw. Biplanar osteotomy is then performed from medial to lateral (paralleling the PTS), and from distal to proximal, deep to the patellar tendon and preserving the tibial tubercle to avoid significant changes in patellar height. A 1 cm cortical hinge is maintained laterally to avoid fracture. Osteotomes are then sequentially placed to open the osteotomy gap to the desired degree of correction. At this point, the ratio between the anterior and posterior osteotomy gaps may be adjusted to enable a small change in PTS. The posterior gap is preferentially opened to allow a decrease in PTS, thereby protecting the ACL graft.[36] Following verification of the desired amount of correction by intraoperative fluoroscopy, the osteotomy is secured with a locking plate. Careful plate placement is necessary to permit drilling of the ACL tibial tunnel, and to maintain adjustments to the PTS. After the plate is secured, the tibial tunnel is drilled, and the ACL graft is passed and fixed according to the surgeon's protocol. When performing OTT technique, the authors fix the graft with 2 Richards staples on the femoral side and an interference screw on the tibial side. When performing AM portal drilling, the femoral side is secured with continuous loop suspensory fixation.[37] Finally, bone grafting of the osteotomy site is performed per surgeon preference (**Figs. 5** and **6**).

Postoperative rehabilitation

Patients undergoing combined ACLR and HTO are placed in a hinged knee brace, with immediate range of motion permitted as tolerated. Non-weight-bearing is maintained for 4 weeks, with progressive weight-bearing from 4 to 6 weeks, and full weight-bearing at 6 weeks provided there is radiographic evidence of osteotomy healing. Return to sport (RTS) testing is performed at 9 months postoperatively, with full RTS dictated by patient progression and comfort level.

Outcomes and complications

Studies have demonstrated combined ACLR and MOW-HTO or LCW-HTO to be viable treatment options for appropriately selected patients with varus and ACL-deficient knees. A 2013 study reported significant improvements in patient-reported outcomes (PROs) and no cases of revision in their prospective study of 32 patients undergoing combined ACLR and LCW-HTO at mean 6.5-year follow-up.[23] Similarly, a retrospective study of 24 patients undergoing ACLR and MOW-HTO found significant improvements in Lysholm and Tegner scores as well as mechanical femorotibial angle, no cases of nonunion or loss of fixation, and full knee range of motion at mean 5.2-year follow-up.[38] A more recent study with mean 12-year follow-up reported significant improvements in IKDC and Visual Analog Scale scores with 2 cases of revision in 21 patients who underwent combined ACLR, MOW-HTO, and chondral resurfacing for moderate-to-severe medial OA.[39] Finally, a retrospective review of 35 patients treated with

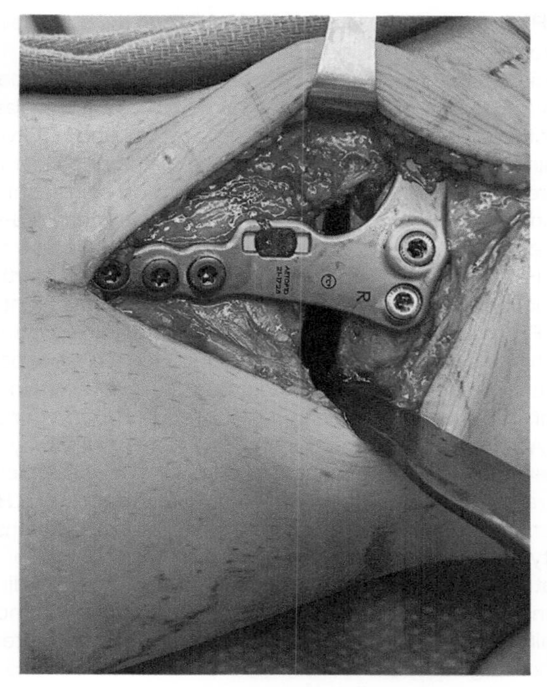

Fig. 5. Intraoperative photo demonstrating MOW-HTO with plate fixation.

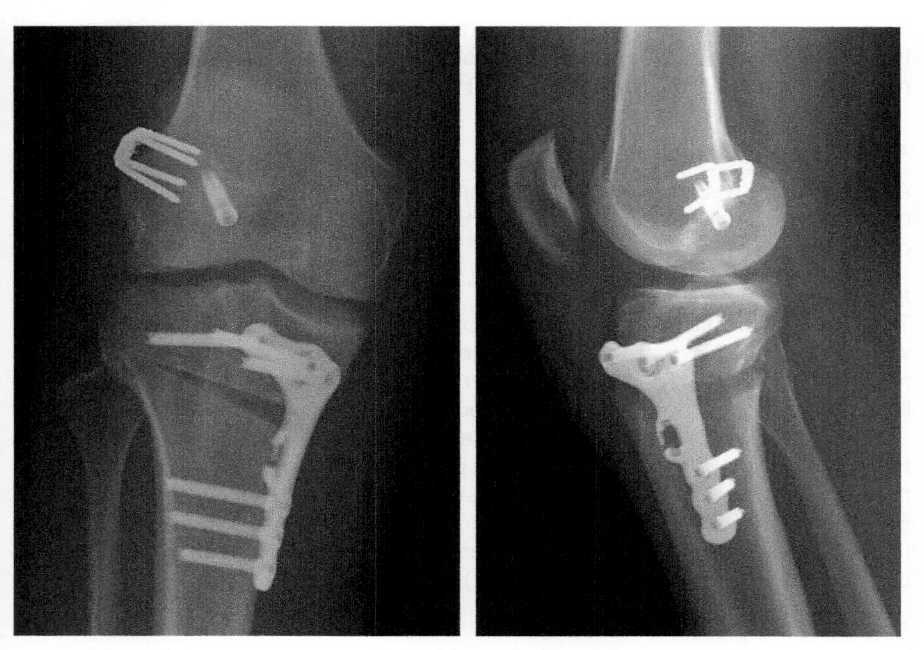

Fig. 6. Postoperative AP and lateral radiographs demonstrating MOW-HTO in setting of revision ACLR.

ACLR and MOW-HTO noted an 80% rate of RTS (31% at the same level) with 3 failures at mean 10-year follow-up.[40]

While ACL-deficient patients with combined instability and varus benefit from simultaneous ACLR and HTO, some patients may be candidates for isolated HTO without ACLR. A retrospective study of 26 patients undergoing isolated HTO versus 26 patients undergoing combined ACLR and HTO for medial OA with concomitant ACL deficiency found similar improvements in pain and instability with no significant difference in OA progression or complication rate between the 2 groups at mean 5.8-year follow-up.[41] Similarly, a more recent retrospective study examined the outcomes of 79 patients undergoing isolated HTO, HTO with simultaneous ACL or PCL reconstruction, or isolated ligament reconstruction. The authors reported significant improvements in knee stability with comparable PROs in all groups, although inferior stability was noted in the first group.[42] Notably, the patients in the first group were older, while the patients in the third group had significantly less varus than the other groups. As a result, these and other authors advocate for performing single-stage ACLR and HTO in younger patients with combined varus, ACL insufficiency, and instability. Conversely, they recommend isolated HTO in older patients with medial OA, chronic ACL insufficiency, and a chief complaint of pain rather than instability, with the option of staged ACLR if instability persists.[31,42] However, it is important to note that these recommendations are limited by a lack of high-quality, randomized comparative studies.

Complication rates following HTO vary from 0%[25] to 41%[43] depending on the severity of complication and type of osteotomy performed. The most common complications include cortical hinge fracture, symptomatic implant, loss of correction, nonunion/delayed union, and surgical site infection.[43] Peroneal nerve injury is also reported in 6% of patients undergoing LCW-HTO.[44] In a randomized comparative study of LCW-HTO versus MOW-HTO for medial knee OA, MOW was associated with a significantly higher rate of complications than LCW (38% vs 9%), yet LCW patients had a significantly increased rate of conversion to total knee arthroplasty (22% vs 8%) at 6-year follow-up.[44] Finally, progression of OA is not uncommon following combined HTO and ACLR, with rates varying from 22% at 6-year follow-up[23] to 39% at 10-year follow-up.[39]

Anterior Closing Wedge Osteotomy

Anterior closing wedge (ACW) HTO is an option for addressing increased PTS. Biomechanical studies have demonstrated that ACW-HTO can reduce the PTS and decrease in-situ forces on the ACL graft.[45,46]

Indications

The current indication for ACW-HTO is patients undergoing second revision ACLR with an elevated PTS more than 12°. Several contraindications have been described for performing ACW-HTO. ACW-HTO can provide some correction to coronal malalignment if an asymmetric wedge is resected; however, it is technically demanding and less effective compared to the correction achieved by a MOW-HTO or LCW-HTO. Therefore, ACW-HTO should not be performed in the setting of significant varus deformity (>5°) and severe tibiofemoral osteoarthritis (Kellgren-Lawrence grade IV).[47] Baseline knee hyperextension greater than 10° is a contraindication for ACW-HTO as the anterior correction may exacerbate genu recurvatum alignment. Relative contraindications include obesity (BMI >30 kg/m^2) and active smokers.[48]

Surgical technique

Various surgical techniques for performing ACW-HTO have been described, which are primarily distinguished by management of the tibial tubercle. ACW-HTO can be performed either proximally, distally, or through the level of tibial tubercle with a tubercle osteotomy. The tibial tubercle osteotomy (TTO) technique minimizes the risk of iatrogenic injury to the patellar tendon and allows for control over the tubercle, which can be distalized to preserve the length of the extensor mechanism. However, utilizing the TTO necessitates a prolonged postoperative recovery with delayed mobilization to allow for healing of the osteotomy site.[49] Alternatively, an HTO performed proximal or distal to the tubercle avoids the need for TTO. A proximal osteotomy has the advantage of improved healing potential of the proximal tibial cancellous bone, but can result in patella alta if the proximal tibia is over-shortened.[50,51] A distal osteotomy avoids altering the mechanical alignment of the knee extensor mechanism and allows more options for fixation, but relies on achieving osseous union through meta-diaphyseal bone.[52]

The osteotomy should be planned with a goal of correction to the average native PTS of 5° to 8°.[50] The senior author prefers the transtuberosity technique for performing ACW-HTO.[53] The procedure is performed with the patient supine through an anteromedial incision, incorporating the previous ACLR incision when possible. A tourniquet is placed but typically not inflated during osteotomy to allow for monitoring of bleeding. The TTO is performed first to protect the patellar tendon and visualize the proximal tibia. Converging guide pins are inserted and advanced to the posterior tibial cortex according to the planned correction, with the proximal pin placed approximately 5 cm distal to the anterior joint line. The HTO is performed with the knee in flexion to protect the posterior neurovascular structures. An oscillating saw is used to perform the osteotomy, with the final posterior 1 cm of the osteotomy performed using an osteotome for greater control. The bone wedge is removed and can be used for bone tunnel grafting if performing a staged revision ACLR. Reduction is performed by bringing the knee into extension and applying gentle manual pressure until the osteotomy is closed. The posterior tibial cortex can be perforated with a small drill bit to mobilize the osteotomy site without fully compromising the posterior hinge. Multiple options for fixation of the osteotomy are available including Richards staples, dynamic compression plating, pre-contoured proximal tibial plating, and patient specific instrumentation.[52] If concomitant or staged ACLR is planned, consideration should be made for tibial tunnel placement when placing fixation. When performed, concomitant ACLR is completed as described in the previous section, with graft harvest performed prior to the osteotomy. Of note, bone-patella tendon-bone autograft cannot be harvested when a transtuberosity TTO technique is used.

Postoperative rehabilitation

A period of non-weight-bearing is recommended to allow for healing of the osteotomy site, with transition to partial weight-bearing from around 4 to 6 weeks. Immediate active and passive range of motion with quadriceps activation exercises is permitted; however, it is critical that bracing is maintained to prevent hyperextension and development of recurvatum deformity. Closed chain exercises can be incorporated once weight-bearing is permitted, followed by light-impact activities at approximately 12 weeks. Return to activities and sport is typically achieved around 3 to 4 months unless performed simultaneously with revision ACLR.

Outcomes and complications

Reported outcome data for ACW-HTO in the literature are limited to case series without long-term follow-up. However, these studies have demonstrated improved radiographic and subjective outcomes.[13] The first series of 5 patients undergoing ACW-HTO combined with revision ACLR was published in 2014 and reported an average correction PTS of 5° with significantly improved PROs and no cases of graft failure.[9] A recent retrospective series of 58 ACL-deficient knees undergoing ACW-HTO reported a significant decrease in mean PTS from an average of 14.6° to 6.5°.[13] When compared with a series of 18 patients who underwent combined ACW-HTO and MOW-HTO, there was a significantly lower final PTS with isolated sagittal corrections (6.4° verses 8.1°), as well as a significant inverse correlation between the amount of sagittal and coronal correction.[13] A recent systematic review of the literature found favorable outcomes with no reported cases of recurrent ACL graft failure.[14] There is interest around the role for ACW-HTO in primary ACLR, though this remains highly debated.[21]

Complications have been reported after ACW-HTO. Hinge fracture of the posterior tibia is a critical complication which can compromise both the correction and healing potential of the fracture site. The small proximal segment and inability to access the posterior tibia through the standard anteromedial surgical approach presents a challenge for achieving fixation when a hinge fracture occurs.[48] Fluoroscopic guidance should be utilized during the surgical procedure to avoid extending the osteotomy through the posterior tibial cortex, and the oscillating saw should be cooled frequently during the osteotomy to mitigate the risk of nonunion secondary to osteonecrosis.[54]

As discussed, anterior closing correction can create a recurvatum deformity, particularly in patients with baseline knee hyperextension.[49] Overcorrection must be avoided to prevent gait imbalance and increased forces across the PCL. Similarly, failure to maintain or restore the length of the extensor mechanism when performing a surpratubercle or transtubercle ACW-HTO can result in patella alta deformity. Baseline standing radiographs should be obtained during preoperative planning and supratubercle osteotomy should be avoided in patients with baseline patella alta. Other potential complications reported in the literature include neurovascular injury, coronal plane malalignment, compartment syndrome, nonunion, and pseudoarthrosis.[50]

SUMMARY

As the number of primary ACLRs continues to rise, it is important to identify and address factors associated with failure. Sagittal and coronal knee malalignments play a substantial role in ACL graft failure, and identifying coronal and sagittal imbalance is crucial in ACLR. When performed under proper indications, MOW-HTO, LCW-HTO, and ACW-HTO have shown promise in correcting malalignment and improving outcomes in the revision setting. Moving forward, clinical research is needed to address the role of osteotomy procedures in the primary setting to protect against subsequent graft failure in patients.

CLINICS CARE POINTS

- Evidence have shown the benefit of high tibial osteotomy (HTO) to address coronal and sagittal malalignment in ACLR.
- High tibial osteotomy via a medial opening wedge (MOW) or a lateral closing wedge (LCW) has demonstrated efficacy in unloading the medial compartment via lateral translation of the lower limb mechanical axis.
- Anterior closing wedge (ACW) HTO is an option for addressing increased PTS.

DISCLOSURE

The authors have no relevant commercial or financial conflicts of interest.

REFERENCES

1. Liukkonen RJ, Ponkilainen VT, Reito A. Revision rates after primary ACL reconstruction performed between 1969 and 2018: a systematic review and metaregression analysis. Orthop J Sports Med 2022;10(8). 23259671221110191.
2. Shen X, Qin Y, Zuo J, et al. A systematic review of risk factors for anterior cruciate ligament reconstruction failure. Int J Sports Med 2021;42(8):682–93.
3. van de Pol GJ, Arnold MP, Verdonschot N, et al. Varus alignment leads to increased forces in the anterior cruciate ligament. Am J Sports Med 2009; 37(3):481–7.
4. Kim SJ, Moon HK, Chun YM, et al. Is correctional osteotomy crucial in primary varus knees undergoing anterior cruciate ligament reconstruction? Clin Orthop Relat Res 2011;469(5):1421–6.
5. Naudie DD, Amendola A, Fowler PJ. Opening wedge high tibial osteotomy for symptomatic hyperextension-varus thrust. Am J Sports Med 2004;32(1):60–70.
6. Zhao D, Pan JK, Lin FZ, et al. Risk factors for revision or rerupture after anterior cruciate ligament reconstruction: a systematic review and meta-analysis. Am J Sports Med 2023;51(11):3053–75.
7. Giffin JR, Vogrin TM, Zantop T, et al. Effects of increasing tibial slope on the biomechanics of the knee. Am J Sports Med 2004;32(2):376–82.
8. Lee CC, Youm YS, Cho SD, et al. Does Posterior Tibial Slope Affect Graft Rupture Following Anterior Cruciate Ligament Reconstruction? Arthroscopy 2018;34(7): 2152–5.
9. Sonnery-Cottet B, Mogos S, Thaunat M, et al. Proximal tibial anterior closing wedge osteotomy in repeat revision of anterior cruciate ligament reconstruction. Am J Sports Med 2014;42(8):1873–80.
10. Winkler PW, Chan CK, Lucidi GA, et al. Increasing the posterior tibial slope lowers in situ forces in the native ACL primarily at deep flexion angles. J Orthop Res 2022;41(7):1430–8.
11. Marriott K, Birmingham TB, Kean CO, et al. Five-year changes in gait biomechanics after concomitant high tibial osteotomy and ACL reconstruction in patients with medial knee osteoarthritis. Am J Sports Med 2015;43(9):2277–85.
12. Gupta A, Tejpal T, Shanmugaraj A, et al. Surgical techniques, outcomes, indications, and complications of simultaneous high tibial osteotomy and anterior cruciate ligament revision surgery: a systematic review. HSS J 2019;15(2):176–84.
13. Weiler A, Gwinner C, Wagner M, et al. Significant slope reduction in ACL deficiency can be achieved both by anterior closing-wedge and medial open-wedge high tibial osteotomies: early experiences in 76 cases. Knee Surg Sports Traumatol Arthrosc 2022;30(6):1967–75.
14. Bosco F, Giustra F, Giai Via R, et al. Could anterior closed-wedge high tibial osteotomy be a viable option in patients with high posterior tibial slope who undergo anterior cruciate ligament reconstruction? A systematic review and meta-analysis. Eur J Orthop Surg Traumatol 2022;33(6):2201–14.
15. Kraeutler MJ, Welton KL, McCarty EC, et al. Revision anterior cruciate ligament reconstruction. J Bone Joint Surg Am 2017;99(19):1689–96.
16. Osti L, Buda M, Osti R, et al. Preoperative planning for ACL revision surgery. Sports Med Arthrosc Rev 2017;25(1):19–29.

17. Allen CR, Giffin JR, Harner CD. Revision anterior cruciate ligament reconstruction. Orthop Clin North Am 2003;34(1):79–98.
18. Erickson BJ, Cvetanovich GL, Frank RM, et al. Revision ACL reconstruction: a critical analysis review. JBJS Rev 2017;5(6):e1.
19. Paley D, Herzenberg JE, Tetsworth K, et al. Deformity planning for frontal and sagittal plane corrective osteotomies. Orthop Clin North Am 1994;25(3):425–65.
20. Murray R, Winkler PW, Shaikh HS, et al. High tibial osteotomy for varus deformity of the knee. J Am Acad Orthop Surg Glob Res Rev 2021;5(7):e21.00141.
21. Nazzal EM, Zsidai B, Pujol O, et al. Considerations of the posterior tibial slope in anterior cruciate ligament reconstruction: a scoping review. Current Reviews in Musculoskeletal Medicine 2022;15(4):291–9.
22. Akoto R, Alm L, Drenck TC, et al. Slope-correction osteotomy with lateral extra-articular tenodesis and revision anterior cruciate ligament reconstruction is highly effective in treating high-grade anterior knee laxity. Am J Sports Med 2020;48(14):3478–85.
23. Zaffagnini S, Bonanzinga T, Grassi A, et al. Combined ACL reconstruction and closing-wedge HTO for varus angulated ACL-deficient knees. Knee Surg Sports Traumatol Arthrosc 2013;21(4):934–41.
24. Noyes FR, Barber-Westin SD, Hewett TE. High tibial osteotomy and ligament reconstruction for varus angulated anterior cruciate ligament-deficient knees. Am J Sports Med 2000;28(3):282–96.
25. Stride D, Wang J, Horner NS, et al. Indications and outcomes of simultaneous high tibial osteotomy and ACL reconstruction. Knee Surg Sports Traumatol Arthrosc 2019;27(4):1320–31.
26. Noyes FR, Barber-Westin SD. Anterior cruciate ligament revision reconstruction: results using a quadriceps tendon-patellar bone autograft. Am J Sports Med 2006;34(4):553–64.
27. Won HH, Chang CB, Je MS, et al. Coronal limb alignment and indications for high tibial osteotomy in patients undergoing revision ACL reconstruction. Clin Orthop Relat Res 2013;471(11):3504–11.
28. Tischer T, Paul J, Pape D, et al. The impact of osseous malalignment and realignment procedures in knee ligament surgery: a systematic review of the clinical evidence. Orthop J Sports Med 2017;5(3). 2325967117697287.
29. Klek M, Dhawan A. The role of high tibial osteotomy in acl reconstruction in knees with coronal and sagittal plane deformity. Curr Rev Musculoskelet Med 2019;12(4):466–71.
30. Toofan H, Tabatabaei Irani P, Ghadimi E, et al. Simultaneous arthroscopic anterior cruciate ligament reconstruction using double suspensory technique and medial open-wedge, high tibial osteotomy. Arthroscopy Techniques. 2022;11(12):e2357–64.
31. Cantivalli A, Rosso F, Bonasia DE, et al. high tibial osteotomy and anterior cruciate ligament reconstruction/revision. Clin Sports Med 2019;38(3):417–33.
32. Lu J, Tang S, Wang Y, et al. Clinical outcomes of closing- and opening-wedge high tibial osteotomy for treatment of anteromedial unicompartmental knee osteoarthritis. J Knee Surg 2019;32(8):758–63.
33. van Raaij TM, Brouwer RW. Proximal tibial valgus osteotomy: lateral closing wedge. JBJS Essent Surg Tech 2015;5(4):e26.
34. Luites JW, Brinkman JM, Wymenga AB, et al. Fixation stability of opening- versus closing-wedge high tibial osteotomy: a randomised clinical trial using radiostereometry. J Bone Joint Surg Br 2009;91(11):1459–65.

35. Ducat A, Sariali E, Lebel B, et al. Posterior tibial slope changes after opening- and closing-wedge high tibial osteotomy: a comparative prospective multicenter study. Orthop Traumatol Surg Res 2012;98(1):68–74.
36. Alaia MJ, Kaplan DJ, Mannino BJ, et al. Tibial sagittal slope in anterior cruciate ligament injury and treatment. J Am Acad Orthop Surg 2021;29(21):e1045–56.
37. Hughes JD, Vaswani R, Gibbs CM, et al. Anterior cruciate ligament reconstruction with a partial-thickness quadriceps tendon graft secured with a continuous-loop fixation device. Arthrosc Tech 2020;9(5):e603–9.
38. Jin C, Song EK, Jin QH, et al. Outcomes of simultaneous high tibial osteotomy and anterior cruciate ligament reconstruction in anterior cruciate ligament deficient knee with osteoarthritis. BMC Musculoskelet Disord 2018;19(1):228.
39. Schuster P, Schlumberger M, Mayer P, et al. Excellent long-term results in combined high tibial osteotomy, anterior cruciate ligament reconstruction and chondral resurfacing in patients with severe osteoarthritis and varus alignment. Knee Surg Sports Traumatol Arthrosc 2020;28(4):1085–91.
40. Schneider A, Gaillard R, Gunst S, et al. Combined ACL reconstruction and opening wedge high tibial osteotomy at 10-year follow-up: excellent laxity control but uncertain return to high level sport. Knee Surg Sports Traumatol Arthrosc 2020; 28(3):960–8.
41. Mehl J, Paul J, Feucht MJ, et al. ACL deficiency and varus osteoarthritis: high tibial osteotomy alone or combined with ACL reconstruction? Arch Orthop Trauma Surg 2017;137(2):233–40.
42. Kim JS, Park SB, Choi HG, et al. Is there any benefit in the combined ligament reconstruction with osteotomy compared to ligament reconstruction or osteotomy alone?: Comparative outcome analysis according to the degree of medial compartment osteoarthritis with anterior or posterior cruciate ligament insufficiency. Arch Orthop Trauma Surg 2022;143(7):3677–89.
43. Yabuuchi K, Kondo E, Onodera J, et al. Clinical outcomes and complications during and after medial open-wedge high tibial osteotomy using a locking plate: a 3- to 7-year follow-up study. Orthop J Sports Med 2020;8(6). 2325967120922535.
44. Duivenvoorden T, Brouwer RW, Baan A, et al. Comparison of closing-wedge and opening-wedge high tibial osteotomy for medial compartment osteoarthritis of the knee: a randomized controlled trial with a six-year follow-up. J Bone Joint Surg Am 2014;96(17):1425–32.
45. Imhoff FB, Mehl J, Comer BJ, et al. Slope-reducing tibial osteotomy decreases ACL-graft forces and anterior tibial translation under axial load. Knee Surg Sports Traumatol Arthrosc 2019;27(10):3381–9.
46. Yamaguchi KT, Cheung EC, Markolf KL, et al. Effects of anterior closing wedge tibial osteotomy on anterior cruciate ligament force and knee kinematics. Am J Sports Med 2018;46(2):370–7.
47. Shekhar A, Tapasvi S, van Heerwaarden R. Anterior closing wedge osteotomy for failed anterior cruciate ligament reconstruction: state of the art. JAAOS Global Research & Reviews 2022;6(9):e2200044.
48. Vadhera AS, Knapik DM, Gursoy S, et al. Current concepts in anterior tibial closing wedge osteotomies for anterior cruciate ligament deficient knees. Curr Rev Musculoskelet Med 2021;14(6):485–92.
49. DePhillipo NN, Kennedy MI, Dekker TJ, et al. Anterior closing wedge proximal tibial osteotomy for slope correction in failed ACL reconstructions. Arthrosc Tech 2019;8(5):e451–7.
50. Geers K, Ormseth B, Garrone A, et al. Anterior closing wedge proximal tibial osteotomy and revision anterior cruciate ligament reconstruction with quadriceps

tendon autograft. Video Journal of Sports Medicine 2021;1(5). 26350254211022758.

51. Floyd ER, Carlson GB, Monson J, et al. Tibial tubercle preserving anterior closing wedge proximal tibial osteotomy and ACL tunnel bone grafting for increased posterior tibial slope in failed ACL reconstructions. Arthrosc Tech 2021;10(10): e2221–8.
52. Ganokroj P, Peebles AM, Mologne MS, et al. Anterior closing-wedge high tibial slope-correcting osteotomy using patient-specific preoperative planning software for failed anterior cruciate ligament reconstruction. Arthrosc Tech 2022; 11(11):e1989–95.
53. Zsidai B, Özbek EA, Engler ID, et al. Slope-reducing high tibial osteotomy and over-the-top anterior cruciate ligament reconstruction with achilles tendon allograft in multiple failed anterior cruciate ligament reconstruction. Arthrosc Tech 2022;11(11):e2021–8.
54. Hees T, Petersen W. Anterior closing-wedge osteotomy for posterior slope correction. Arthrosc Tech 2018;7(11):e1079–87.

Surgical Techniques in Primary ACL Reconstruction

Getting It Right the First Time

Sahil Dadoo, BS[a,*], Zachary J. Herman, MD[a],
Jonathan D. Hughes, MD[a,b]

KEYWORDS

• ACL reconstruction (ACLR) • Graft selection • Tunnel techniques • Graft fixation
• ACLR in skeletally immature

KEY POINTS

- The approach to anterior cruciate ligament reconstruction (ACLR) should be individualized, focusing on a patient's unique anatomy and restoration of the knee to its native state.
- Graft choices include autografts (hamstring tendon, bone-patella tendon-bone, and quadriceps tendon) and allografts, each with unique advantages and disadvantages based on patient factors and goals.
- Nonanatomic femoral and tibial tunnel placement can increase the risk of graft failure following ACLR.
- Graft fixation method is influenced by several factors including surgeon preference, experience, cost, and ease of use.
- Special consideration should be given to ACLR in the skeletally immature and high-risk populations.

INTRODUCTION

The ideal anterior cruciate ligament reconstruction (ACLR) is an individualized approach that factors in a patient's unique anatomy and attempts to restore the structures of the knee to their native state.[1] Surgeons are tasked with difficult decisions during surgical planning, including selecting the ideal graft for the patient, determining the best techniques for anatomic tunnel placement, and using special considerations for the adolescent and older athlete populations. This article is focused on the background, trends, and outcomes in the literature surrounding these decisions for primary ACLR.

[a] Department of Orthopaedic Surgery, UPMC Freddie Fu Sports Medicine Center, University of Pittsburgh, 3200 S. Water Street, Pittsburgh, PA 15203, USA; [b] Department of Orthopaedics, Institute of Clinical Sciences, Sahlgrenska Academy, University of Gothenburg, Gothenburg, Sweden
* Corresponding author. 3200 South Water Street, Pittsburgh, PA 15203.
E-mail address: sahildadoo@gmail.com

Clin Sports Med 43 (2024) 399–412
https://doi.org/10.1016/j.csm.2023.08.007
0278-5919/24/

Trends in Graft Selection

The ideal graft choice for ACLR has been an important focus of research during the last several decades. Options for graft choice can be broadly split into autografts and allografts. Autograft choices include hamstring tendon (HT), bone-patella tendon-bone (BPTB), and quadriceps tendon (QT) with or without bone block. Allograft tissue choices can be split into soft-tissue allografts and allografts with bone blocks. Soft-tissue allografts include the hamstrings, tibialis anterior, tibialis posterior, peroneal tendons, and iliotibial (IT) band. Allografts with bone blocks include BPTB, Achilles tendon, and quadriceps tendon.[2]

Historically among the autograft choices, BPTB was the most commonly used autograft after its introduction in 1963 and still remains the most popular choice among high-level athletes.[3] The HT was introduced in the 1980s and has now become the most popular tendon worldwide, currently being used in more than 50% of primary ACLR cases.[4] Yet, during the last decade, there have been signs of declining use of HT and increasing use of the QT, with studies showing QT use in 2.5% of all ACLRs in 2010, and 11% of all ACLRs in 2014.[5,6] The QT was first introduced in the late 1970s as an alternative to the BPTB autograft due to its larger size and more robust mass[7]; however, due to initial studies demonstrating worse clinical outcomes, it originally remained unpopular. Although long-term follow-up data on QT use in ACLR is sparse, the graft continues to grow in popularity. Several short-term follow-up studies exist and demonstrate comparable clinical, functional, and patient-reported outcomes (PROs) to BPTB and HT autografts.[5,8] Finally, allograft use has increased during the past 20 years, with large database studies in the last decade showing allograft is being used in 40% to 45% of ACLR cases.[9] Allograft use is especially becoming more popular in revision ACL surgeries (20%–51% of revision cases) due to avoidance of additional donor site morbidity.[10]

PATIENT EVALUATION OVERVIEW

Evaluation of a suspected ACL-injured knee should include a thorough history and physical examination. Imaging evaluation includes plain radiographs to evaluate for bony pathology and/or the presence of a Segond fracture. Full-length lower limb radiographs can additionally be obtained to assess for standing malalignment, which can increase stress of the native ACL and ACL graft after ACLR.[11] Magnetic resonance imaging (MRI) should be obtained to confirm the ACL tear, evaluate bone contusion patterns, and look for concomitant injuries to meniscal, chondral, and/or ligamentous structures.

Lateral meniscus (LM) tears are the most common secondary pathologic condition in acute ACL tears, whereas medial meniscus (MM) tears are the most common secondary pathologic condition in chronic ACL tears.[12] If present, these tears must be addressed preferentially with meniscal repair versus resection to reduce the risk of long-term complications such as knee osteoarthritis (OA).[13] In addition, although MM root tears are rare and usually degenerative in nature, LM root tears are commonly traumatic in nature and occur in 7% to 12% of ACL injuries.[14] Studies have shown that LM root tears further reduce knee stability in ACL-deficient knees and that repair of these tears can restore both antero-posterior and rotatory knee stability.[14,15] RAMP lesions of the MM are gaining increased attention due to their association with ACL injuries. Although high-level evidence is lacking, the literature generally recommends repair of unstable RAMP lesions, whereas stable RAMP lesions can achieve equivalent outcomes following surgical repair and trephination and abrasion.[16]

Articular cartilage injury occurs at a rate of 16% to 46% in the setting of acute ACL tears, and studies have demonstrated an increase in PROs after combined ACLR with osteochondral autograft transplantation or autologous chondrocyte implantation.[17] Finally, large database studies have demonstrated multiligament reconstructions account for 8% of all knee-ligament reconstructions.[18] MCL injuries in particular are often overlooked, with evidence suggesting MCL injuries are present in up to 67% of ACL injuries.[19] If found on imaging or intraoperative examination, concomitant ligamentous injury should be addressed with reconstruction and/or repair, based on the grade and severity of injury.

GRAFT SELECTION AND ASSOCIATED OUTCOMES

Bone-Patella Tendon-Bone

BPTB autograft has long been considered the gold-standard graft choice for ACLR due to positive short-term and long-term clinical outcomes, such as 83% return to sport (RTS) rate at 4-year follow-up and 9% failure rate at 17-year follow-up.[20,21] Advantages of BPTB autograft include faster bone tunnel incorporation due to the bone-to-bone healing and more consistency in graft size when compared with other autograft choices.[22,23] Further, biomechanical studies of the BPTB graft have shown higher ultimate loads to failure and increased tensile strength when compared with the native ACL and HT graft.[24]

Although outcomes with BPTB autograft are excellent, there are complications associated with BPTB autografts that have led to a recent decline in its use. The most commonly reported disadvantages include anterior knee pain, with reported rates as high as 55%, patellar tendon rupture, patellar fracture, and tibio-femoral osteoarthritis (OA).[21,25,26] As a result, BPTB autograft is relatively contraindicated in patients with preexisting anterior knee pain or those who have to kneel more frequently for profession or sport (eg, wrestlers, mechanics, and plumbers).[23]

Hamstring Tendon

The use of the HT autograft increased in popularity due to adverse outcomes and complications associated with BPTB use.[4] Although demonstrating greater cross-sectional area, increased biomechanical strength, and higher loads to failure than BPTB in cadaveric studies,[23] it has also been shown to have comparable rates of RTS and PROs compared with BPTB autograft.[27] Rates of residual anterior knee laxity following HT autograft ACLR are low,[28] and HT has proven the most cost-effective method of surgery for ACLR when compared with BPTB and allograft choices.[29]

Still, there are concerns regarding the use of HT autograft given increasing literature showing higher failure rates when compared with other autografts.[30] A recent randomized controlled trial comparing HT and BPTB autografts demonstrated comparable PROs and rates of return to preinjury activity level at 5-year follow-up; however, a significant difference in failure rates (15% for HT vs 4% for BPTB).[31] Other studies have similarly demonstrated failure rates greater than 10% following ACLR with HT autograft, especially in younger patients.[32] Another concern regarding the use of HT autograft is the increased tunnel widening seen following its use.[33] Although the cause and clinical relevance of this is largely unknown, it has been shown to influence the techniques needed for revision ACLR surgery, including the decision to complete the revision ACLR in 1 or 2 stages. In general, HT autograft should be avoided in younger patients, especially female athletes, and athletes that require significant hamstring strength for stability and function (eg, judo, wrestlers, and so forth).

Quadriceps Tendon

In the last several years, the QT has become an increasingly popular choice for both primary and revision ACLR due to the versatility of the graft and complications associated with other autograft choices.[7,34] Short-term outcomes following ACLR with QT have been positive, demonstrating comparable PROs and postoperative knee laxity, and lower rates of complications and donor site morbidity when compared with HT and BPTB autografts.[5] One of the important advantages of QT use for ACLR is the ability to harvest a more robust tendon than other autografts, with studies showing QT harvest results in 50% greater mass than BPTB and similar ultimate loads to failure when compared with a 6-strand HT.[23]

As with all graft choices, there are some disadvantages to using the QT. Due to the large vascular supply of the quadriceps, postoperative hematoma is a potential complication. Weakness of the quadriceps muscles and inferior knee extensor strength has also been reported after QT use, yet conflicting evidence exists.[35] Finally, quadriceps tendon rupture is a very rare complication of QT use, occurring in 0.7% of cases.[36]

Allograft

Advantages of allograft use include shorter operation times, preservation of autogenous tissue, and avoidance of donor site morbidity.[2] Allograft sizes tend to be more predictable and have comparable strength to autograft tissue at the time of ACLR.[37] In addition, allografts have been shown to be an effective graft choice in older patients, with recent studies showing an 8.0% failure rate and acceptable PROs in patients aged older than 40 years.[38]

Although well tolerated in older adults, one important disadvantage of allograft use is the increased failure rate, up to 40%, observed in younger athletes.[39] A recent randomized controlled trial comparing allografts and autografts at minimum 10-year follow-up found similar PROs and postoperative knee stability between the 2 groups; however, a 3-fold increase in failure rates following allograft use (26.5% vs 8.3%, respectively) was found.[40] Other disadvantages of allograft use include increased incorporation time, variability in irradiation technique resulting in differing tensile properties, higher cost, and historical increased risk of infection.[2] Despite these disadvantages, allograft remains a popular choice among older, lower demand, patients and in revision ACLR settings.[10]

Authors' Preferred Approach

The authors' preferred approach to graft selection is based on patient age and activity-related indications. In younger, higher demand patients aged 18 to 29 years, the preferred graft choice is BPTB or QT, unless patient preference, extensor mechanism insufficiency, and/or prior contralateral ACL-R graft use dictates the need for HT. In patients aged 30 to 40 years, any autograft is generally indicated for patients who desire return to high-demand activities; however, allograft may be considered for those with lower activity levels. In patients aged 40 years or older, allograft is preferentially considered.

TECHNIQUES IN ANTERIOR CRUCIATE LIGAMENT RECONSTRUCTION

Femoral Tunnel Techniques

Anatomic placement of the femoral tunnel is crucial to restore knee kinematics, prevent graft impingement or overconstraint of the knee, and improve rotatory knee instability postoperatively (**Fig. 1**).[41] It has been demonstrated that anatomic femoral tunnel placement reproduces function of the native ACL better than isometric placement,

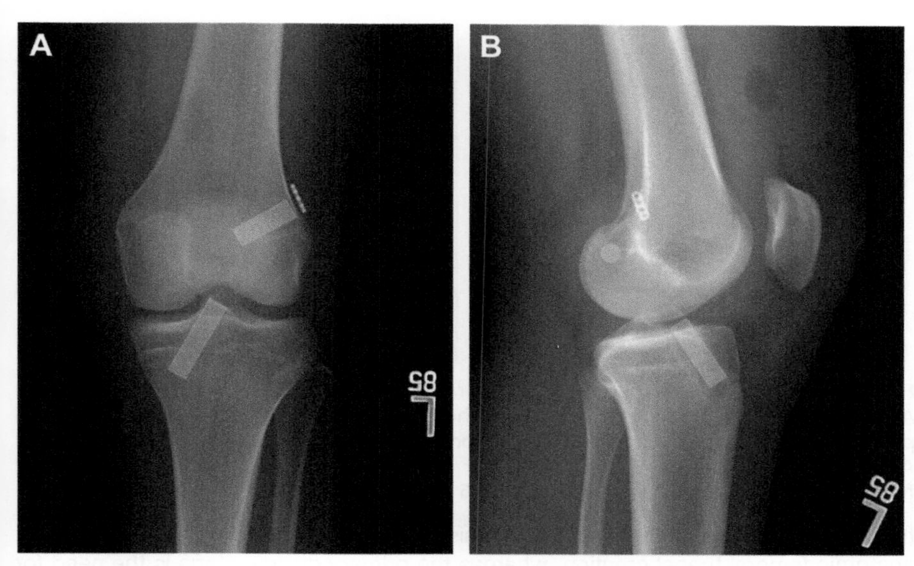

Fig. 1. Postoperative anatomic tunnel placement (highlighted in yellow) after primary ACLR in the (*A*) anterior-posterior and (*B*) lateral views.

where the femoral tunnel is located high in the femoral notch.[42] This is because the anatomic footprint of the ACL is located more distally and posteriorly, with the intercondylar and bifurcate ridges demarking the anteromedial (AM) and posterolateral bundles (**Fig. 2**). Anatomic ACLR is aimed at identifying the patient's unique anatomy and landmarks, and recreating the native anatomy of the ACL.[43] However, doing so requires individualizing the approach to ACLR tunnel placement because the size and location of the ACL femoral and tibial insertion sites can vary markedly among patients.[44] One of the most common causes of graft failure after ACLR is improper placement of the femoral tunnel.[45] A recent study determined that femoral tunnels placed too anterior and too proximal were independent risk factors for revision ACLR.[46] It has also been found that low-volume surgeons place their femoral tunnels significantly more anterior and proximal than high-volume surgeons, which can lead to increased risk of revision ACLR.[46,47] Therefore, it is critical to properly visualize the anatomic ACL footprint to ensure adequate posterior placement of the femoral tunnel.

Historically during the last 2 decades, the most common approach for creating the femoral tunnel was the transtibial (TT) approach, where the femoral tunnel is created via the tibial tunnel. However, there has been a decrease in the rate of TT drilling and an increase in the rate of drilling via the AM portal due to studies demonstrating that the TT technique results in a femoral tunnel that is too anterior and therefore nonanatomic.[48] A recent study found that patients who underwent ACLR with the TT technique had 2.49 higher odds of subsequent ipsilateral knee surgery.[49] Benefits of the AM portal technique include more anatomic and horizontal placement of the femoral tunnel (independent of graft type) as well as superior short-term outcomes and patient satisfaction, possibly due to the decreased risk of revision ACLR and subsequent knee surgery.[50] Retrograde drilling via an outside-in approach is another technique used to create anatomic placement of the femoral tunnel. The technique involves arthroscopically identifying the bifurcate and intercondylar ridges, placing the tunnel guide in appropriate anatomic position, and drilling the femoral tunnel from the cortex into

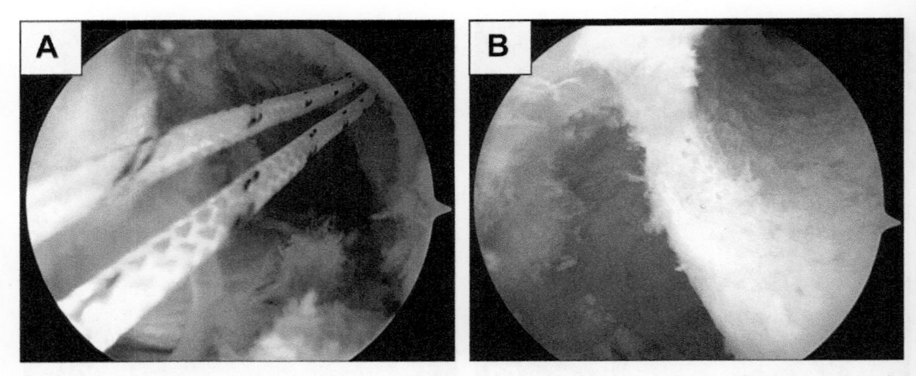

Fig. 2. Intraoperative view of anatomic femoral tunnel placement in a left knee ACLR. (*A*) Anteroposterior view of femoral notch from the AL portal, with an anatomic femoral tunnel placed distal and posterior on the lateral femoral condyle with draw sutures for the planned ACL graft placement. (*B*) View of posterior lateral femoral condyle showing anatomic femoral tunnel placement at maximum 4 to 6 mm anterior to posterior condylar wall.

the joint.[51] The primary advantage of this technique is allowing for independent anatomic femoral tunnel creation, whereas the primary disadvantage is the need for a second incision, which results in increased surgical site morbidity and worse cosmesis.[50]

Tibial Tunnel Techniques

Although extensive research exists on anatomic femoral tunnel techniques, less attention has been given to the placement of tibial tunnels in ACLR. Similar to femoral tunnel placement, knowledge of the native ACL anatomy is crucial for proper graft positioning, and malposition of the either tunnel can increase the risk of adverse outcomes. A recent study found that anterior femoral tunnel placement was associated with cartilaginous changes postoperatively, whereas posterior tibial tunnels were associated with an increased risk of bucket-handle meniscus tears.[52]

Optimal visualization of the tibial footprint is necessary for tibial tunnel placement, which can be aided by placing a high anterolateral (AL) portal. The most reliable landmark of tibial ACL insertion is the remnant stump (**Fig. 3**). In addition, the tibial spine,

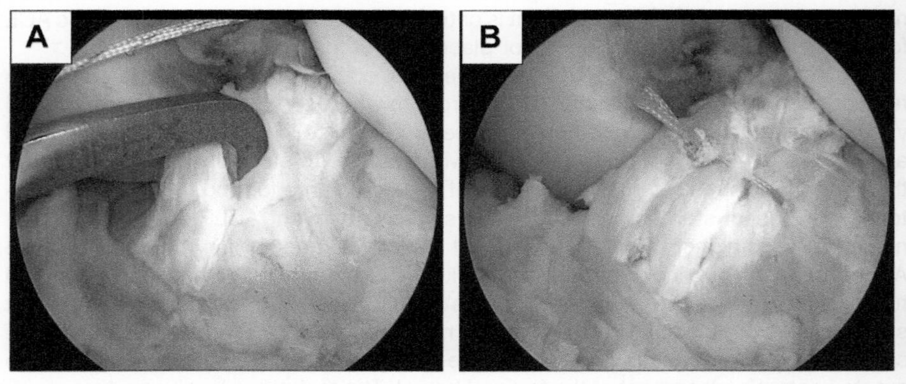

Fig. 3. Intraoperative view of anatomic tibial tunnel placement and tibial stump preservation. (*A*) Tibial drill guide through center of ACL remnant stump. (*B*) ACLR tendon in anatomic location through center of tibial stump.

intermeniscal ligament, and anterior horn of the LM can be used as landmarks for tibial tunnel placement.[53] The tibial tunnel is usually drilled at 50 to 55° in the sagittal plane from the center of the footprint intra-articularly to a point medial to the tibial tubercle and proximal to the hamstring insertion at the pes anserinus.[54] In the coronal plane, the tunnel should be placed at an angle less than 75° (ideal 60–65°) with respect to the medial joint line of the tibia.[55] In general, restoring native ACL anatomy and preventing impingement is key during tibial drilling. A target restoration of 50% to 80% of the native tibial insertion site has been proposed in order to match the cross-sectional area of the graft to the average midsubstance size of the native ACL.[56]

Fixation Techniques

Just as variance exists in graft choice and tunnel placement, fixation techniques in ACLR are numerous and can be divided anatomically based on aperture and suspensory fixations, with both options available on femoral and tibial sides. Aperture, or intratunnel, fixation methods use graft-to-bone interference screw or bone plug fixation. Advantages include minimal graft elongation, less graft-tunnel motion, and greater tensile strength, with the potential for more stability in the long-term.[57,58] However, disadvantages include bone-screw divergence, inappropriate insertion depth, possible tunnel blow-out, and damage to the bone-graft junction.[59,60] Suspensory, or extratunnel, fixation methods are numerous and include cortical buttons, fixed loop devices, adjustable loop devices, screw and washer, and cortical plate and screw. Advantages of suspensory fixation include increased graft durability, ease of use, and simplification in revision settings.[59] Disadvantages include implant breakage, loosening of adjustable devices, and tunnel widening.[59] Despite the numerous fixation techniques, no clear consensus in outcomes after ACLR exists, with suspensory and aperture fixation demonstrating equivalent PROs and functional outcomes.[61] Overall, choice of graft fixation is influenced by several factors including, surgeon preference, experience, cost, and ease of use. Further research is needed to elucidate the superiority of one fixation method over another.

Authors' Preferred Approach

The authors' preferred approach is to begin with a high AL portal for complete visualization of the anatomic tibial footprint. A spinal needle can then be placed for creation of an AM portal, which is used to drill the femoral tunnel. The AM portal technique is advantageous because it allows for maximum visualization of the anatomic femoral footprint, to ensure posterior femoral tunnel placement without the risk of "breaking through" the posterior condylar wall. For graft fixation, the authors recommend using either fixed suspensory fixation or interference screws in an isolated or combined fashion. Further, although no standardized protocols for graft tensioning exist, the authors prefer to fix the graft in near full extension with slight posterior drawer force applied.

CONSIDERATIONS FOR SPECIAL POPULATIONS

Anterior Cruciate Ligament Reconstruction in the Skeletally Immature

Special consideration should be given to ACLR in the skeletally immature (<12/13 years old in girls; <14 years old in boys)[62] population. In recent years, there has been an increase in ACL ruptures and subsequent ACLR in skeletally immature patients, likely due to an increased athletic activity and sport specialization in this population.[63] Originally, treatment was foregone or delayed until skeletal maturity due to the risk of physeal injury and growth disturbance. However, nonsurgical or delayed surgical management has been associated with poor outcomes including recurrent instability, increased meniscal and chondral damage, and decreased return to athletic participation.[64] As such, techniques have been developed to address ACL ruptures in pediatric patients without violating the physis. Examples include over-the-top IT band autografting and all-epiphyseal fixation techniques.

The intra-articular and extra-articular IT band, over-the-top reconstruction was first described around 2000.[65] The central portion of the IT band is harvested proximally and left attached to Gerdy tubercle. The graft is brought through the knee in an over-the-top-position posteriorly and is passed under the intermeniscal ligament anteriorly within an epiphyseal groove on the tibia. The graft is fixed with suture to the intermuscular septum and periosteum on the femur and to the periosteum on the tibia. Advantages include avoidance of the physes and ease in revision settings (no tunnels; all other autograft sources intact).[64] This method has proven successful, with improved PROs, high rates of RTS, and low incidence of complication.[66,67]

Another option for ACLR in the skeletally immature population is the all-epiphyseal technique originally described in 2004[68] with subsequent modifications reported.[69] It uses hamstring or quadriceps tendon autograft and all-epiphyseal sockets with epiphyseal fixation. Published data show that the technique provides promising results in terms of PROs and return to activity, whereas maintaining low rates of complication including physeal compromise and growth disturbance.[70] Recent studies comparing IT band over-the-top and all-epiphyseal techniques for ACLR in skeletally immature patients have concluded that both techniques are safe and successful with comparable complication (including rerupture) rates between the 2 groups. The incidence of overgrowth was found to be more common in the all-epiphyseal group, whereas angular deformity was more common in the over-the-top group.[71]

The undulating nature of the physis can result in placement of nonanatomic tunnels, thereby increasing the risk of future graft rupture. Therefore, especially in all-epiphyseal techniques, it remains important to visualize the anatomic ACL footprint and ensure anatomic tunnel placement.

High-Risk Populations—Role of Anterolateral Procedures?

Younger age, higher activity levels, and patients with generalized joint hyperlaxity are well-known risk factors for ACLR failure.[72] In these patients, particular attention to the optimal graft choice, anatomic tunnel placement, and consideration for additional procedures such as lateral extra-articular tenodesis (LET) can improve clinical outcomes. Indications for LET include younger patients (<25 years old), grade 2 or higher pivot shift, hyperextension greater than 10°, and generalized ligamentous laxity.[32]

The STABILITY I Trial was a randomized clinical trial, which examined the influence of adding LET to primary HT ACLR in high-risk individuals as indicated above. This study determined the addition of LET resulted in a significantly reduced rate of graft rupture (11% vs 4%, $P < .001$).[32] Currently, the STABILITY II Trial is an ongoing government-funded clinical trial aimed at elucidating the risk of reinjury in young, active, high-risk patients undergoing ACLR using BPTB or QT autograft with or without LET. Patients aged 14 to 25 years old with a first-time ACL rupture who participate in pivoting sports and/or have generalized joint hyperlaxity are randomized to receive either BPTB or QT autograft, with or without LET, in a 1:1:1:1 ratio.

Due to the current lack of high-level literature regarding the influence of LET in primary ACL-R with QT or BPTB, the authors reserve the use of LET in primary ACLR settings to patients enrolled in the STABILITY II study. In the setting of revision or multiple revision ACLR, LET may be indicated in patients with high-grade rotatory instability, where no other identifiable causes of ACLR failure exist (eg, tunnel malposition or increased posterior tibial slope).

SUMMARY

The ideal primary ACLR is an individualized approach that factors in a patient's anatomy, characteristics, and desires to restore knee kinematics and function. Special attention should be given when choosing the appropriate graft for a patient, considering the biomechanics, advantages, and potential disadvantages or complications of each graft that could affect a patient's quality of life and return to activity postoperatively. Although evidence is limited regarding the superiority of certain techniques over others, understanding tunnel placement and fixation methods is critical in terms of intraoperative preparedness. Finally, unique populations such as skeletally immature patients or older athletes should be given the appropriate care and considerations when planning, in order to avoid serious complication. There is no "one size fits all" approach to primary ACLR, and each case requires a thorough understanding of the above topics to develop the most appropriate plan for each patient.

CLINICS CARE POINTS

- The ideal approach for primary ACLR is an individualized, anatomy-based approach that aims to restore knee kinematics to its native state.
- Several graft choices exist for ACLR, including autograft and allograft, that have unique advantages and disadvantages when factoring in a patient's lifestyle, occupation, and desires for future RTS/activity.
- The placement of anatomic tunnels through the native femoral and tibial ACL footprints is of paramount importance, and various techniques can be used to achieve this goal.
- Young patients with higher activity levels are at an increased risk for ACLR failure, and special attention must be given in these patients to avoid damage to open physes and ensure adequate postoperative rotatory knee stability.

DISCLOSURE

The authors have no relevant commercial or financial conflicts of interest.

REFERENCES

1. Araujo PH, Kfuri Junior M, Ohashi B, et al. Individualized ACL reconstruction. Knee Surg Sports Traumatol Arthrosc 2014;22(9):1966–75.
2. Hulet C, Sonnery-Cottet B, Stevenson C, et al. The use of allograft tendons in primary ACL reconstruction. Knee Surg Sports Traumatol Arthrosc 2019;27(6):1754–70.
3. Erickson BJ, Harris JD, Fillingham YA, et al. Anterior cruciate ligament reconstruction practice patterns by NFL and NCAA football team physicians. Arthroscopy 2014;30(6):731–8.
4. Arnold MP, Calcei JG, Vogel N, et al. ACL Study Group survey reveals the evolution of anterior cruciate ligament reconstruction graft choice over the past three decades. Knee Surg Sports Traumatol Arthrosc 2021;29(11):3871–6.
5. Slone HS, Romine SE, Premkumar A, et al. Quadriceps tendon autograft for anterior cruciate ligament reconstruction: a comprehensive review of current literature and systematic review of clinical results. Arthroscopy 2015;31(3):541–54.
6. Lee S, Seong SC, Jo CH, et al. Anterior cruciate ligament reconstruction with use of autologous quadriceps tendon graft. J Bone Joint Surg Am 2007;89(Suppl 3):116–26.

7. Diermeier T, Tisherman R, Hughes J, et al. Quadriceps tendon anterior cruciate ligament reconstruction. Knee Surg Sports Traumatol Arthrosc 2020;28(8): 2644–56.
8. Fulkerson JP, Langeland R. An alternative cruciate reconstruction graft: the central quadriceps tendon. Arthroscopy 1995;11(2):252–4.
9. Maletis GB, Inacio MC, Funahashi TT. Analysis of 16,192 anterior cruciate ligament reconstructions from a community-based registry. Am J Sports Med 2013;41(9):2090–8.
10. Condello V, Zdanowicz U, Di Matteo B, et al. Allograft tendons are a safe and effective option for revision ACL reconstruction: a clinical review. Knee Surg Sports Traumatol Arthrosc 2019;27(6):1771–81.
11. Klek M, Dhawan A. The Role of High Tibial Osteotomy in ACL Reconstruction in Knees with Coronal and Sagittal Plane Deformity. Curr Rev Musculoskelet Med 2019;12(4):466–71.
12. Millett PJ, Willis AA, Warren RF. Associated injuries in pediatric and adolescent anterior cruciate ligament tears: does a delay in treatment increase the risk of meniscal tear? Arthroscopy 2002;18(9):955–9.
13. Weber J, Koch M, Angele P, et al. The role of meniscal repair for prevention of early onset of osteoarthritis. J Exp Orthop 2018;5(1):10.
14. Tang X, Marshall B, Wang JH, et al. Lateral Meniscal Posterior Root Repair With Anterior Cruciate Ligament Reconstruction Better Restores Knee Stability. Am J Sports Med 2019;47(1):59–65.
15. Shybut TB, Vega CE, Haddad J, et al. Effect of lateral meniscal root tear on the stability of the anterior cruciate ligament-deficient knee. Am J Sports Med 2015;43(4):905–11.
16. Bumberger A, Koller U, Hofbauer M, et al. Ramp lesions are frequently missed in ACL-deficient knees and should be repaired in case of instability. Knee Surg Sports Traumatol Arthrosc 2020;28(3):840–54.
17. Brophy RH, Zeltser D, Wright RW, et al. Anterior cruciate ligament reconstruction and concomitant articular cartilage injury: incidence and treatment. Arthroscopy 2010;26(1):112–20.
18. Lind M, Menhert F, Pedersen AB. The first results from the Danish ACL reconstruction registry: epidemiologic and 2 year follow-up results from 5,818 knee ligament reconstructions. Knee Surg Sports Traumatol Arthrosc 2009;17(2):117–24.
19. Willinger L, Balendra G, Pai V, et al. High incidence of superficial and deep medial collateral ligament injuries in 'isolated' anterior cruciate ligament ruptures: a long overlooked injury. Knee Surg Sports Traumatol Arthrosc 2022;30(1): 167–75.
20. Rauck RC, Apostolakos JM, Nwachukwu BU, et al. Return to Sport After Bone-Patellar Tendon-Bone Autograft ACL Reconstruction in High School-Aged Athletes. Orthop J Sports Med 2021;9(6). https://doi.org/10.1177/23259671211011510. 23259671211011510.
21. Sajovic M, Stropnik D, Skaza K. Long-term comparison of semitendinosus and gracilis tendon versus patellar tendon autografts for anterior cruciate ligament reconstruction: a 17-year follow-up of a randomized controlled trial. Am J Sports Med 2018;46(8):1800–8.
22. Park MJ, Lee MC, Seong SC. A comparative study of the healing of tendon autograft and tendon-bone autograft using patellar tendon in rabbits. Int Orthop 2001; 25(1):35–9.

23. Buerba R. Graft selection in contemporary anterior cruciate ligament reconstruction. J Am Acad Orthop Surg Glob Res Rev 2021;5(10). https://doi.org/10.5435/JAAOSGlobal-D-21-00230.
24. Staubli HU, Schatzmann L, Brunner P, et al. Mechanical tensile properties of the quadriceps tendon and patellar ligament in young adults. Am J Sports Med 1999;27(1):27–34.
25. Benner RW, Shelbourne KD, Freeman H. Infections and patellar tendon ruptures after anterior cruciate ligament reconstruction: a comparison of ipsilateral and contralateral patellar tendon autografts. Am J Sports Med 2011;39(3):519–25.
26. Lee GH, McCulloch P, Cole BJ, et al. The incidence of acute patellar tendon harvest complications for anterior cruciate ligament reconstruction. Arthroscopy 2008;24(2):162–6.
27. Chen W, Li H, Chen Y, et al. Bone-patellar tendon-bone autografts versus hamstring autografts using the same suspensory fixations in acl reconstruction: a systematic review and meta-analysis. Orthop J Sports Med 2019;7(11). https://doi.org/10.1177/2325967119885314. 2325967119885314.
28. Ahlden M, Kartus J, Ejerhed L, et al. Knee laxity measurements after anterior cruciate ligament reconstruction, using either bone-patellar-tendon-bone or hamstring tendon autografts, with special emphasis on comparison over time. Knee Surg Sports Traumatol Arthrosc 2009;17(9):1117–24.
29. Genuario JW, Faucett SC, Boublik M, et al. A cost-effectiveness analysis comparing 3 anterior cruciate ligament graft types: bone-patellar tendon-bone autograft, hamstring autograft, and allograft. Am J Sports Med 2012;40(2):307–14.
30. Samuelsen BT, Webster KE, Johnson NR, et al. Hamstring autograft versus patellar tendon autograft for acl reconstruction: is there a difference in graft failure rate? a meta-analysis of 47,613 patients. Clin Orthop Relat Res 2017;475(10):2459–68.
31. Mohtadi NG, Chan DS. A randomized clinical trial comparing patellar tendon, hamstring tendon, and double-bundle acl reconstructions: patient-reported and clinical outcomes at 5-year follow-up. J Bone Joint Surg Am 2019;101(11):949–60.
32. Getgood AMJ, Bryant DM, Litchfield R, et al. Lateral extra-articular tenodesis reduces failure of hamstring tendon autograft anterior cruciate ligament reconstruction: 2-year outcomes from the stability study randomized clinical trial. Am J Sports Med 2020;48(2):285–97.
33. L'Insalata JC, Klatt B, Fu FH, et al. Tunnel expansion following anterior cruciate ligament reconstruction: a comparison of hamstring and patellar tendon autografts. Knee Surg Sports Traumatol Arthrosc 1997;5(4):234–8.
34. Winkler PW, Vivacqua T, Thomassen S, et al. Quadriceps tendon autograft is becoming increasingly popular in revision ACL reconstruction. Knee Surg Sports Traumatol Arthrosc 2022;30(1):149–60.
35. Cohen D, Slawaska-Eng D, Almasri M, et al. Quadricep ACL Reconstruction Techniques and Outcomes: an Updated Scoping Review of the Quadricep Tendon. Curr Rev Musculoskelet Med 2021;14(6):462–74.
36. Singh H, Glassman I, Sheean A, et al. Less than 1% risk of donor-site quadriceps tendon rupture post-ACL reconstruction with quadriceps tendon autograft: a systematic review. Knee Surg Sports Traumatol Arthrosc 2022. https://doi.org/10.1007/s00167-022-07175-0.

37. Vyas D, Rabuck SJ, Harner CD. Allograft anterior cruciate ligament reconstruction: indications, techniques, and outcomes. J Orthop Sports Phys Ther 2012; 42(3):196–207.
38. Sylvia SM, Perrone GS, Stone JA, et al. The majority of patients aged 40 and older having allograft anterior cruciate ligament reconstruction achieve a patient acceptable symptomatic state. Arthroscopy 2022;38(5):1537–43.
39. Cruz AI Jr, Beck JJ, Ellington MD, et al. Failure rates of autograft and allograft acl reconstruction in patients 19 years of age and younger: a systematic review and meta-analysis. JB JS Open Access 2020;5(4). https://doi.org/10.2106/JBJS.OA.20.00106.
40. Bottoni CR, Smith EL, Shaha J, et al. Autograft versus allograft anterior cruciate ligament reconstruction: a prospective, randomized clinical study with a minimum 10-year follow-up. Am J Sports Med 2015;43(10):2501–9.
41. Zantop T, Diermann N, Schumacher T, et al. Anatomical and nonanatomical double-bundle anterior cruciate ligament reconstruction: importance of femoral tunnel location on knee kinematics. Am J Sports Med 2008;36(4):678–85.
42. Musahl V, Plakseychuk A, VanScyoc A, et al. Varying femoral tunnels between the anatomical footprint and isometric positions: effect on kinematics of the anterior cruciate ligament-reconstructed knee. Am J Sports Med 2005;33(5):712–8.
43. Fu FH, van Eck CF, Tashman S, et al. Anatomic anterior cruciate ligament reconstruction: a changing paradigm. Knee Surg Sports Traumatol Arthrosc 2015; 23(3):640–8.
44. Kopf S, Pombo MW, Szczodry M, et al. Size variability of the human anterior cruciate ligament insertion sites. Am J Sports Med 2011;39(1):108–13.
45. Jaecker V, Zapf T, Naendrup JH, et al. High non-anatomic tunnel position rates in ACL reconstruction failure using both transtibial and anteromedial tunnel drilling techniques. Arch Orthop Trauma Surg 2017;137(9):1293–9.
46. Byrne KJ, Hughes JD, Gibbs C, et al. Non-anatomic tunnel position increases the risk of revision anterior cruciate ligament reconstruction. Knee Surg Sports Traumatol Arthrosc 2022;30(4):1388–95.
47. Hughes JD, Gibbs CM, Almast A, et al. More anatomic tunnel placement for anterior cruciate ligament reconstruction by surgeons with high volume compared to low volume. Knee Surg Sports Traumatol Arthrosc 2022;30(6):2014–9.
48. Tibor L, Chan PH, Funahashi TT, et al. Surgical Technique Trends in Primary ACL Reconstruction from 2007 to 2014. J Bone Joint Surg Am 2016;98(13):1079–89.
49. Duffee A, Magnussen RA, Pedroza AD, et al. Transtibial ACL femoral tunnel preparation increases odds of repeat ipsilateral knee surgery. J Bone Joint Surg Am 2013;95(22):2035–42.
50. Robin BN, Jani SS, Marvil SC, et al. Advantages and Disadvantages of Transtibial, Anteromedial Portal, and Outside-In Femoral Tunnel Drilling in Single-Bundle Anterior Cruciate Ligament Reconstruction: A Systematic Review. Arthroscopy 2015;31(7):1412–7.
51. Espejo-Baena A, Espejo-Reina A. Anatomic outside-in anterior cruciate ligament reconstruction using a suspension device for femoral fixation. Arthrosc Tech 2014;3(2):e265–9.
52. Chiba D, Tsuda E, Tsukada H, et al. Tunnel malpositions in anterior cruciate ligament risk cartilaginous changes and bucket-handle meniscal tear: Arthroscopic survey in both primary and revision surgery. J Orthop Sci 2017;22(5):892–7.
53. Ferretti M, Doca D, Ingham SM, et al. Bony and soft tissue landmarks of the ACL tibial insertion site: an anatomical study. Knee Surg Sports Traumatol Arthrosc 2012;20(1):62–8.

54. Burnham JM, Malempati CS, Carpiaux A, et al. Anatomic Femoral and Tibial Tunnel Placement During Anterior Cruciate Ligament Reconstruction: Anteromedial Portal All-Inside and Outside-In Techniques. Arthrosc Tech 2017;6(2):e275–82.
55. Howell SM, Hull ML. Checkpoints for judging tunnel and anterior cruciate ligament graft placement. J Knee Surg 2009;22(2):161–70.
56. Fox MA, Engler ID, Zsidai BT, et al. Anatomic anterior cruciate ligament reconstruction: Freddie Fu's paradigm. J isakos 2022. https://doi.org/10.1016/j.jisako.2022.08.003.
57. Ishibashi Y, Rudy TW, Livesay GA, et al. The effect of anterior cruciate ligament graft fixation site at the tibia on knee stability: evaluation using a robotic testing system. Arthroscopy 1997;13(2):177–82.
58. Tsuda E, Fukuda Y, Loh JC, et al. The effect of soft-tissue graft fixation in anterior cruciate ligament reconstruction on graft-tunnel motion under anterior tibial loading. Arthroscopy 2002;18(9):960–7.
59. Zeng C, Lei G, Gao S, et al. Methods and devices for graft fixation in anterior cruciate ligament reconstruction. Review. Cochrane Database Syst Rev. 2018; 2018(6):CD010730.
60. Crum RJ, de Sa D, Kanakamedala AC, et al. Aperture and Suspensory Fixation Equally Efficacious for Quadriceps Tendon Graft Fixation in Primary ACL Reconstruction: A Systematic Review. J Knee Surg 2020;33(7):704–21.
61. Brand J Jr, Weiler A, Caborn DN, et al. Graft fixation in cruciate ligament reconstruction. Am J Sports Med 2000;28(5):761–74.
62. Kelly PM, Diméglio A. Lower-limb growth: how predictable are predictions? J Child Orthop 2008;2(6):407–15.
63. Beck NA, Lawrence JTR, Nordin JD, et al. ACL Tears in School-Aged Children and Adolescents Over 20 Years. Pediatrics 2017;139(3). https://doi.org/10.1542/peds.2016-1877.
64. Fabricant PD, Kocher MS. Management of ACL Injuries in Children and Adolescents. J Bone Joint Surg Am 2017;99(7):600–12.
65. Micheli LJ, Rask B, Gerberg L. Anterior cruciate ligament reconstruction in patients who are prepubescent. Clin Orthop Relat Res 1999;364:40–7.
66. Wren TL, Beltran V, Katzel MJ, et al. Iliotibial Band Autograft Provides the Fastest Recovery of Knee Extensor Mechanism Function in Pediatric Anterior Cruciate Ligament Reconstruction. Int J Environ Res Public Health 2021;18(14). https://doi.org/10.3390/ijerph18147492.
67. Willimon SC, Jones CR, Herzog MM, et al. Micheli Anterior Cruciate Ligament Reconstruction in Skeletally Immature Youths:A Retrospective Case Series With a Mean 3-Year Follow-up. Am J Sports Med 2015;43(12):2974–81.
68. Anderson AF. Transepiphyseal replacement of the anterior cruciate ligament using quadruple hamstring grafts in skeletally immature patients. J Bone Joint Surg Am 2004;86-A Suppl 1(Pt 2):201–9.
69. Cruz AI Jr. Fabricant PD, McGraw M, Rozell JC, Ganley TJ, Wells L. All-Epiphyseal ACL Reconstruction in Children: Review of Safety and Early Complications. J Pediatr Orthop 2017;37(3):204–9.
70. Fourman MS, Hassan SG, Roach JW, et al. Anatomic all-epiphyseal ACL reconstruction with "inside-out" femoral tunnel placement in immature patients yields high return to sport rates and functional outcome scores a minimum of 24 months after reconstruction. Knee Surg Sports Traumatol Arthrosc 2021;29(12):4251–60.
71. Wong SE, Feeley BT, Pandya NK. Comparing Outcomes Between the Over-the-Top and All-Epiphyseal Techniques for Physeal-Sparing ACL Reconstruction: A

Narrative Review. Orthop J Sports Med 2019;7(3). https://doi.org/10.1177/2325967119833689. 2325967119833689.

72. Kaeding CC, Pedroza AD, Reinke EK, et al. Risk Factors and Predictors of Subsequent ACL Injury in Either Knee After ACL Reconstruction: Prospective Analysis of 2488 Primary ACL Reconstructions From the MOON Cohort. Am J Sports Med 2015;43(7):1583–90.

Lateral Extra-Articular Tenodesis and Anterolateral Procedures

Bertrand Sonnery-Cottet, MD, PhD[a], Alessandro Carrozzo, MD[b,*]

KEYWORDS

- Anterior cruciate ligament (ACL) • ACL reconstruction
- Lateral extra-articular tenodesis • Anterolateral ligament (ALL) • ALL reconstruction
- Lateral extra-articular procedures

KEY POINTS

- Combined injuries involving the anterior cruciate ligament (ACL) and anterolateral structures have been found to result in greater rotational instability, necessitating a reevaluation of lateral extra-articular procedures (LEAPs).
- LEAPs show promising results in certain populations and warrant consideration as a valuable adjunct to ACL reconstruction (ACLR) to achieve satisfactory outcomes, particularly in high-risk populations.
- The addition of LEAPs, such as nonanatomic lateral extra-articular tenodesis or anatomic anterolateral ligament reconstruction, to ACLR has demonstrated significant advantages in specific patient populations.

INTRODUCTION

Slocum and Larson stated that "one of the most fascinating facets of the problem of knee ligament injuries is rotatory instability" and focused on the occurrence of this phenomenon in anterior cruciate ligament (ACL)-deficient knees.[1] A few years later, Galway and Macintosh described the pivot-shift test as a means to detect anterolateral rotatory instability (ALRI).[2] Even during those early years, anterolateral structures were acknowledged as secondary stabilizers to the ACL in managing ALRI.[2–4] Consequently, some surgeons have proposed lateral extra-articular procedures (LEAPs) as a solution to rotational instability. Lemaire provided the first account of lateral extra-articular tenodesis (LET) in the literature, which was subsequently followed by publications from pioneer knee surgeons such as Macintosh, Losee, Arnold and Coker,

[a] Orthopaedic Surgery, Centre Orthopédique Santy, FIFA Medical Centre of Excellence, Groupe Ramsay-Générale de Santé, Hôpital Privé Jean Mermoz, Lyon, France; [b] Orthopedic Unit, Sant'Andrea University Hospital, La Sapienza University, Rome, Italy
* Corresponding author.
E-mail address: alessandrocarrozzo27@gmail.com

Clin Sports Med 43 (2024) 413–431
https://doi.org/10.1016/j.csm.2023.08.008 sportsmed.theclinics.com
0278-5919/24/

Ellison, Andrews, and others, who presented various surgical techniques based on lateral tenodesis for rotational control of the tibia, either as stand-alone procedures or in conjunction with intra-articular ACL reconstructions (ACLRs).[3,5]

LEAPs enjoyed popularity until the late 1980s, when the American Orthopedic Society for Sports Medicine organized a consensus conference in Snowmass, Colorado, inviting the leading knee surgeons of that time. The experts at the Snowmass conference concluded that LEAPs did not offer significant advantages over isolated intra-articular reconstructions. Furthermore, they highlighted the increased morbidity, elevated risk of complications, and late onset of osteoarthritis (OA) associated with LEAPs.[6] Consequently, in response to this consensus and with the advent of arthroscopic intra-articular ACLR, LEAPs were nearly universally abandoned.[7]

Nevertheless, subsequent research confirmed the synergistic role of anterolateral structures in conjunction with the ACL in controlling anterolateral rotational stability.[8–12] Combined injuries involving the ACL and anterolateral structures were found to result in greater anterolateral rotational instability than isolated ACL injuries and were reported to occur in approximately 90% of patients with acute ACL rupture.[13–15]

Moreover, the remarkable identification of the anterolateral ligament (ALL) by Steven Claes and colleagues sparked renewed interest in previously disregarded extra-articular lateral procedures.[16] This renewed interest became imperative due to the growing number of reports indicating a failure rate exceeding 20% after isolated ACLR in high-risk populations.[17–19] Despite significant advancements in surgical techniques, hardware, and rehabilitation for ACLR, unacceptable postoperative persistence of rotational instability and the pivot-shift phenomenon remain prevalent.[20–22] This postoperative rotational instability correlates with poor clinical outcomes, graft failure, and the subsequent need for revision surgery.[22,23]

Recently, the International Anterolateral Complex Consensus Group Meeting established indications for combining LET with ACLR.[24] These indications include revision ACLR (R-ACLR), high-grade rotational laxity (grade 2 or 3 pivot shift), generalized ligamentous laxity, genu recurvatum exceeding 10°, and young patients (<25 year old) returning to contact pivoting sports.

In light of these developments, it is clear that a reevaluation of LEAPs and their potential benefits is warranted given the challenges of achieving satisfactory results with isolated ACL reconstruction in certain populations.

SURGICAL TECHNIQUES

The purpose of this section is to illustrate the surgical techniques of the most commonly reported LEAP techniques in the literature. Both nonanatomic reconstruction techniques, such as LETs, and anatomic ALL reconstruction techniques will be analyzed.

LATERAL EXTRA-ARTICULAR TENODESIS

Modified Lemaire

The addition of the modified Lemaire to ACLR has been shown with Level 1 evidence to reduce anterolateral rotational laxity, clinically relevant reduction in graft rupture, and persistent rotational laxity at 2 years after surgery.[22] This technique is now widely used worldwide, and both biomechanical and clinical studies have supported its efficacy.[25,26]

The leg is positioned with the knee in approximately 90° of flexion. A 5-cm longitudinal incision is then made centered on the lateral femoral epicondyle (**Fig. 1**A). The subcutaneous tissue is dissected down to the iliotibial band (ITB), whose posterior border is identified. From the posterior half of the ITB, a 9-cm long by 1-cm wide strip

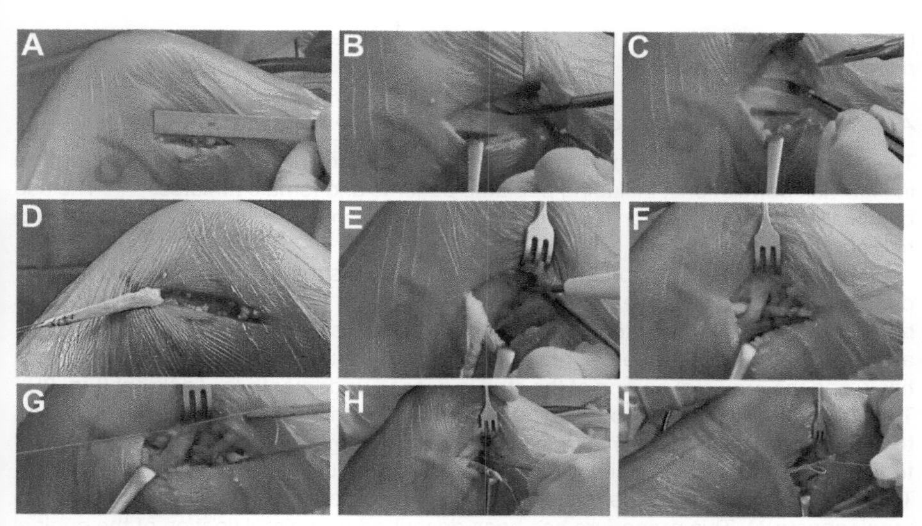

Fig. 1. Modified Lemaire performed on a left knee. (*A*) A 5-cm skin incision; (*B*) From the posterior half of the ITB, a 1-cm wide strip is dissected, leaving the distal attachment to Gerdy's tubercle intact; (*C*) Identification of the fat pad for proximal harvest extension to ensure a sufficiently long ITB graft; (*D*) The deep attachments to the vastus lateralis are released, and the free end is whip sutured with #0 nonabsorbable suture; (*E*) The fat pad is released to identify the insertion point for the LET; (*F*) The ITB graft is then passed under the FCL from distal to proximal; (*G*) The incisions around the LCL are then closed to prevent fluid extravasation; (*H*) At the insertion point for the LET, proximal and posterior to the lateral epicondyle, a 2.6-mm drill is used to drill the cortex, followed by insertion of a 2.6-mm knotless suture anchor; (*I*) The whip-stitched graft is passed through a loop of the suture anchor, and the graft is fixed near the extension.

is dissected, leaving the distal attachment to Gerdy's tubercle intact (**Fig. 1**B). Extending the incision proximally beyond the fat pad ensures that the graft will be long enough (**Fig. 1**C). The deep attachments to the vastus lateralis are released, and the free end is whip sutured with #0 nonabsorbable suture (**Fig. 1**D). The inferior portion of the ITB is then released to ensure that it can be closed at the end of the procedure. The fat pad is also released to identify the insertion point for the LET (**Fig. 1**E). The fibular collateral ligament (FCL) is then identified by applying varus tension, and an incision is made anteriorly and posteriorly to its proximal portion. The ITB graft is then passed under the FCL from distal to proximal using a right-angled clamp (**Fig. 1**F). The incisions around the LCL are then closed to prevent fluid extravasation (**Fig. 1**G). At this point, a vancomycin dressing is applied over the surgical exposure of the lateral surface of the knee. ACLR is then performed. Performing an out-in technique to create the femoral tunnel will facilitate the prevention of tunnel collision with that of the LET.

A variety of systems can be used for femoral fixation: staples, fixation in a bone tunnel with an interference screw, or systems that use smaller tunnels as suture anchors. The previously marked insertion point for the extra-articular tenodesis proximal and posterior to the lateral epicondyle is identified. A 2.6-mm drill is used to drill the cortex, followed by insertion of a 2.6-mm knotless suture anchor (**Fig. 1**H). Importantly, the angle of the drill and anchor can be adjusted to ensure that tunnel convergence is avoided. The whip-stitched graft is then passed through a loop of the suture anchor and fixed near the extension (**Fig. 1**I). This avoids fixation of the tibia in external rotation. The graft is then sutured back onto itself, and the fat pad is closed with a number

0 absorbable suture. The ITB is then closed with the same suture, aided by prior release of its lower portion.

Arnold-Coker Modification of the McIntosh Technique

This technique has been shown in the literature to reduce the risk of ACL graft rupture in high-risk populations, including pediatric patients and female athletes.[27–29] The use of this all-soft-tissue fixation technique has not been shown to increase the long-term risk of OA.[30]

With the knee in 90° flexion, a 10- to 12-cm incision is made from the lateral femoral condyle to Gerdy's tubercle. The ITB is exposed, and a 1-cm wide, 13-cm long strip is harvested from approximately 3 cm anterior to the posterior border, leaving its distal attachment to Gerdy's tubercle intact (**Fig. 2**A). The fibular collateral ligament is identified, and the proximal portion of the strip is passed underneath the ligament (**Fig. 2**B). The tibia is held in maximal external rotation, and the strip is then reflected and sutured to itself under tension with the knee at 90° flexion using absorbable periosteal #2 sutures placed at the level of Gerdy's tubercle and lateral collateral ligament (**Fig. 2**C, D). This allows for maximum shortening of the fascial strip and, ultimately, tightness of the repair construct. This procedure has been described as a simplification of the original technique of MacIntosh and Darby, which instead involves the creation of an osteoperiosteal tunnel posterior to the femoral attachment of the fibular collateral ligament, through which a strip of the ITB is passed before being looped through the lateral intermuscular septum and sutured back onto itself at Gerdy's tubercle with the knee flexed to 90° and held in external rotation.

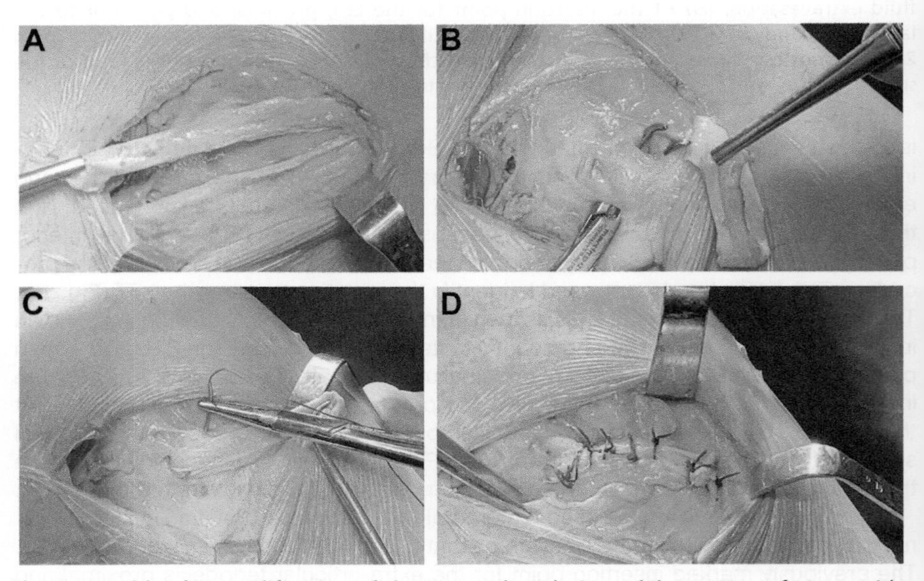

Fig. 2. Arnold-Coker modification of the McIntosh technique. (*A*) An ITB graft 1 cm wide, 13 cm long is harvested from approximately 3 cm anterior to the posterior border, leaving its distal attachment to Gerdy's tubercle intact; (*B*) The fibular collateral ligament is identified, and the proximal portion of the strip is passed underneath the ligament; (*C*) The strip is then reflected and sutured to itself under tension with the knee at 90° flexion using absorbable periosteal #2 sutures placed at the level of Gerdy's tubercle and lateral collateral ligament; (*D*) Final appearance. (*Courtesy of* Edoardo Monaco, MD, Associate Professor.)

Marcacci–Zaffagnini Technique

This technique allows intra-articular reconstruction of the ACL and LET using a single continuous hamstring graft and is a valuable choice for young active or skeletally immature patients.[31,32]

The semitendinosus and gracilis tendons are harvested and left attached at their distal insertions. The tendons are sutured together with #2 nonabsorbable sutures. The tibial tunnel is prepared under arthroscopy. Then, a 3- to 5-cm longitudinal incision is made on the lateral aspect of the knee, just proximal to the lateral femoral epicondyle. The iliotibial band is divided in its posterior third and retracted anteriorly. Using electrocautery and scissors, the lateral aspect of the thigh is dissected to reach the lateral intermuscular septum. Once the lateral intermuscular septum is clearly identified, the posterior aspect of the joint capsule can be reached by passing over this structure. The correct over-the-top position is found by palpating the posterior tubercle of the lateral femoral condyle with a finger. A curved Kelly clamp is passed from the anteromedial portal into the notch, and the tip is placed against the posterior portion of the capsule as proximal as possible. Once the tip of the clamp can be palpated from the lateral aspect of the femur, it is pushed through the thin posterior layer of the knee capsule to reach the previously prepared posterior space. A suture loop is placed in the tip of the clamp, which is then retrieved from the tibial tunnel. The semitendinosus and gracilis tendon grafts are then passed through the knee joint.

When the graft is removed from the lateral incision, a groove is made in the lateral aspect of the femur just proximal to the lateral condyle to reach a more isometric position. The graft is tensioned with the knee at approximately 90° and the foot externally rotated, and two barbed staples are used to secure the combined gracilis and semitendinosus tendons to the lateral femoral cortex in the groove. A 2-cm skin incision is made just below Gerdy's tubercle and on the anterolateral fascia. The remaining graft is pulled down and stapled below Gerdy's tubercle to the lateral aspect of the tibia. This technique can also be performed in a physeal-sparing variant. Tibial tunnel and staple fixation can be performed in a physeal-sparing manner by monitoring with intraoperative radiographs (**Fig. 3**).[33]

Kocher–Micheli Technique

This ITB-based technique has been proposed in the pediatric population, combining ACLR with LET without the need to perform bone tunneling for either ACL or LET reconstruction.

An incision of approximately 6 cm is made obliquely from the lateral joint line to the superior border of the ITB. The ITB is dissected proximally under the skin using a curved meniscotome or a specific tendon harvester. The graft should be approximately 18 cm long, whereas the width should begin 1 cm distally and increase progressively to 3 cm proximally. The ITB is left attached distally at Gerdy's tubercle. Dissection is performed distally to separate the ITB from the joint capsule and lateral patellar retinaculum. The free proximal end of the ITB is then tubularized with a #2 nonabsorbable suture. A 2 to 0 braided absorbable suture is then used to tubularize the remaining graft from where it passes over the lateral femoral condyle. The over-the-top position on the femur and the over-the-front position under the intermeniscal ligament are identified. Under arthroscopic assistance, the free end of the ITB graft is passed through the over-the-top position and out of the anteromedial portal using a full-length clamp or a two-incision rear entry guide. A second incision of approximately 4.5 cm is made over the proximal medial aspect of the tibia in the region of the pes anserinus. The dissection is carried through the subcutaneous tissue to the periosteum. From this incision, a curved clamp

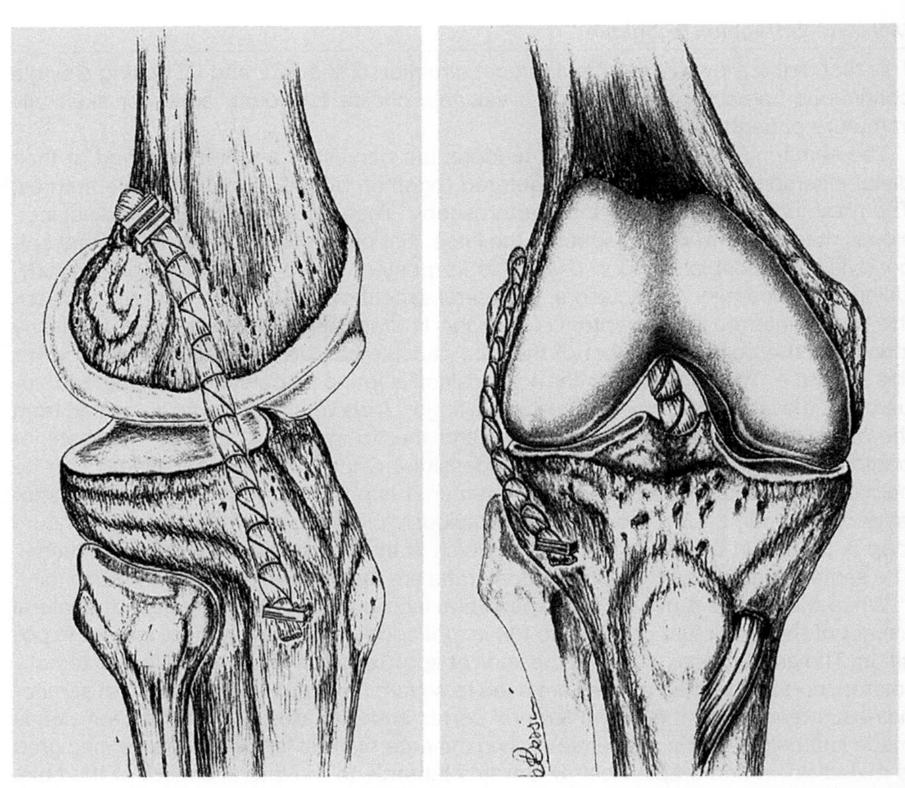

Fig. 3. The "over-the-top" Marcacci–Zaffagnini ACL + LET technique. (*From* Marcacci M, Zaffagnini S, Iacono F, Neri MP, Loreti I, Petitto A. Arthroscopic intra- and extra-articular anterior cruciate ligament reconstruction with gracilis and semitendinosus tendons. Knee Surg Sports Traumatol Arthrosc. 1998;6(2):68-75.)

is inserted into the joint below the intermeniscal ligament. A small groove is made in the anteromedial aspect of the proximal tibial epiphysis under the intermeniscal ligament using a curved rat tail rasp to bring the tibial graft placement more posteriorly. The free end of the graft is then passed through the joint, under the intermeniscal ligament in the anteromedial epiphyseal groove, and out through the medial tibial incision. On the femoral side, the graft is fixed through the lateral incision with the knee in 90° flexion and 15° external rotation using mattress sutures to the lateral femoral condyle at the insertion of the lateral intermuscular septum for extra-articular reconstruction. The tibial side is then fixed through the medial incision with the knee in 20° of flexion, and tension is applied to the graft. A periosteal incision is made distal to the proximal tibial physis as verified by fluoroscopy. A depression is made in the proximal medial tibial metaphyseal cortex, and the graft is sutured to the periosteum at the rough edges with mattress sutures (**Fig. 4**).[34,35]

ANTEROLATERAL LIGAMENT RECONSTRUCTIONS

Numerous authors have documented various technical approaches to ALL reconstruction (ALLR) using different grafts, with the most commonly used being a gracilis autograft.[36–39] The gracilis tendon may be a more appropriate graft choice for LEAPs

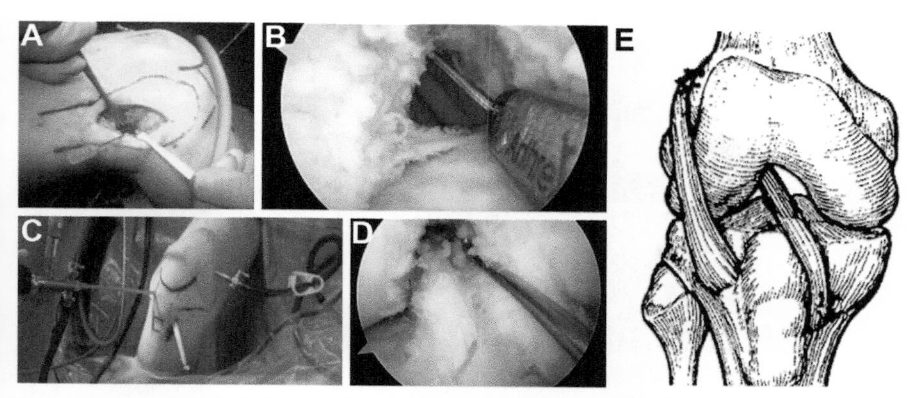

Fig. 4. Kocher–Micheli technique for combining intra-articular ACL reconstruction and LET. (*A*) Lateral incision: a spinal needle is directed through the capsule using an outside-in approach to keep the graft proximal to the capsule and high in the notch; (*B*) A suture passer is used to direct the sutures at the end of the graft; (*C*) The graft is passed through the capsule and out of the tibial incision; (*D*) Iliotibial band graft positioned intra-articularly in the knee joint; (*E*) Appearance of the Kocher–Micheli technique. (*From* [*A–D*] Willimon SC, Jones CR, Herzog MM, et al. Micheli Anterior Cruciate Ligament Reconstruction in Skeletally Immature Youths: A Retrospective Case Series With a Mean 3-Year Follow-up. Am J Sports Med. 2015;43(12):2974–2981. https://doi.org/10.1177/0363546515608477); [*E*] Kocher MS, Garg S, Micheli LJ. Physeal sparing reconstruction of the anterior cruciate ligament in skeletally immature prepubescent children and adolescents. J Bone Joint Surg Am. 2005;87(11):2371-2379. doi:10.2106/JBJS.D.02802.)

due to its quasistatic properties similar to the ALL and low-energy dissipation and permanent deformation under dynamic loads with respect to ITB.[40] These techniques offer advantages over LET procedures by closely replicating the anatomic structure of the ALL, thereby achieving biomechanics that more closely resemble the native ligament. ALLR can be accomplished through independent tunnel placement, separate from that used for ACLR. This is particularly applicable when using an in-out or transtibial technique for femoral tunnel drilling. Graft fixation, typically using a doubled gracilis tendon, can be achieved using screws,[39] anchors[36] or knotless soft anchors.[41] The utilization of the latter has recently gained attention in knee surgery, as it facilitates graft fixation while minimizing tunnel convergence through the creation of small bone tunnels. However, the author's personal preference is performing combined ACL and ALLR using a continuous semitendinosus and gracilis autograft.

Authors' Preferred Technique

The efficacy of this technique has been demonstrated in mitigating postoperative residual knee instability and reducing failure rates across various at-risk populations, such as young patients involved in pivoting sports and elite athletes.[42–45] In addition, this technique provides protection for meniscal sutures without leading to overconstraint.[46–48]

The patient is positioned in a supine manner on the operating table in a standard arthroscopy position. Before applying the povidone-iodine-coated cutaneous drape, three bony landmarks are identified: the head of the fibula, Gerdy's tubercle, and the lateral epicondyle. Two stab incisions, spaced approximately 2 cm apart, are made approximately 1 cm distal to the joint line between Gerdy's tubercle and the fibular head. Another stab incision is created slightly posterior and proximal to the lateral epicondyle on the femur (**Fig. 5**A). To create the bony tunnel on the tibia, a

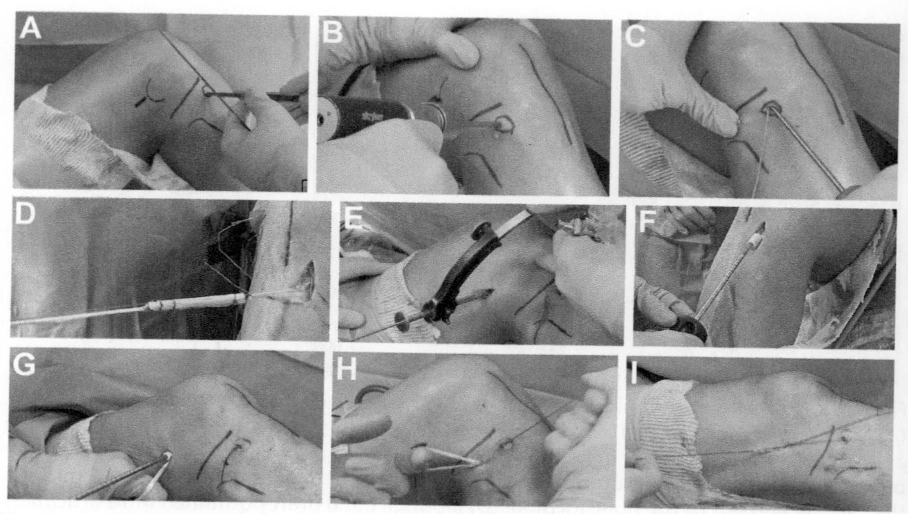

Fig. 5. Combined ACL + ALL reconstruction with hamstring tendon autograft. (*A*) Two stab incisions are made between Gerdy's tubercle and the fibular head. Another stab incision is created slightly posterior and proximal to the lateral epicondyle on the femur; (*B*) A 4.5-mm drill is used to create the bony tunnel on the tibia; (*C*) A suture is passed to form a loop to shuttle the ALL graft; (*D*) Final appearance of the ACL + ALL graft; (*E*) An outside-in approach is used to insert a guidewire from the ALL isometric point on the lateral epicondyle to the intra-articular femoral origin of the ACL; (*F*) An interference screw is inserted into the tibial tunnel using a nitinol guidewire; (*G*) With the knee in 30° of flexion, the femoral interference screw is placed; (*H*) The arthroscopic grasper is passed beneath the iliotibial band once again, bringing the gracilis graft back proximally and out through the proximal incision; (*I*) The sutures securing the ACL graft proximally are looped around the ALL graft and tied with the knee fully extended and in neutral rotation. (*Courtesy of* Dr Bertrand Sonnery–Cottet.)

4.5-mm drill is used, and the tunnel entrances are widened to facilitate graft passage (**Fig. 5**B). Subsequently, the two tunnels are connected subcortically using a right-angled clamp. A suture (No. 2 Ethibond; Ethicon, Somerville, NJ) is passed to form a loop for later ALL graft shuttling (**Fig. 5**C). To ensure the nonisometry of the ALL graft, the knee is taken through its range of motion, with the graft held taut in extension and slack in flexion. The semitendinosus and gracilis tendons are harvested using an open-ended tendon stripper (pigtail hamstring tendon [HT] stripper; Arthrex, Naples, FL). Initially, the attachment sites for both tendons are preserved. The gracilis tendon is then whip-stitched using a nonabsorbable suture. The semitendinosus tendon is measured from its insertion and marked using a skin marker at specific distances, namely, 4 and 10 cm for female patients and 5 and 11 cm for male patients. The gracilis tendon is subsequently incised from its base of insertion and sutured onto the semitendinosus tendon, starting at the proximal mark and concluding at the distal mark, using multiple No. 1 nonabsorbable sutures (Ethicon). A No. 2 ultra-high molecular weight polyethylene wire is placed on the semitendinosus tendon at the distal mark, and the graft is folded onto itself, secured with No. 1 nonabsorbable sutures at the proximal mark. The graft is then tripled over itself and tagged with No. 1 nonabsorbable sutures to form a tubularized graft. Consequently, an ACL graft is created, consisting of three parts semitendinosus and one part gracilis (**Fig. 5**D). The ALL graft extends distally from the gracilis portion of the graft. Proper sizing of the graft is verified. Using arthroscopic assistance, the femoral ACL tunnel is established. The drill guide is positioned intra-articularly at the femoral origin of the ACL. Subsequently, the drill guide is placed on the lateral femoral cortex, aligning with the predetermined optimal point for ALL isometry. An outside-in approach is used to insert a guidewire from the ALL isometric point on the lateral epicondyle to the femoral origin of the ACL (**Fig. 5**E). Once the guidewire is in place, an appropriately sized hole for the ACL is drilled. The tibial ACL tunnel is created in a manner that preserves the ACL remnant. The tibial guide is positioned at a 55° angle, starting from the external cortex and extending into the ACL insertion. Sequential reaming is conducted, initially using a 6-mm reamer followed by the previously determined size reamer for the ACL. A suture passer is inserted into the femoral tunnel and threaded transtibial through the tibial tunnel. The suture is used to shuttle the ACL-ALL graft transtibial into and out of the femoral tunnel. An interference screw, matching the size of the ACL graft, is inserted into the tibial tunnel using a nitinol guidewire (**Fig. 5**F). With the knee positioned at 30° of flexion, a femoral interference screw, also matching the size of the ACL graft, is placed into the femoral tunnel using a nitinol guidewire (**Fig. 5**G). The suture connected to the gracilis tendon is shuttled to the posterior bone tunnel beneath the ITB through an arthroscopic grasper. Subsequently, the gracilis graft is shuttled through the tibial bone tunnel using the previously passed suture. The arthroscopic grasper is passed beneath the ITB once again, bringing the gracilis graft back proximally and out through the proximal incision (**Fig. 5**H). The sutures securing the ACL graft proximally are then looped around the ALL graft and tied once more with the knee fully extended and in neutral rotation (**Fig. 5**I).

CLINICAL RESULTS

Significant advantages in performing LET or ALLR have been demonstrated in specific populations.

Pediatric Patients

Monaco and colleagues[27] conducted a comparative study including 111 pediatric patients with a mean follow-up of 43.8 months. Forty patients underwent isolated ACLR with hamstring autografts, and 71 had risk factors for rerupture and received ACLR with hamstring autografts + Coker-Arnold LET. The addition of LET to ACLR was associated with a significantly lower graft rupture rate than ACLR alone (0.0% vs 15.0%, respectively; odds ratio [OR], 15.91; P = .012) and with significantly better knee stability (pivot-shift grade 3: 0.0% vs 11.4%, respectively; P = .021) (side-to-side anteroposterior laxity difference 0.5 mm: 0.0% vs 17.1%, respectively; P = .003) and Tegner activity scores (7 vs 6, respectively; P = .010).

Perelli and colleagues[49] conducted a multicenter cohort study comparing skeletally immature patients receiving isolated ACLR with HT with patients receiving a combined modified Lemaire LET. The final population was composed of 66 patients with a mean age of 13.8 years. Patients receiving the combined procedure had a significantly lower ACL failure rate (14.7% vs 6.3%; P = .021) and better anteroposterior stability as well as better rotational stability. There was no difference between the two groups in the Pedi-IKDC and pediatric functional activity brief scale (Pedi-FABS) scores.

Kocher and colleagues[50] published their results with the largest case series currently available in the literature. They included 240 patients with Tanner stage I–II and a mean follow-up of 25.8 months. These patients underwent combined intra- and extra-articular reconstruction using the Kocher–Micheli technique with a single fascia lata graft without hardware fixation. Patients treated with this technique demonstrated excellent Pedi-IKDC and Lysholm patient reported outcome measures (PROM) scores, return to sport with a mean Tegner score of 7.8, and a 4% failure rate.

Young Patients

Getgood and coauthors[22] published the 2-year outcomes of the multicenter randomized clinical trial STABILITY. They included 589 patients with ACL deficiency who were randomly allocated to undergo single-bundle HT autograft ACLR alone or combined with modified Lemaire LET. They reported the clinical failure rate, defined as an asymmetric pivot shift, and graft rupture rate, defined as evidence of a graft tear on MRI or confirmed during revision surgery. In the isolated ACLR group, 40% of patients experienced clinical failure compared with 25% of ACLR + LET patients (relative risk reduction [RRR], 0.38; 95% CI, 0.21–0.52; $P < .0001$). In addition, graft rupture occurred in 11% in the ACLR group compared with 4% in the ACL + LET group (RRR, 0.67; 95% CI, 0.36–0.83; $P < .001$). At 3 months, patients in the isolated ACLR group had less pain as measured by the P4 ($P = .003$) and KOOS ($P = .007$), with KOOS pain persisting in favor of the ACLR group to 6 months ($P = .02$), but no clinically important differences in patient-reported outcome measures were found between the groups at other time points.

Patients with Ligamentous Hyperlaxity

Helito and colleagues[51] conducted a cohort study in which 90 patients undergoing ACLR with ligamentous hyperlaxity were evaluated. Sixty patients received isolated ACLR, and 30 patients also received ALLR. At a mean follow-up of 29.6 months, patients who received the combined procedure showed better anteroposterior clinical stability as assessed by KT-1000 arthrometer ($P = .02$), better rotational stability as assessed by the pivot-shift test ($P = .03$), and a lower reconstruction failure rate (21.7% vs 3.3%; $P = .03$). There were no differences in PROMs.

Patients Participating in Pivoting Sports

Sonnery-Cottet and colleagues[44] conducted a prospective study including young patients involved in pivot sports who underwent primary ACLR with a bone–patellar tendon–bone (BPTB) graft, quadrupled HT graft, or HT graft combined with ALLR. Five hundred two patients (mean age, 22.4 years) with a mean follow-up of 38.4 months were included. At the mean follow-up, the graft failure rate in patients receiving ACLR + ALLR was 2.5 times less than that in patients receiving ACLR alone with BPTB grafts (hazard ratio [HR], 0.393; 95% CI, 0.153–0.953) and 3.1 times less than that in patients receiving ACLR alone with HT grafts (HR, 0.327; 95% CI, 0.130–0.758), with no significant difference in the graft failure rate between patients receiving HT and BPTB grafts. Nevertheless, ACLR + ALLR was associated with higher odds of returning to preinjury levels of sport than the 4HT graft (OR, 1.938; 95% CI, 1.174–3.224) but not the BPTB graft (OR, 1.460; 95% CI, 0.813–2.613).

In a recent propensity-matched study conducted by Pioger and colleagues,[52] clinical outcomes following ACLR were compared between two groups: ACLR with BPTB autografts and combined ACLR + ALLR with HT autografts. The study involved a large cohort of patients, with a total of 1009 matched pairs and a median follow-up of 101.3 months. The findings revealed that patients in the ACLR alone group were three times more likely to experience graft failure than those in the combined ACLR + ALLR group (HR, 3.554 [95% CI, 1.744–7.243]; $P = .0005$). In addition, there was a significantly higher reoperation rate in the isolated ACLR group than in the combined ACLR + ALLR group (20.5% vs 8.9%; $P < .0001$). Based on these results, the authors concluded that patients who underwent isolated ACLR with BPTB autografts had significantly poorer graft survival and overall reoperation-free survival than those who underwent combined ACLR + ALLR with HT autografts.

Borque and colleagues[53] conducted a cohort study including 455 elite athletes who underwent ACLR alone (n = 338) or combined with modified Lemaire (n = 117). In the ACLR alone group, 9.5% of patients experienced ACL graft failure, compared with 3.4% in the ACLR + LET group (P = .045).

Guy and colleagues conducted a study on elite skiers from the French ski team. The authors analyzed 81 ACLR procedures; 50 were isolated, and 31 were combined with a LEAP, which was performed using modified Lemaire or ALLR. Graft rupture rates were 34.0% in the ACLR alone group and 6.5% in the ACLR + LEAP group. Multivariable analysis demonstrated that adding a LEAP was associated with a significant reduction in the risk of ACL graft rupture relative to ACLR alone (HR, 5.286 [95% CI, 1.068–26.149]; P = .0412). Age (HR, 1.114; P = .1157), sex (HR, 1.573; P = .3743), and ACL graft type (HR, 1.417; P = .5394) were not significant risk factors.

Hopper and colleagues[42] recently conducted a cohort study to determine the risk factors for graft failure in professional athletes undergoing ACLR. The authors included a total of 342 athletes with a mean follow-up of 100.2 months (range, 24–215 months). Out of these, 31 patients (9.1%) experienced graft failures, requiring revision surgery due to symptomatic instability. The rate of graft failure was significantly higher in cases where ACLR was not combined with a LEAP (15.5% vs 6.0%; P = .0105) and in athletes aged 21 years or younger (13.8% vs 6.6%; P = .0290). A multivariate analysis using a Cox model revealed that athletes who underwent isolated ACLR were at a 2.678-fold higher risk of ACL graft rupture (HR, 2.678 [95% CI, 1.173–4.837], P = .0164) than those who underwent ACLR combined with a LEAP. Furthermore, athletes younger than 21 years had a 2.381-fold higher risk of graft failure (HR, 2.381 [95% CI, 1.313–5.463]; P = .0068) than athletes older than 21 years. Sex, sport, and graft type did not show significant associations with graft failure.

Female Athletes

Vadalà and colleagues[29] conducted a prospective comparative study of female athletes undergoing isolated ACLR with HT grafting or combined ACLR + Coker-Arnold LET. At a mean 44.6-month follow-up, there were no graft failures at the last follow-up, but residual positive glide was found in 57.1% of the isolated group and in 18.6% of the combined procedures group.

Chronic Lesions

Helito and colleagues[54] conducted a cohort study to evaluate the results of combined ACL and ALLR in patients with chronic ACL injuries. They compared 33 patients who underwent combined ACLR + ALLR with 68 patients who underwent isolated HT ACLR. At a median follow-up of 25 months, 7.3% of the isolated ACLR patients experienced graft failure compared with none of the patients in the combined procedure group. Patients who received the combined procedure also had better KT-1000 scores (P = .048) and a lower rate of pivot shift on physical examination: 9.1% positive versus 35.3% in the isolated ACLR group (P = .011). In terms of PROMs, patients who received the combined procedure had better results on both the IKDC (P = .0013) and Lysholm (P < .0001) scores.

Revision Anterior Cruciate Ligament Reconstruction

Saithna and colleagues[55] recently conducted a review to determine whether the combination of a LEAP) with R-ACLR offers significant advantages over isolated R-ACLR. Eight comparative studies were included, most of which reported more favorable outcomes with the combined procedures. Failure rates after R-ACLR + LEAP ranged from 0% to 13%, whereas those after isolated R-ACLR ranged from 4.4% to 21.4%. The difference in postoperative side-to-side anteroposterior laxity was also lower with R-ACLR + LEAP (1.3–3.9 mm) than with isolated R-ACLR (1.8–5.9 mm). High-grade pivot shift was less common in patients who underwent R-ACLR + LEAP (0%–11.1%) than in those who underwent isolated R-ACLR (10.2%–23.8%). However, no consistent differences were found between the two approaches regarding return to sports or PROMs.

DISCUSSION

This review examined the LEAPs (LET and ALLR) commonly found in the literature. These techniques aim to address residual knee instability after ACLR, and their biomechanical effectiveness has been well documented.[26] The functional benefits of these procedures have been confirmed in vivo, as the addition of a LEAP significantly improves stability and reduces the risk of graft rupture in various populations at risk.

The rationale for adding these procedures to ACLR is based on several factors. First, the peripheral structures have a longer and more efficient lever arm than the central structures, making them more effective in controlling rotation. Second, LEAPs have a protective effect on the intra-articular graft. This effect was first demonstrated by Engebretsen and colleagues[56] in a biomechanical study where they showed an average 43% reduction in stress on the ACL graft. Engebretsen's findings were later confirmed by Draganich and colleagues[57] and more recently by Marom and colleagues,[58] who showed that LET reduced ACL graft force by up to 80% under applied rotational loads. This load sharing has a protective effect with particular emphasis on the initial postoperative period of integration and remodeling of the reconstructed ACL: the addition of a LEAP results in better graft healing and integration as assessed by MRI.[59] LEAPs are also intended to treat tears of secondary restraints, whose injuries result in increased rotational instability and pivot shift.[2–4]

Biomechanical studies indicate that both LET and ALLR restore normal kinematics and can significantly reduce residual anterolateral rotational instability in isolated ACL-reconstructed knees when an anterolateral reconstruction is present.[25,26,60,61] A meta-analysis conducted by Ra and colleagues[62] investigated the clinical outcomes of patients who underwent ALLR or LET, concluding that anterior stability was comparatively inferior with combined ACLR using LET compared with ALLR. However, rotational stability and PROMs did not differ significantly between the two procedures.

In a more recent systematic review and meta-analysis by Na and colleagues,[63] the efficacy of LEAPs in primary ACLR was analyzed. The authors found that compared with isolated ACLR, combined ACLR with LEAPs resulted in improved pivot-shift grades and graft failure rates, regardless of the LEAP technique. A limited, marginal improvement in PROMs was observed in patients who underwent LEAPs combined with ACLR. In contrast to ALLR, patients who underwent LET combined with ACLR had an increased risk of knee stiffness and adverse events.

In the context of R-ACLR, Rayes and colleagues[64] matched 36 patients and compared patients who received R-ACLR with HT + ALLR with patients who received R-ACLR with BPTB + modified Lemaire LET. At a mean follow-up of 5 years, there were no significant differences in the rate of graft rupture (HT-ALL, 0%; BPTB-Lemaire, 11.1%; $P = .13$) or reinterventions (HT-ALL, 8.3%; BPTB-Lemaire, 22.2%; $P = .23$). No specific complications related to LEAPs were observed in either group. In addition, there were no significant differences in knee laxity parameters, return to sports, or clinical scores between the groups at final follow-up, except for the Tegner

Activity Scale score (HT-ALL, 6.4; BPTB-Lemaire, 7.3; P = .03). Overall, the literature does not provide clear guidance on which LEAP to choose. Careful consideration of patient characteristics and surgeon expertise is necessary.

Although combining ACLR with an LEAP shows promising results in terms of knee stability and decreased graft rupture rate, there are concerns about the risk of over-constraint.[65–71] Some studies have reported higher rates of lateral tibiofemoral arthritis, but these findings were confounded by other factors such as meniscectomy and transtibial femoral tunnel positioning.[65,66,72] Long-term follow-up studies have not consistently demonstrated an increased risk of OA with the addition of LEAPs. Ferretti and colleagues[30] reported that the addition of a Coker-Arnold LET to an anatomically placed ACLR did not increase the risk of OA at a mean follow-up of 10 years. Similarly, Marcacci and colleagues[73] and Zaffagnini and colleagues[74,75] did not observe an increased risk of OA with the addition of LEAPs using the Marcacci–Zaffagnini technique in studies with a 20-year follow-up. Recently, Shatrov and colleagues[48] evaluated the incidence of OA with isolated ACLR versus ACLR + ALLR at medium-term follow-up. The patients were matched based on additional risk factors for developing OA, and a total of 80 patients (42 ACLR + ALLR and 38 isolated ACLR) were analyzed with a mean follow-up of 104 months. The authors found no significant difference between groups for joint space narrowing in the medial or lateral tibiofemoral compartment. In addition, they highlighted that lateral meniscal tears increased the risk of lateral tibiofemoral narrowing by nearly five times (OR, 4.9; 95% CI, 1.547–19.367; P = .0123). In skeletally immature patients, concerns about overstrain are even greater, but there are limited data on postoperative deformities in patients who have undergone ACLR + LEAPs. In a recent review,[76] valgus deformities were reported, but the number of cases was very small, and there are few reports in the literature of postoperative deformities in patients who received ACLR + LEAP.[31,77] However, these postoperative deformities cannot be attributed with certainty to the LEAP rather than the ACLR itself.

SUMMARY

The addition of LEAPs, such as nonanatomic LET or anatomic ALLR, to ACLR has demonstrated significant advantages in specific patient populations. Clinical results from various studies have consistently shown improved knee stability, reduced graft rupture rates, and better patient-reported outcomes with the use of LEAPs in ACLR.

CLINICS CARE POINTS

- Lateral extra-articular procedure (LEAP) techniques, including lateral extra-articular tenodesis (LET) and anterolateral ligament reconstruction (ALLR), restore normal knee kinematics and significantly reduce residual anterior laxity after isolated anterior cruciate ligament reconstruction (ACLR).
- The protective effect of LEAPs on the intra-articular graft results in improved graft healing and integration and reduced stress on the ACL graft, leading to better postoperative outcomes.
- LEAPs have shown evidence of improving clinical stability, reducing graft failure rates, and yielding equal or better patient-reported outcome measures in patients at high risk for persistent instability after ACLR or graft rupture. These populations include skeletally immature patients, patients with ligamentous hyperlaxity, female athletes, athletes participating in pivoting sports, elite athletes, patients with chronic ACL injury, and patients requiring revision ACLR.

- The choice between LET and ALLR depends on the specific patient population and surgeon's preference, as the current literature does not provide strong recommendations regarding the selection of LEAP technique.
- Further research is needed to better understand the long-term outcomes, potential complications, and optimal selection of LEAP techniques in different patient populations.

REFERENCES

1. Slocum DB, Larson RL. Rotatory instability of the knee. Its pathogenesis and a clinical test to demonstrate its presence. J Bone Joint Surg Am 1968;50(2): 211–25.
2. Galway HR, MacIntosh DL. The lateral pivot shift: a symptom and sign of anterior cruciate ligament insufficiency. Clin Orthop Relat Res 1980;147:45–50.
3. Slette EL, Mikula JD, Schon JM, et al. Biomechanical Results of Lateral Extra-articular Tenodesis Procedures of the Knee: A Systematic Review. Arthroscopy 2016;32(12):2592–611.
4. Hughston JC, Andrews JR, Cross MJ, et al. Classification of knee ligament instabilities. Part II. The lateral compartment. J Bone Joint Surg Am 1976;58(2):173–9.
5. Ferretti A, Monaco E, Carrozzo A. Extra-Articular Reconstructions in ACL-Deficient Knee. In: Ferretti A, editor. Anterolateral rotatory instability in ACL-deficient knee. Champaign, IL: Springer; 2022. p. 117–31.
6. Pearl AJ, Bergfeld JA. Extra-articular reconstruction in the anterior cruciate ligament deficient knee. Snowmass: AOSSM; 2014. 19890900210.
7. Ferretti A. Extra-articular reconstruction in the anterior cruciate ligament deficient knee: a commentary. Joints 2014;2(1):41–7.
8. yang Song G, Zhang H, qian WQ, et al. Risk Factors Associated With Grade 3 Pivot Shift After Acute Anterior Cruciate Ligament Injuries. Am J Sports Med 2016;44(2):362–9.
9. Song GY, Zhang H, Wu G, et al. Patients with high-grade pivot-shift phenomenon are associated with higher prevalence of anterolateral ligament injury after acute anterior cruciate ligament injuries. Knee Surg Sports Traumatol Arthrosc 2017; 25(4):1111–6.
10. Monaco E, Fabbri M, Mazza D, et al. The Effect of Sequential Tearing of the Anterior Cruciate and Anterolateral Ligament on Anterior Translation and the Pivot-Shift Phenomenon: A Cadaveric Study Using Navigation. Arthroscopy 2018; 34(4):1009–14.
11. Sonnery-Cottet B, Daggett M, Fayard JM, et al. Anterolateral Ligament Expert Group consensus paper on the management of internal rotation and instability of the anterior cruciate ligament - deficient knee. J Orthop Traumatol 2017; 18(2):91–106.
12. Ferretti A, Monaco E, Gaj E, et al. Risk Factors for Grade 3 Pivot Shift in Knees With Acute Anterior Cruciate Ligament Injuries: A Comprehensive Evaluation of the Importance of Osseous and Soft Tissue Parameters From the SANTI Study Group. Am J Sports Med 2020;48(10).
13. Terry GC, Norwood LA, Hughston JC, et al. How iliotibial tract injuries of the knee combine with acute anterior cruciate ligament tears to influence abnormal anterior tibial displacement. Am J Sports Med 1993;21(1):55–60.
14. Ferretti A, Monaco E, Fabbri M, et al. Prevalence and Classification of Injuries of Anterolateral Complex in Acute Anterior Cruciate Ligament Tears. Arthroscopy 2017;33(1):147–54.

15. Ferretti A, Monaco E, Redler A, et al. High Prevalence of Anterolateral Ligament Abnormalities on MRI in Knees With Acute Anterior Cruciate Ligament Injuries: A Case-Control Series From the SANTI Study Group. Orthop J Sports Med 2019; 7(6). 232596711985291.
16. Claes S, Vereecke E, Maes M, et al. Anatomy of the anterolateral ligament of the knee. J Anat 2013;223(4):321–8.
17. Webster KE, Feller JA. Exploring the High Reinjury Rate in Younger Patients Undergoing Anterior Cruciate Ligament Reconstruction. Am J Sports Med 2016; 44(11):2827–32.
18. Webster KE, Feller JA, Leigh WB, et al. Younger patients are at increased risk for graft rupture and contralateral injury after anterior cruciate ligament reconstruction. Am J Sports Med 2014;42(3):641–7.
19. Grassi A, Kim C, Marcheggiani Muccioli GM, et al. What Is the Mid-term Failure Rate of Revision ACL Reconstruction? A Systematic Review. Clin Orthop Relat Res 2017;475(10):2484–99.
20. Prodromos CC, Joyce BT, Shi K, et al. A meta-analysis of stability after anterior cruciate ligament reconstruction as a function of hamstring versus patellar tendon graft and fixation type. Arthroscopy 2005;21(10):1202.
21. Mohtadi NG, Chan DS, Dainty KN, et al. Patellar tendon versus hamstring tendon autograft for anterior cruciate ligament rupture in adults. Cochrane Database Syst Rev 2011;2011(9):CD005960.
22. Getgood AMJ, Bryant DM, Litchfield R, et al. Lateral Extra-articular Tenodesis Reduces Failure of Hamstring Tendon Autograft Anterior Cruciate Ligament Reconstruction: 2-Year Outcomes From the STABILITY Study Randomized Clinical Trial. Am J Sports Med 2020;48(2):285–97.
23. Ayeni OR, Chahal M, Tran MN, et al. Pivot shift as an outcome measure for ACL reconstruction: a systematic review. Knee Surg Sports Traumatol Arthrosc 2012; 20(4):767–77.
24. Getgood A, Brown C, Lording T, et al. The anterolateral complex of the knee: results from the International ALC Consensus Group Meeting. Knee Surg Sports Traumatol Arthrosc 2019;27(1):166–76.
25. Delaloye JR, Hartog C, Blatter S, et al. Anterolateral Ligament Reconstruction and Modified Lemaire Lateral Extra-Articular Tenodesis Similarly Improve Knee Stability After Anterior Cruciate Ligament Reconstruction: A Biomechanical Study. Arthroscopy 2020;36(7):1942–50.
26. van der Wal WA, Meijer DT, Hoogeslag RAG, et al. The iliotibial band is the main secondary stabilizer for anterolateral rotatory instability and both a lemaire tenodesis and anterolateral ligament reconstruction can restore native knee kinematics in the ACL reconstructed knee. a systematic review of biomechanical cadaveric studies. Arthroscopy 2023. https://doi.org/10.1016/j.arthro.2023.05.005.
27. Monaco E, Carrozzo A, Saithna A, et al. Isolated ACL Reconstruction Versus ACL Reconstruction Combined With Lateral Extra-articular Tenodesis: A Comparative Study of Clinical Outcomes in Adolescent Patients. Am J Sports Med 2022; 50(12).
28. Guzzini M, Mazza D, Fabbri M, et al. Extra-articular tenodesis combined with an anterior cruciate ligament reconstruction in acute anterior cruciate ligament tear in elite female football players. Int Orthop 2016;40(10):2091–6.
29. Vadalà AP, Iorio R, De Carli A, et al. An extra-articular procedure improves the clinical outcome in anterior cruciate ligament reconstruction with hamstrings in female athletes. Int Orthop 2013;37(2):187–92.

30. Ferretti A, Monaco E, Ponzo A, et al. Combined Intra-articular and Extra-articular Reconstruction in Anterior Cruciate Ligament–Deficient Knee: 25 Years Later. Arthroscopy 2016;32(10):2039–47.
31. Roberti di Sarsina T, Macchiarola L, Signorelli C, et al. Anterior cruciate ligament reconstruction with an all-epiphyseal "over-the-top" technique is safe and shows low rate of failure in skeletally immature athletes. Knee Surg Sports Traumatol Arthrosc 2019;27(2):498–506.
32. Zaffagnini S, Lucidi GA, Macchiarola L, et al. The 25-year experience of over-the-top ACL reconstruction plus extra-articular lateral tenodesis with hamstring tendon grafts: the story so far. J Exp Orthop 2023;10(1):36.
33. Marcacci M, Zaffagnini S, Iacono F, et al. Arthroscopic intra- and extra-articular anterior cruciate ligament reconstruction with gracilis and semitendinosus tendons. Knee Surg Sports Traumatol Arthrosc 1998;6(2):68–75.
34. Willimon SC, Jones CR, Herzog MM, et al. Micheli Anterior Cruciate Ligament Reconstruction in Skeletally Immature Youths: A Retrospective Case Series With a Mean 3-Year Follow-up. Am J Sports Med 2015;43(12):2974–81.
35. Kocher MS, Garg S, Micheli LJ. Physeal sparing reconstruction of the anterior cruciate ligament in skeletally immature prepubescent children and adolescents. J Bone Joint Surg Am 2005;87(11):2371–9.
36. Helito CP, Bonadio MB, Gobbi RG, et al. Combined Intra- and Extra-articular Reconstruction of the Anterior Cruciate Ligament: The Reconstruction of the Knee Anterolateral Ligament. Arthrosc Tech 2015;4(3):e239–44.
37. Sonnery-Cottet B, Barbosa NC, Tuteja S, et al. Minimally Invasive Anterolateral Ligament Reconstruction in the Setting of Anterior Cruciate Ligament Injury. Arthrosc Tech 2016;5(1):e211–5.
38. Ferretti A, Monaco E, Fabbri M, et al. The Fascia Lata Anterolateral Tenodesis Technique. Arthrosc Tech 2017;6(1):e81–6.
39. Chahla J, Menge TJ, Mitchell JJ, et al. Anterolateral Ligament Reconstruction Technique: An Anatomic-Based Approach. Arthrosc Tech 2016;5(3):e453–7.
40. Taylan O, Slane J, van Beek N, et al. Characterizing the viscoelastic properties of the anterolateral ligament and grafts commonly used in its reconstruction. Clin Biomech 2023;104:105949.
41. Mesnier T, Cavaignac M, Marot V, et al. Knee Anterolateral Ligament Reconstruction With Knotless Soft Anchor: Shallow Fixation Prevents Tunnel Convergence. Arthrosc Tech 2022;11(4):e511–6.
42. Hopper GP, Pioger C, Philippe C, et al. Risk Factors for Anterior Cruciate Ligament Graft Failure in Professional Athletes: An Analysis of 342 Patients With a Mean Follow-up of 100 Months From the SANTI Study Group. Am J Sports Med 2022;50(12):3218–27.
43. Guy S, Fayard JM, Saithna A, et al. Risk of Graft Rupture After Adding a Lateral Extra-articular Procedure at the Time of ACL Reconstruction: A Retrospective Comparative Study of Elite Alpine Skiers From the French National Team. Am J Sports Med 2022;50(6).
44. Sonnery-Cottet B, Saithna A, Cavalier M, et al. Anterolateral Ligament Reconstruction Is Associated With Significantly Reduced ACL Graft Rupture Rates at a Minimum Follow-up of 2 Years: A Prospective Comparative Study of 502 Patients From the SANTI Study Group. Am J Sports Med 2017;45(7):1547–57.
45. Rosenstiel N, Praz C, Ouanezar H, et al. Combined Anterior Cruciate and Anterolateral Ligament Reconstruction in the Professional Athlete: Clinical Outcomes From the Scientific Anterior Cruciate Ligament Network International Study Group

in a Series of 70 Patients With a Minimum Follow-Up of 2 Years. Arthroscopy 2019;35(3):885–92.
46. Gousopoulos L, Hopper GP, Saithna A, et al. Suture Hook Versus All-Inside Repair for Longitudinal Tears of the Posterior Horn of the Medial Meniscus Concomitant to Anterior Cruciate Ligament Reconstruction: A Matched-Pair Analysis From the SANTI Study Group. Am J Sports Med 2022;50(9):2357–66.
47. El Helou A, Gousopoulos L, Shatrov J, et al. Failure Rates of Repaired Bucket-Handle Tears of the Medial Meniscus Concomitant With Anterior Cruciate Ligament Reconstruction: A Cohort Study of 253 Patients From the SANTI Study Group With a Mean Follow-up of 94 Months. Am J Sports Med 2023;51(3): 585–95.
48. Shatrov J, Freychet B, Hopper GP, et al. Radiographic Incidence of Knee Osteoarthritis After Isolated ACL Reconstruction Versus Combined ACL and ALL Reconstruction: A Prospective Matched Study From the SANTI Study Group. Am J Sports Med 2023. 3635465231168899.
49. Perelli S, Costa GG, Terron VM, et al. Combined Anterior Cruciate Ligament Reconstruction and Modified Lemaire Lateral Extra-articular Tenodesis Better Restores Knee Stability and Reduces Failure Rates Than Isolated Anterior Cruciate Ligament Reconstruction in Skeletally Immature Patients. Am J Sports Med 2022; 50(14):3778–85.
50. Kocher MS, Heyworth BE, Fabricant PD, et al. Outcomes of physeal-sparing ACL reconstruction with iliotibial band autograft in skeletally immature prepubescent children. Journal of Bone and Joint Surgery - American 2018;100(13):1087–94.
51. Helito CP, Sobrado MF, Giglio PN, et al. Combined Reconstruction of the Anterolateral Ligament in Patients With Anterior Cruciate Ligament Injury and Ligamentous Hyperlaxity Leads to Better Clinical Stability and a Lower Failure Rate Than Isolated Anterior Cruciate Ligament Reconstruction. Arthroscopy 2019;35(9): 2648–54.
52. Pioger C, Gousopoulos L, Hopper GP, et al. Clinical Outcomes After Combined ACL and Anterolateral Ligament Reconstruction Versus Isolated ACL Reconstruction With Bone-Patellar Tendon-Bone Grafts: A Matched-Pair Analysis of 2018 Patients From the SANTI Study Group. Am J Sports Med 2022;50(13): 3493–501.
53. Borque KA, Jones M, Laughlin MS, et al. Effect of Lateral Extra-articular Tenodesis on the Rate of Revision Anterior Cruciate Ligament Reconstruction in Elite Athletes. Am J Sports Med 2022;50(13):3487–92.
54. Helito CP, Camargo DB, Sobrado MF, et al. Combined reconstruction of the anterolateral ligament in chronic ACL injuries leads to better clinical outcomes than isolated ACL reconstruction. Knee Surg Sports Traumatol Arthrosc 2018;26(12): 3652–9.
55. Saithna A, Monaco E, Carrozzo A, et al. Anterior Cruciate Ligament Revision Plus Lateral Extra-Articular Procedure Results in Superior Stability and Lower Failure Rates Than Does Isolated Anterior Cruciate Ligament Revision but Shows No Difference in Patient-Reported Outcomes or Return to Sports. Arthroscopy 2023; 39(4):1088–98.
56. Engebretsen L, Lew WD, Lewis JL, et al. The effect of an iliotibial tenodesis on intraarticular graft forces and knee joint motion. Am J Sports Med 1990;18(2): 169–76.
57. Draganich LF, Reider B, Ling M, et al. An in vitro study of an intraarticular and extraarticular reconstruction in the anterior cruciate ligament deficient knee. Am J Sports Med 1990;18(3):262–6.

58. Marom N, Ouanezar H, Jahandar H, et al. Lateral Extra-articular Tenodesis Reduces Anterior Cruciate Ligament Graft Force and Anterior Tibial Translation in Response to Applied Pivoting and Anterior Drawer Loads. Am J Sports Med 2020;48(13):3183–93.
59. Cavaignac E, Mesnier T, Marot V, et al. Effect of Lateral Extra-articular Tenodesis on Anterior Cruciate Ligament Graft Incorporation. Orthop J Sports Med 2020; 8(11). 2325967120960097.
60. Gibbs CM, Hughes JD, Popchak AJ, et al. Anterior cruciate ligament reconstruction with lateral extraarticular tenodesis better restores native knee kinematics in combined ACL and meniscal injury. Knee Surg Sports Traumatol Arthrosc 2022; 30(1):131–8.
61. Inderhaug E, Stephen JM, Williams A, et al. Anterolateral Tenodesis or Anterolateral Ligament Complex Reconstruction: Effect of Flexion Angle at Graft Fixation When Combined With ACL Reconstruction. Am J Sports Med 2017;45(13): 3089–97.
62. Ra HJ, Kim JH, Lee DH. Comparative clinical outcomes of anterolateral ligament reconstruction versus lateral extra-articular tenodesis in combination with anterior cruciate ligament reconstruction: systematic review and meta-analysis. Arch Orthop Trauma Surg 2020;140(7):923–31.
63. Na BR, Kwak WK, Seo HY, et al. Clinical Outcomes of Anterolateral Ligament Reconstruction or Lateral Extra-articular Tenodesis Combined With Primary ACL Reconstruction: A Systematic Review With Meta-analysis. Orthop J Sports Med 2021;9(9). 23259671211023100.
64. Rayes J, Ouanezar H, Haidar IM, et al. Revision Anterior Cruciate Ligament Reconstruction Using Bone-Patellar Tendon-Bone Graft Combined With Modified Lemaire Technique Versus Hamstring Graft Combined With Anterolateral Ligament Reconstruction: A Clinical Comparative Matched Study With a Mean Follow-up of 5 Years From The SANTI Study Group. Am J Sports Med 2022; 50(2):395–403.
65. Castoldi M, Magnussen RA, Gunst S, et al. A Randomized Controlled Trial of Bone-Patellar Tendon-Bone Anterior Cruciate Ligament Reconstruction With and Without Lateral Extra-articular Tenodesis: 19-Year Clinical and Radiological Follow-up. Am J Sports Med 2020;48(7):1665–72.
66. Cohen M, Amaro JT, Ejnisman B, et al. Anterior cruciate ligament reconstruction after 10 to 15 years: association between meniscectomy and osteoarthrosis. Arthroscopy 2007;23(6):629–34.
67. Geeslin AG, Moatshe G, Chahla J, et al. Anterolateral Knee Extra-articular Stabilizers: A Robotic Study Comparing Anterolateral Ligament Reconstruction and Modified Lemaire Lateral Extra-articular Tenodesis. Am J Sports Med 2018; 46(3):607–16.
68. Neri T, Dabirrahmani D, Beach A, et al. Different anterolateral procedures have variable impact on knee kinematics and stability when performed in combination with anterior cruciate ligament reconstruction. J ISAKOS 2021;6(2):74–81.
69. Neri T, Cadman J, Beach A, et al. Lateral tenodesis procedures increase lateral compartment pressures more than anterolateral ligament reconstruction, when performed in combination with ACL reconstruction: a pilot biomechanical study. J ISAKOS 2021;6(2):66–73.
70. O'Brien SJ, Warren RF, Pavlov H, et al. Reconstruction of the chronically insufficient anterior cruciate ligament with the central third of the patellar ligament. J Bone Joint Surg Am 1991;73(2):278–86.

71. Strum GM, Fox JM, Ferkel RD, et al. Intraarticular versus intraarticular and extra-articular reconstruction for chronic anterior cruciate ligament instability. Clin Orthop Relat Res 1989;245:188–98.
72. Cinque ME, Kunze KN, Williams BT, et al. Higher Incidence of Radiographic Posttraumatic Osteoarthritis With Transtibial Femoral Tunnel Positioning Compared With Anteromedial Femoral Tunnel Positioning During Anterior Cruciate Ligament Reconstruction: A Systematic Review and Meta-analysis. Am J Sports Med 2022; 50(1):255–63.
73. Marcacci M, Zaffagnini S, Giordano G, et al. Anterior cruciate ligament reconstruction associated with extra-articular tenodesis: A prospective clinical and radiographic evaluation with 10- to 13-year follow-up. Am J Sports Med 2009; 37(4):707–14.
74. Zaffagnini S, Marcacci M, Lo Presti M, et al. Prospective and randomized evaluation of ACL reconstruction with three techniques: a clinical and radiographic evaluation at 5 years follow-up. Knee Surg Sports Traumatol Arthrosc 2006; 14(11):1060–9.
75. Zaffagnini S, Marcheggiani Muccioli GM, Grassi A, et al. Over-the-top ACL Reconstruction Plus Extra-articular Lateral Tenodesis With Hamstring Tendon Grafts: Prospective Evaluation With 20-Year Minimum Follow-up. Am J Sports Med 2017;45(14):3233–42.
76. Carrozzo A, Monaco E, Saithna A, et al. Clinical Outcomes of Combined Anterior Cruciate Ligament Reconstruction and Lateral Extra-articular Tenodesis Procedures in Skeletally Immature Patients: A Systematic Review From the SANTI Study Group. J Pediatr Orthop 2023;43(1):24–30.
77. Wilson PL, Wyatt CW, Wagner KJ, et al. Combined Transphyseal and Lateral Extra-articular Pediatric Anterior Cruciate Ligament Reconstruction: A Novel Technique to Reduce ACL Reinjury While Allowing for Growth. Am J Sports Med 2019;47(14):3356–64.

Anterior Cruciate Ligament Repair—Here to Stay or History Repeating Itself?

Seth L. Sherman, MD[a,*], Yazdan Raji, MD[a], Jacob G. Calcei, MD[b], Mark F. Sherman, MD[c]

KEYWORDS

- ACL repair • Healing potential • Techniques • Selection criteria • Outcomes • Complications

KEY POINTS

- Primary anterior cruciate ligament (ACL) repair is regaining interest as an alternative treatment option for acute and subacute ACL injuries, aiming to preserve the native ligament and promote biological healing.
- New surgical techniques such as dynamic intraligamentary stabilization, suture tape augmentation, suture anchor repair, and bridge-enhanced ACL repair are showing promising results concerning postoperative stability and function.
- Patient selection is a key step in the preoperative planning stages when considering primary ACL repair.
- Although primary ACL repair techniques show promising early results, further robust research, including longer term follow-up, higher level randomized studies, and comparative analyses against traditional reconstruction methods, is necessary to define its effectiveness as a potential treatment alternative.

INTRODUCTION

Anterior cruciate ligament (ACL) injuries continue to be a prevalent concern among athletes and those with an active lifestyle. The management strategies for ACL injuries have long been debated with current standard practice advocating for ACL reconstruction using various graft options. Historically, the ACL has been deemed to have poor healing capacity, even in the setting of direct primary repair. This has primarily been attributed to the variation in blood supply of the cruciate ligaments relative to

[a] Department of Orthopaedic Surgery, Stanford University School of Medicine, 450 Broadway, MC 6342, Pavilion C, Redwood City, CA 94063, USA; [b] University Hospitals Drusinsky Sports Medicine Institute, Case Western Reserve University School of Medicine, 11100 Euclid Avenue, Hanna House 6th Floor, Cleveland, OH 44106, USA; [c] Richmond University Medical Center, 2052 Richmond Road, Staten Island, NY 10306, USA
* Corresponding author. Department of Orthopaedic Surgery, Stanford University School of Medicine, 450 Broadway, MC 6342, Pavilion C, Redwood City, CA 94063.
E-mail address: shermans@stanford.edu

Clin Sports Med 43 (2024) 433–448
https://doi.org/10.1016/j.csm.2023.09.001
sportsmed.theclinics.com

the collateral ligaments as well as the exposure to synovial fluid in the intra-articular space.[1–3] However, there has been a resurgence of interest in ACL repair techniques as potential treatment alternatives in recent years.

HISTORICAL PERSPECTIVE ON ANTERIOR CRUCIATE LIGAMENT REPAIR

Historical primary ACL repair techniques included surgery within the first week after injury using 4 nonabsorbable U-sutures in the ligament stump pulled through 2 drill holes in the femur and tibia as described by the Palmer technique in 1938.[4] Primary ACL repair was initially introduced for acute ACL injuries in a military cohort by Feagin and colleagues.[5] Although the study presented notable diagnostic findings of acute ACL injuries, their results of the primary ACL repair were less convincing with 17 of 32 patients sustaining significant reinjury after this procedure at 5-year follow-up.[5] Similarly, Engebresten and colleagues reported a 25% failure rate after primary ACL repair in a study with a mean 6-year follow-up.[6] Additional literature continued to demonstrate poor outcomes following primary ACL repair with ACL retears ranging from 30% to 50%.[7–9] However, Sherman and colleagues presented promising results in their study on primary ACL repair using the Marshall multiple suture technique, particularly within a subset of older patients with proximal ACL avulsions, skiers, concomitant low-grade medial collateral ligament tear, as well as those without ligamentous laxity.[10] This subgroup has laid the groundwork for the resurgence of interest in primary ACL techniques. These findings also led to the development of Sherman Classification System, which describes ACL tears based on location of the tear: type I (ACL soft tissue avulsion off the femoral insertion); type II (tear through the substance of the upper one-third of the ACL); type III (midsubstance tear); and type IV (distal tear).[10]

POTENTIAL ADVANTAGES OF PRIMARY ANTERIOR CRUCIATE LIGAMENT REPAIR

When performed successfully, ACL repairs can take advantage of maintaining the intrinsic proprioceptive fibers of the ACL, which provide spatial feedback and dynamic stability.[11,12] Karpeli and colleagues highlights the influence of ACL deficiency on neuromuscular control of the knee, affecting central processing and efferent motor signaling as evidenced by functional MRI, suggesting that this injury extends beyond a musculoskeletal concern.[13] Previous studies have indicated that the injured ACL stump retains physiologically normal mechanoreceptors for approximately 3 months postinjury.[14–17] Additionally, in a study assessing functional outcomes and proprioception following ACL reconstruction based on extent of the remnant tibial stump, Lee and colleagues demonstrated significant improvement in proprioception in the group with greater than 20% remnant ACL stump as compared with the group with less than 20% remnant ACL.[18] Such findings support the rationale for primary repair to preserve native proprioception following injury and surgery.

Furthermore, arthroscopic primary ACL repair is less invasive as compared with ACL reconstruction, which requires graft harvest and larger intraosseous tunnels. Arthrofibrosis is a common complication following ACL reconstruction with an incidence between 4% and 38%.[19,20] A retrospective case-control study by van der List and colleagues compared postoperative range of motion (ROM) following primary repair and reconstruction techniques. The study demonstrated significantly higher ROM in the primary repair group at 1 week and 1 month postoperatively without any changes in the complication profile as compared with the ACL reconstruction group.[21] The adoption of ACL repair in appropriately selected patients may allow for an expedited rehabilitation protocol and ultimately earlier return to sport. However, these latter points require higher levels of evidence from prospective comparative studies and longer term follow-up before making these conclusions.

It is obvious that primary ACL repair does not have graft site morbidity as seen in ACL reconstruction.[22] Specifically, autograft harvesting is associated with cutaneous hypoesthesia related to the infrapatellar branches of the saphenous nerve, unesthetic scars, and notably anterior knee pain, which is seen more commonly in bone-patellar tendon-bone (BPTB) and quadriceps tendon autografts. BPTB autograft has been linked with patellar tendon shortening and subsequent patella baja, leading anterior knee pain with kneeling and increased incidence of patellofemoral pathologic condition, namely osteoarthritis (OA).[23,24] These issues can be avoided with ACL primary repair.

Finally, the radiographic prevalence of OA after ACL reconstruction has been reported to range between 10% and 90%.[25,26] Barenius and colleagues observed that medial compartment OA was seen most frequently, with a 3-fold increased prevalence of OA after an ACL reconstruction as opposed to contralateral healthy knees.[27] Li and colleagues reported on predictors of radiographic knee OA after ACL reconstruction, and noted earlier medial meniscectomy, grade 2 or greater medial chondrosis, length of follow-up, and body mass index were the best predictors of OA following ACL reconstruction.[28] Although the evidence is not yet clear on whether primary ACL repair will reduce the long-term risk of OA progression versus surgical reconstruction, this is an area of active research and of critical importance.

CURRENT TECHNIQUES

Dynamic Intraligamentary Stabilization

The dynamic intraligamentary stabilization (DIS) device was developed to stabilize the knee during the self-healing period by preventing sagittal plane translation. Kohl and colleagues assessed the efficacy of the DIS technique in a sheep animal model using imaging, biomechanical, and histologic evaluations at 3 months postoperatively.[29] The technique involved marrow stimulation at the femoral footprint, creation of anteromedial tibial and posterolateral femoral notch osseous tunnels, insertion of the threaded sleeve on the tibial side, and passage of the braided wire through the joint and secured to the femur using suspensory fixation.[29] At the end point of the study, all repairs were well defined with ligament continuity on MRI, and histologic analysis indicating scar formation at the ends of the transected ligament with hypercellularity and neovascularization.[29] Kohl and colleagues subsequently performed this technique on human cadaveric knees comparing sagittal plane stability relative to that of the intact ACL, ruptured ACL, and primary ACL repair. The study demonstrated mean laxity values improved for DIS at initial stabilization and following 50 motion cycles, with values lower than that of the intact ligament.[30] Haberli and colleagues also set out to assess the biomechanical stability of human cadaveric ACL repairs using the DIS technique in a dynamic loading scenario.[31] Their findings showed that the anteroposterior (AP) translation of the knee at different flexion angles (0°, 30°, 60°, and 90°) did not significantly differ between the precyclical and postcyclical loading test time points, indicating comparable biomechanical stability after the repair.[31] Similarly, Schliemann and colleagues demonstrated that ACL repair using DIS showed no difference in anterior translation in knees with either 60 N or 80 N of preload as compared with ACL-intact knees.[32] Eggli and colleagues then applied the DIS technique to a series of 10 physically active patients with an ACL rupture, in which the procedure was performed within a median of 9.9 days and allowed to return to sport at 5 months postoperatively.[33] Overall, there was only 1 rerupture at 5 months postoperatively with the remaining 9 patients demonstrating excellent median Lysholm, International Knee Documentation Committee (IKDC), Tegner and satisfaction scores as well as acceptable sagittal plane translation.[33] The results of this study was later corroborated by Henle and colleagues in a separate case series of 278 patients undergoing primary ACL repair using the DIS technique and continued to demonstrate excellent 12-month postoperative Lysholm, IKDC, Tegner, and satisfaction scores as well as AP translation.[34] Other retrospective clinical studies involving primary ACL with DIS device have noted similar improvement in patient-reported outcomes, satisfaction rates, and AP translation at 1-year follow-up with a 6.5% rerupture rate and an 18% reoperation rate.[35,36] Most importantly, one study reports a 60% hardware removal of the tibial screw.[36] Finally, in a prospective study of patients undergoing DIS following acute ACL injuries, Krismer and colleagues reported a 9.5% rerupture rate, identifying negative predictive factors of pursuing competitive sporting activities with a Tegner preinjury score greater than 7 and midsubstance ACL rupture location.[37] Notably, the authors remarked that the ACL rerupture rate decreased to 3.9% when those risk factors were absent.[37]

Suture Tape Augmentation

Independent suture tape reinforcement (ISTR) is an ACL repair technique that involves introduction of a bridging intra-articular ultra-high-strength suture tape. This suture tape is suspensory femoral fixation, knotless bone anchor fixation to the proximal tibia, and a looped wire to maintain the position of the distal ACL stump at its femoral footprint.[38,39] This technique is generally indicated for acute proximal ACL avulsions that are nonretracted and deemed to have acceptable quality based on clinical evaluation.[38,39] Heusdens and colleagues reported the first case series of proximal ACL rupture treated with the ISTR technique with 2-year follow-up. In this study of 42 consecutive patients, all Knee Injury and Osteoarthritis Outcome Score (KOOS) subscales and Visual Analogue Scale (VAS) scores improved significantly relative to preoperative scores with the largest improvement at 3 months postoperatively.[40] There was a reduction in the Marx activity level at 2-year follow-up with an overall 4.8% rerupture rate.[40] Similarly, McKay and colleagues reported significant improvements in all KOOS and Western Ontario and McMaster osteoarthritis index scores postoperatively in their case series of 68 patients, with the majority of the improvements being observed at 3 months postoperatively[41] There were 4 reported reoperations with only 1 associated with a rerupture.[41] Overall, the initial findings from clinical studies evaluating the ISTR technique suggest its potential relevance as a treatment option for acute proximal ACL ruptures; however, future randomized studies are needed in order to directly compare with standard ACL reconstruction options.

Suture Anchor Primary Anterior Cruciate Ligament Repair

Previous discussions have focused on the various repair options available for proximal ACL ruptures. DiFelice and colleagues described a proximal tear repair technique with passage of a running, locking No. 2 TigerWire (Arthrex) in the anteromedial bundle distal stump and a similar No. 2 FiberWire (Arthrex) in the posterolateral bundle.[42] The limbs from each suture are subsequently passed through two 4.75-mm Bio-Composite SwiveLock suture anchors (Arthrex) and inserted into the footprint of each respective ACL bundle.[42] In this cohort of 11 consecutive patients, 10 out of 11 patients reported good subjective and objective outcomes including Lysholm, Tegner activity, and IKDC scores at a minimum 2-year follow-up.[42] In a biomechanical study, van der List and colleagues assessed the postoperative gap formation and maximum failure load following primary ACL repair with suture button fixation or suture anchor fixation.[43] Gap formation was approximately 1 mm after 100 cycles with an overall maximum failure load of 243 N and no significant difference between fixation methods.[43] Then using a similar technique in a clinical study, van der List and colleagues compared postoperative ROM and complications of proximal ACL avulsion tear repair using suture anchors and standard ACL reconstruction techniques, and showed higher ROM with the repair group at 1-week and 1-month postoperatively with a trend toward few complications as compared with reconstruction group.[21] Vermeijden and colleagues and Jonkergouw and colleagues published similar results in larger retrospective case series for primary repair of proximal ACL tears using suture anchor fixation with notable improvements in IKDC, Lysholm, modified Cincinnati, and Tegner activity scores at a minimum 2-year follow-up.[44,45] Notably, Jonkergouw and colleagues identified patient age less than 21 years as a risk factor for failure (37.0%) as compared with 22 to 35 years and greater than 35 years age groups (4.2% and 3.2%, both $P < .005$).[45] In another retrospective clinical study, Hoffman and colleagues investigated the long-term outcomes of ACL suture anchor repair of acute proximal femoral avulsion tears, showing a mean Lysholm score of 85.3, modified Cincinnati score of 83.8, and IKDC score of 87.3 and a retear rate of 8.3%, consistent with previous literature.[46] Additionally, Liao assessed the effectiveness of primary arthroscopic repair using the suture anchor pulley technique for partial proximal ACL tears, with a mean Lysholm score of 91.5 and a mean IKDC Subjective score of 88.1 suggesting that this technique is an effective treatment option.[47] Finally, DeFelice and colleagues assessed the midterm clinical outcomes of a previous cohort of primary ACL repair using the suture anchor technique at a minimum of 5-year follow-up, and reported excellent postoperative mean Lysholm, modified Cincinnati, Tegner, and IKDC subjective scores with a 9% failure rate, which took place at 3 months postoperatively.[48] The collective outcomes of primary suture anchor fixation of proximal avulsion tears have been encouraging in this carefully selected subset of patients with excellent tissue quality but long-term, prospective, comparative studies are essential to determine its role and indication in the broader scope of procedures.

Bridge-Enhanced Anterior Cruciate Ligament Repair

Bridge-Enhanced ACL repair (BEAR) involves suture repair of acute ACL ruptures that is supplemented with a biological extracellular matrix (ECM) scaffold between the torn ligament stumps to stimulate fibrovascular scar formation.[49,50] The scaffold is manufactured from bovine tissue and processed into a slurry of ECM proteins, predominately composed of collagen.[51] In a histologic porcine model, Proffen and colleagues set out to determine features that correlated with mechanical properties of healing ACL with reconstruction and Bioenhanced repair techniques.[52] The results demonstrated cellular organization subscore, yield load, maximum load, and linear stiffness were predictive of ACL healing in Bioehanced technique at 6 months postoperatively, whereas collagen subscore was predictive at 12 months postrepair.[52] In preclinical animal studies, Bridge-Enhanced Repair technique had shown similar mechanical properties to ACL reconstruction grafts with less posttraumatic arthritis.[53] In a prospective randomized clinical trial, Murray and colleagues set out to assess the noninferiority of BEAR in terms of functional outcomes and AP laxity as compared with traditional ACL reconstruction techniques.[54] At 2-year follow-up, BEAR was found to meet noninferiority criteria for IKDC and side-to-side AP laxity when compared with ACL reconstruction.[54] There was no significant difference in ACL reinjury between the groups, although the study was only powered to detect differences in the IKDC Subjective Score.[54] Collectively, these studies have demonstrated promising results for BEAR and suggest prospective, long-term studies are warranted for this technique.

CURRENT SYSTEMATIC REVIEWS AND META-ANALYSES

There are numerous compilation studies in this field to provide valuable insights into the efficacy and outcomes of ACL primary repair (**Table 1**). A systematic review by Cao and colleagues highlights that biological enhancement methods lead to decreased sagittal translation and improved patient-reported outcomes when compared with the ACL repair group alone, hence showing promise as a viable option for arthroscopic primary repair.[55] Internal brace augmentation, as demonstrated in the systematic review by Wilson and colleagues also presents encouraging results with improved KOOS, Lysholm, and IKDC scores as well as satisfactory AP laxity (mean side-to-side difference of 1.2 mm).[56] Li conducted a meta-analysis showing ACL repair had comparable outcomes to reconstruction in select patients in regards to Tegner, Lysholm, Lachman, and KT-1000 testing.[57] Vermeijden and colleagues also conducted a proportion meta-analysis of 13 studies with 418 patients that underwent primary repair of proximal ACL tears using suture augmentation, and showed an overall failure rate of 8% with good to excellent functional outcomes.[58] In a systematic review and meta-analysis of recent studies, van der List and colleagues assessed the effectiveness of various ACL repair techniques and showed that while primary repair with dynamic augmentation led to more reoperations relative to other repair techniques, there were no differences in patient-reported outcomes among the groups.[59] Houck and colleagues and Papalia and colleagues also examined the clinical outcomes of primary arthroscopic ACL repair in their respective systematic reviews, and report improvement in postoperative outcomes.[60,61] However, the authors comment that the data is inconsistent and should be interpreted with caution.[60,61] Nwachukwu and colleagues conducted an updated systematic review, which again indicated improvements in the postoperative patient-reported outcomes following primary ACL repair; however, the findings also noted that proximal ruptures treated with repairs had a revision rate of 12.9% and an overall total reoperation of 18.2%.[62] Conversely, van Eck and colleagues suggests that internal bracing and repair of proximal ACL tears show better healing potential relative to distal or midsubstance tears but further research is needed.[63] Finally, although there is significant focus on the development of surgical techniques for ACL treatment alternatives, there is currently a paucity of high-level evidence for postoperative ACL repair rehabilitation protocol as evidenced by Hourston and colleagues[64] and can be an area of further investigation for future studies. Overall, these studies provide valuable insights into the evolving landscape of ACL primary repair and highlight the importance of patient selection, rehabilitation, and continued research to optimize outcomes.

REPAIR VERSUS RECONSTRUCTION COMPARATIVE ANALYSIS

Several studies have contributed to the ongoing debate regarding the choice between ACL repair and reconstruction (**Table 2**). Hoogeslag and colleagues conducted a randomized controlled clinical trial comparing repair using dynamic augmented suture repair technique and single bundle hamstring autograft reconstruction and reported 2-year follow-up clinical results.[65] They found that ACL repair resulted in similar subjective and objective outcomes compared with reconstruction with no significant difference in IKDC subjective score and similar ipsilateral ACL failure, suggesting that repair can be a viable option.[65] A 5-year follow-up study was performed by the same study group, which illustrated similar IKDC Subjective Score and ipsilateral ACL failure between the 2 cohorts, suggesting that repair can be a viable option.[66] Similarly, Murray and colleagues conducted a prospective randomized clinical trial comparing bridge-enhanced ACL repair to hamstring autograft reconstruction and

Table 1
Detailed list of systematic reviews of primary anterior cruciate ligament repair

Reference	Title	Journal	Level of Evidence	Main Conclusion
Cao et al,[55] 2022	Biological enhancement methods may be a viable option for ACL arthroscopic primary repair - A systematic review	Orthopedics & Traumatology, Surgery & Research	III	Biological-enhanced ACL repair may be a superior option to ACL primary repair alone
Wilson et al,[56] 2022	Anterior cruciate ligament repair with internal brace augmentation: A systematic review	The Knee	III	ACL repair with internal brace augmentation shows promising results
Li,[57] 2022	Efficacy of Repair for ACL Injury: A Meta analysis of Randomized Controlled Trials	International Journal of Sports Medicine	II	ACL repair shows comparable outcomes to reconstruction for select patients
Vermeijden et al,[58] 2022	Primary repair with suture augmentation for proximal anterior cruciate ligament tears: A systematic review with meta-analysis	The Knee	III	Primary repair with suture augmentation may be a valuable treatment option for proximal ACL tears
Hourston et al,[64] 2022	A systematic review of anterior cruciate ligament primary repair rehabilitation	Journal of Clinical Orthopedics and Trauma	III	Rehabilitation after ACL primary repair is an important aspect of patient management in of further investigation
van der List et al,[59] 2020	Arthroscopic primary repair of proximal anterior cruciate ligament tears seems safe but higher level of evidence is needed: a systematic review and meta-analysis of recent literature	Knee Surgery, Sports Traumatology, Arthroscopy	III	Arthroscopic primary repair of proximal ACL tears seems safe but higher level evidence is needed
Houck et al,[60] 2019	Primary Arthroscopic Repair of the Anterior Cruciate Ligament: A Systematic Review of Clinical Outcomes	Arthroscopy	III	Primary arthroscopic ACL repair can lead to good clinical outcomes for select patients
Papalia et al,[61] 2019	Arthroscopic primary repair of the anterior cruciate ligament in adults: a systematic review	British Medical Bulletin	III	Arthroscopic primary repair of the ACL can provide satisfactory results in the short term to midterm

(*continued on next page*)

Table 1
(continued)

Reference	Title	Journal	Level of Evidence	Main Conclusion
Nwachukwu et al,[62] 2019	Anterior Cruciate Ligament Repair Outcomes: An Updated Systematic Review of Recent Literature	Arthroscopy	III	ACL repair outcomes have improved but reconstruction remains the standard treatment
van Eck et al,[63] 2018	Is There a Role for Internal Bracing and Repair of the Anterior Cruciate Ligament? A Systematic Literature Review	American Journal of Sports Medicine	III	Internal bracing and repair of the ACL may have a role in select patients but further research is needed

Table 2
Detailed list of prospective studies on primary anterior cruciate ligament repair

Reference	Title	Journal	Study Design	Level of Evidence	Inclusion Criteria	Exclusion Criteria	Primary Outcome Results
Hoogeslag et al,[66] 2022	Acute Anterior Cruciate Ligament Rupture: Repair or Reconstruction? Five-Year Results of a Randomized Controlled Clinical Trial	American Journal of Sports Medicine	Randomized Controlled Clinical trial	Level I	Acute ACL rupture, age 18–50 y, physically active, no previous ACL injury or surgery	Multiligament injury, revision surgery, meniscus repair	IKDC Subjective Score: Repair 90.2 vs Recon 96.6 ($P = .571$) Ipsilateral failure: Repair 20.8% vs Recon 27.2% ($P = .731$)
Murray et al,[54] 2020	Bridge-Enhanced Anterior Cruciate Ligament Repair Is Not Inferior to Autograft Anterior Cruciate Ligament Reconstruction at 2 y: Results of a Prospective Randomized Clinical Trial	The American Journal of Sports Medicine	Prospective randomized clinical trial	Level I	Acute ACL tear, age 15–50 y, physically active	Previous ACL injury or surgery, meniscus deficiency requiring repair	IKDC Subjective Score: Repair 88.9 vs Recon 84.8 ($P = .15$) AP Knee Laxity: Repair 1.61 mm vs Recon 1.77 mm ($P = .82$) Ipsilateral ACL Surgery: Repair 14.1% vs Recon 5.7% ($P = .32$)
Kösters et al,[67] 2020	Repair With Dynamic Intraligamentary Stabilization vs Primary Reconstruction of Acute Anterior Cruciate Ligament Tears: 2-y Results From a Prospective Randomized Study	American Journal of Sports Medicine	Prospective randomized study	Level II	Acute ACL tear, age 18–50 y, physically active	Previous ACL injury or surgery, meniscus deficiency requiring repair	IKDC Subjective Score ($P = .3783$) Tegner Score ($P = .8815$) Lysholm Score ($P = .1459$) Anterior Tibial Translation: Repair 1.9 mm vs Recon 0.9 mm ($P = .0086$) Ipsilateral ACL Failure: Repair 16.3% vs Recon 12.5% ($P = .432$)

(*continued on next page*)

Table 2
(continued)

Reference	Title	Journal	Study Design	Level of Evidence	Inclusion Criteria	Exclusion Criteria	Primary Outcome Results
Hoogeslag et al,[65] 2019	Acute Anterior Cruciate Ligament Rupture: Repair or Reconstruction? Two-Year Results of a Randomized Controlled Clinical Trial	American Journal of Sports Medicine	Randomized controlled clinical trial	Level I	Acute ACL rupture, age 18–50 y, physically active, no previous ACL injury or surgery	Multi-ligament injury, revision surgery, meniscus repair	IKDC Subjective Score: Repair 95.4 vs Recon 94.3 (*P* = .902) Ipsilateral failure: Repair 8.7% vs Recon 19.0% (*P* = .663)
Sporsheim et al,[68] 2019	Autologous BPTB ACL Reconstruction Results in Lower Failure Rates Than ACL Repair with and without Synthetic Augmentation at 30 y of Follow-up: A Prospective Randomized Study	Journal of Bone and Joint Surgery - American Volume	Prospective randomized study	Level II	Acute ACL tear, age 16–45 y	Previous ACL injury or surgery, meniscus deficiency requiring repair	No difference in Tegner and Lysholm Score Knee Laxity: Lachman (*P* = .79) Pivot shift (*P* = .46) ACL Revision Surgery: Repair 12 vs Recon 1 (*P* = .002)

demonstrated no significant differences in IKDC Subjective Score, knee AP laxity, and subsequent ipsilateral ACL surgery at 2 years, supporting the effectiveness of repair.[54] In contrast, Kösters and colleagues compared repair with DIS to primary reconstruction.[67] They reported superior functional stability in the form of anterior tibial translation (Repair 1.9 mm vs Reconstruction 0.9 mm; $P = .0086$) in the reconstruction group, although patient-reported outcomes were not significantly different between the 2 groups at the 2-year follow-up.[67] Furthermore, Sporsheim and colleagues conducted a long-term follow-up study and found that autologous BPTB ACL reconstruction had lower failure rates compared with ACL repair with or without synthetic augmentation after 30 years.[68] These findings demonstrate the complexity of the decision-making process, with repair showing promise in some studies but reconstruction appearing more favorable in others. Further research is warranted to determine the patient selection criteria in order to optimize outcomes for ACL injury treatment strategies.

PATIENT SELECTION

Proper patient selection is important for success when considering primary ACL repair. Certain factors have been shown to influence the success rate in primary ACL repair in comparison to reconstruction. Specifically, van der List and colleagues reported the positive predictive factors for repairable tears including age greater than 35 years, surgery within 28 days of injury, body mass index less than 26, absence of a lateral meniscus tear, and proximal tear of ACL near the femoral attachment.[69,70]

Conversely, there are specific factors that may negatively affect the success rate of primary ACL repair. One important factor is a more active patient with a Tegner preinjury score greater than 7.[37] The location of the tear is also critical with worse outcomes in patients with a midsubstance ACL tear location and those with damage to the ACL bundles and synovial sheath.[37,71] Finally, younger patients are a negative predictive factor for success in ACL repair.[71] There is emerging evidence suggesting that increased tibial slope may also be a risk factor for failure of primary ACL repair. Further research establishing the patient-specific factors that identify who is best indicated for primary ACL repair will be imperative to the potential success and more widespread adoption of the procedure.

EMERGING TECHNOLOGIES

Techniques and implants continue to evolve as ACL repair is revisited as a plausible option for certain patients with ACL tears. Advancements in suture material, including high-strength tape sutures, collagen-coated sutures, and other suture materials in development such as sutures made of pure woven collagen have and will likely continue to improve the biology and biomechanical potential in ACL repair. Additionally, fixation and augmentation options continue to develop and evolve to maximize the healing potential and strength of ACL repair in order to expand the indications and decrease the negative predictive factors in ACL repair. The obvious benefit of ACL repair is that the patients are able to maintain their own anatomy while avoiding the need to borrow from another area to create a new ACL. Although ACL repair continues to evolve, the biologic augmentation has been introduced to promote the generation of healthy repair tissue. In a small case series, Gobbi and colleagues assessed the effects of a biologic gel consisting of activated platelet-rich plasma and bone marrow aspirate concentrate on preinjury, preoperative and postoperative outcome scores in those undergoing primary ACL repair.[72] The study illustrated good-to-excellent long-term outcomes; however, the rate of secondary ACL insufficiency of

27% was rather alarming. This finding coupled with a lack of a true control group prohibits the assessment of the clinical impact of this augmentation.[72] Nevertheless, the available evidence in this area remains limited, warranting further investigation and research.

SUMMARY

ACL surgery is one of the few remaining procedures in orthopedics where we often have to borrow from one part of the body to give to another. Nonetheless, emerging techniques and technologies surrounding primary ACL repair demonstrate potential for a major change in sports medicine and the treatment of ACL injuries. Primary ACL repairs in acute and subacute settings has shown promising results in older patients with proximal ACL avulsions, skiers, concomitant low-grade medial collateral ligament tear, as well as those without ligamentous laxity. However, further studies are required to procure higher quality long-term evidence. Such investigations should encompass objective testing for rotational stability, radiographic assessment of OA risk, and return to sport safety and efficacy. Finally, head-to-head prospective studies of BEAR and other repairs techniques against the widely used BPTB autograft ACL reconstruction are necessary to ensure their comparative effectiveness. Fortunately, this study is ongoing at present.

CLINICS CARE POINTS

- Patient selection criteria for primary ACL repairs include the following: age > 35 years, surgery within 28 days of injury, a body mass index lower than 26, the absence of a lateral meniscus tear, and a proximal tear of the ACL near the femoral attachment.
- Gap formation and overall maximum failure loads are similar between suture button and suture anchor fixation for primary ACL repair.
- The effects of biologic augmentation in ACL repair has been encouraging in the small case series; however, mid- to long-term comparative studies are necessary to assess the clinical impact of this practice.

DISCLOSURE

The authors have nothing to disclose.

REFERENCES

1. Jack A, Holmes R. Effects of Synovial Fluid on Fibroblasts in Tissue Culture. Clin Orthop Relat Res 1979;138:279–83. Available at: https://journals.lww.com/corr/citation/1979/01000/effects_of_synovial_fluid_on_fibroblasts_in_tissue.40.aspx. Accessed May 21, 2023.
2. Johnson RJ, Beynnon BD, Nichols CE, Renstrom PA. The treatment of injuries of the anterior cruciate ligament. J Bone Joint Surg Am 1992;74(1):140–51.
3. Woo SLY, Vorgin TM, Abramowitch SD. Healing and Repair of Ligament Injuries in the Knee. JAAOS 2000;8(6):364–72. http://journals.lww.com/jaaos.
4. Palmer I. On the injuries to the ligaments of the knee joint. Acta Chir Scand 1938; Suppl(53).
5. Feagin JA, Curl WW. Isolated tear of the anterior cruciate ligament: 5-year follow-up study. Am J Sports Med 1976;4(3):95–100.

6. Engebretsen L, Benum P, Sundalsvoll S. Primary suture of the anterior cruciate ligament a 6-year follow-up of 74 cases. Acta Orthop 1989;60(5):561–4.
7. Odensten M, Lysholm J, Gillquist J. Suture of fresh ruptures of the anterior cruciate ligament: A 5-year follow-up. Acta Orthop Scand 2009;55(3):270–2.
8. Sherman MF, Bonamo JR. Primary repair of the anterior cruciate ligament. Clin Sports Med 1988;7(4):739–50.
9. Strand T, Engesaeter LB, Mølster AO, et al. Knee function following suture of fresh tear of the anterior cruciate ligament. Acta Orthop Scand 2009;55(2):181–4.
10. Sherman MF, Lieber L, Bonamo JR, et al. The long-term followup of primary anterior cruciate ligament repair defining a rationale for augmentation*. Am J Sports Med 1991;19(3):243–55.
11. Barret DS. Proprioception and function after anterior cruciate reconstruction. Journal of Bone and Joint Surgery - Series B 1991;73(5):833–7.
12. Dhillon MS, Bali K, Prabhakar S. Differences among mechanoreceptors in healthy and injured anterior cruciate ligaments and their clinical importance. Muscles Ligaments Tendons J 2012;2(1):38. Available at: http://pmc/articles/PMC3666492/. Accessed May 24, 2023.
13. Kapreli E, Athanasopoulos S, Gliatis J, et al. Anterior cruciate ligament deficiency causes brain plasticity: A functional MRI study. Am J Sports Med 2009;37(12):2419–26.
14. Denti M, Monteleone M, Berardi A, et al. Anterior Cruciate Ligament Mechanoreceptors: Histologic Studies on Lesions and Reconstruction. Clin Orthop Relat Res 1994;308:29–32.
15. Dhillon MS, Bali K, Vasistha RK. Immunohistological evaluation of proprioceptive potential of the residual stump of injured anterior cruciate ligaments (ACL). Int Orthop 2010;34(5):737–41.
16. Georgoulis AD, Pappa L, Moebius U, et al. The presence of proprioceptive mechanoreceptors in the remnants of the ruptured ACL as a possible source of re-innervation of the ACL autograft. Knee Surg Sports Traumatol Arthrosc 2001;9(6):364–8.
17. Ochi M, Iwasa J, Uchio Y, et al. The regeneration of sensory neurones in the reconstruction of the anterior cruciate ligament. J Bone Joint Surg Br 1999;81(5):902–6.
18. Lee BI, Kwon SW, Kim JB, et al. Comparison of Clinical Results According to Amount of Preserved Remnant in Arthroscopic Anterior Cruciate Ligament Reconstruction Using Quadrupled Hamstring Graft. Arthroscopy 2008;24(5):560–8.
19. Ekhtiari S, Horner NS, de Sa D, et al. Arthrofibrosis after ACL reconstruction is best treated in a step-wise approach with early recognition and intervention: a systematic review. Knee Surg Sports Traumatol Arthrosc 2017;25(12):3929–37.
20. Mayr HO, Weig TG, Plitz W. Arthrofibrosis following ACL reconstruction - Reasons and outcome. Arch Orthop Trauma Surg 2004;124(8):518–22.
21. van der List JP, DiFelice GS. Range of motion and complications following primary repair versus reconstruction of the anterior cruciate ligament. Knee 2017;24(4):798–807.
22. Busam ML, Provencher MT, Bach BR. Complications of anterior cruciate ligament reconstruction with bone-patellar tendon-bone constructs: Care and prevention. Am J Sports Med 2008;36(2):379–94.
23. Jarvela T, Paakkala T, Kannus P, et al. The Incidence of Patellofemoral Osteoarthritis and Associated Findings 7 Years After Anterior Cruciate Ligament

Reconstruction with a Bone-Patellar Tendon-Bone Autograft. Am J Sports Med 2001;29(1):18–24.
24. Muellner T, Kaltenbrunner W, Nikolic A, et al. Shortening of the Patellar Tendon After Anterior Cruciate Ligament Reconstruction. Arthrosc J Arthrosc Relat Surg 1998;14(6):592–6.
25. Kessler MA, Behrend H, Henz S, et al. Function, osteoarthritis and activity after ACL-rupture: 11 Years follow-up results of conservative versus reconstructive treatment. Knee Surg Sports Traumatol Arthrosc 2008;16(5):442–8.
26. Lohmander LS, Östenberg A, Englund M, et al. High prevalence of knee osteoarthritis, pain, and functional limitations in female soccer players twelve years after anterior cruciate ligament injury. Arthritis Rheum 2004;50(10):3145–52.
27. Barenius B, Ponzer S, Shalabi A, et al. Increased risk of osteoarthritis after anterior cruciate ligament reconstruction: A 14-year follow-up study of a randomized controlled trial. Am J Sports Med 2014;42(5):1049–57.
28. Li RT, Lorenz S, Xu Y, et al. Predictors of radiographic knee osteoarthritis after anterior cruciate ligament reconstruction. Am J Sports Med 2011;39(12):2595–603.
29. Kohl S, Evangelopoulos DS, Kohlhof H, et al. Anterior crucial ligament rupture: Self-healing through dynamic intraligamentary stabilization technique. Knee Surg Sports Traumatol Arthrosc 2013;21(3):599–605.
30. Kohl S, Evangelopoulos DS, Ahmad SS, et al. A novel technique, dynamic intraligamentary stabilization creates optimal conditions for primary ACL healing: A preliminary biomechanical study. Knee 2014;21(2):477–80.
31. Häberli J, Henle P, Acklin YP, et al. Knee joint kinematics with dynamic augmentation of primary anterior cruciate ligament repair - a biomechanical study. J Exp Orthop 2016;3(1):1–7.
32. Schliemann B, Lenschow S, Domnick C, et al. Knee joint kinematics after dynamic intraligamentary stabilization: cadaveric study on a novel anterior cruciate ligament repair technique. Knee Surg Sports Traumatol Arthrosc 2017;25(4): 1184–90.
33. Eggli S, Kohlhof H, Zumstein M, et al. Dynamic intraligamentary stabilization: novel technique for preserving the ruptured ACL. Knee Surg Sports Traumatol Arthrosc 2015;23(4):1215–21.
34. Henle P, Röder C, Perler G, et al. Dynamic Intraligamentary Stabilization (DIS) for treatment of acute anterior cruciate ligament ruptures: Case series experience of the first three years. BMC Muscoskel Disord 2015;16(1). https://doi.org/10.1186/s12891-015-0484-7.
35. Büchler L, Regli D, Evangelopoulos DS, et al. Functional recovery following primary ACL repair with dynamic intraligamentary stabilization. Knee 2016;23(3): 549–53.
36. Kohl S, Evangelopoulos DS, Schär MO, et al. Dynamic intraligamentary stabilisation: INITIAL EXPERIENCE WITH TREATMENT OF ACUTE ACL RUPTURES. Bone and Joint Journal 2016;98-B(6):793–8.
37. Krismer AM, Gousopoulos L, Kohl S, et al. Factors influencing the success of anterior cruciate ligament repair with dynamic intraligamentary stabilisation. Knee Surg Sports Traumatol Arthrosc 2017;25(12):3923–8.
38. Heitmann M, Dratzidis A, Jagodzinski M, et al. “Ligament bracing” - die augmentierte Kreuzbandnaht: Biomechanische Grundlagen für ein neues Behandlungskonzept. Unfallchirurg 2014;117(7):650–7.
39. Heusdens CHW, Hopper GP, Dossche L, et al. Anterior Cruciate Ligament Repair Using Independent Suture Tape Reinforcement. Arthrosc Tech 2018;7(7): e747–53.

40. Heusdens CHW, Hopper GP, Dossche L, et al. Anterior cruciate ligament repair with Independent Suture Tape Reinforcement: a case series with 2-year follow-up. Knee Surg Sports Traumatol Arthrosc 2019;27(1):60–7.
41. MacKay G, Anthony IC, Jenkins PJ, et al. Anterior Cruciate Ligament Repair Revisited Preliminary Results of Primary Repair with Internal Brace Ligament Augmentation: A Case Series. Orthop Muscular Syst 2015;04(02). https://doi.org/10.4172/2161-0533.1000188.
42. DiFelice GS, Villegas C, Taylor S. Anterior Cruciate Ligament Preservation: Early Results of a Novel Arthroscopic Technique for Suture Anchor Primary Anterior Cruciate Ligament Repair. Arthroscopy 2015;31(11):2162–71.
43. van der List JP, DiFelice GS. Gap formation following primary repair of the anterior cruciate ligament: A biomechanical evaluation. Knee 2017;24(2):243–9.
44. Jonkergouw A, van der List JP, DiFelice GS. Arthroscopic primary repair of proximal anterior cruciate ligament tears: outcomes of the first 56 consecutive patients and the role of additional internal bracing. Knee Surg Sports Traumatol Arthrosc 2019;27(1):21–8.
45. Vermeijden HD, Yang XA, van der List JP, et al. Role of Age on Success of Arthroscopic Primary Repair of Proximal Anterior Cruciate Ligament Tears. Arthroscopy 2021;37(4):1194–201.
46. Hoffmann C, Friederichs J, von Rüden C, et al. Primary single suture anchor re-fixation of anterior cruciate ligament proximal avulsion tears leads to good functional mid-term results: A preliminary study in 12 patients. J Orthop Surg Res 2017;12(1):1–7.
47. Liao W, Zhang Q. Is Primary Arthroscopic Repair Using the Pulley Technique an Effective Treatment for Partial Proximal ACL Tears? Clin Orthop Relat Res 2020; 478(5):1031.
48. DiFelice GS, van der List JP. Clinical Outcomes of Arthroscopic Primary Repair of Proximal Anterior Cruciate Ligament Tears Are Maintained at Mid-term Follow-up. Arthroscopy 2018;34(4):1085–93.
49. Proffen BL, Sieker JT, Murray MM. Bio-enhanced repair of the anterior cruciate ligament. Arthroscopy 2015;31(5):990–7.
50. Vavken P, Fleming BC, Mastrangelo AN, et al. Biomechanical outcomes after bio-enhanced anterior cruciate ligament repair and anterior cruciate ligament reconstruction are equal in a porcine model. Arthroscopy 2012;28(5):672–80.
51. Murray MM, Kiapour AM, Kalish LA, et al. Predictors of Healing Ligament Size and Magnetic Resonance Signal Intensity at 6 Months After Bridge-Enhanced Anterior Cruciate Ligament Repair. Am J Sports Med 2019;47(6):1361–9.
52. Proffen BL, Fleming BC, Murray MM. Histological predictors of maximum failure loads differ between the healing ACL and ACL grafts after 6 and 12 months in vivo. Orthop J Sports Med 2013;1(6). https://doi.org/10.1177/2325967113512457.
53. Murray MM, Fleming BC. Use of a bioactive scaffold to stimulate anterior cruciate ligament healing also minimizes posttraumatic osteoarthritis after surgery. Am J Sports Med 2013;41(8):1762–70.
54. Murray MM, Fleming BC, Badger GJ, et al. Bridge-Enhanced Anterior Cruciate Ligament Repair Is Not Inferior to Autograft Anterior Cruciate Ligament Reconstruction at 2 Years: Results of a Prospective Randomized Clinical Trial. Am J Sports Med 2020;48(6):1305–15.
55. Cao Y, Zhang Z, Song G, et al. Biological enhancement methods may be a viable option for ACL arthroscopic primary repair - A systematic review. Orthop Traumatol Surg Res 2022;108(3). https://doi.org/10.1016/J.OTSR.2022.103227.

56. Wilson WT, Hopper GP, Banger MS, et al. Anterior cruciate ligament repair with internal brace augmentation: A systematic review. Knee 2022;35:192–200.
57. Li Z. Efficacy of Repair for ACL Injury: A Meta-analysis of Randomized Controlled Trials. Int J Sports Med 2022;43(13):1071–83.
58. Vermeijden HD, van der List JP, Benner JL, et al. Primary repair with suture augmentation for proximal anterior cruciate ligament tears: A systematic review with meta-analysis. Knee 2022;38:19–29.
59. van der List JP, Vermeijden HD, Sierevelt IN, et al. Arthroscopic primary repair of proximal anterior cruciate ligament tears seems safe but higher level of evidence is needed: a systematic review and meta-analysis of recent literature. Knee Surg Sports Traumatol Arthrosc 2020;28(6):1946–57.
60. Houck DA, Kraeutler MJ, Belk JW, et al. Primary Arthroscopic Repair of the Anterior Cruciate Ligament: A Systematic Review of Clinical Outcomes. Arthroscopy 2019;35(12):3318–27.
61. Papalia R, Torre G, Papalia G, et al. Arthroscopic primary repair of the anterior cruciate ligament in adults: a systematic review. Br Med Bull 2019;131(1):29–42.
62. Nwachukwu BU, Patel BH, Lu Y, et al. Anterior Cruciate Ligament Repair Outcomes: An Updated Systematic Review of Recent Literature. Arthroscopy 2019;35(7):2233–47.
63. van Eck CF, Limpisvasti O, ElAttrache NS. Is There a Role for Internal Bracing and Repair of the Anterior Cruciate Ligament? A Systematic Literature Review. Am J Sports Med 2018;46(9):2291–8.
64. Hourston GJ, Kankam HK, McDonnell SM. A systematic review of anterior cruciate ligament primary repair rehabilitation. J Clin Orthop Trauma 2022;25. https://doi.org/10.1016/J.JCOT.2022.101774.
65. Hoogeslag RAG, Brouwer RW, Boer BC, et al. Huis in 't Veld R. Acute Anterior Cruciate Ligament Rupture: Repair or Reconstruction? Two-Year Results of a Randomized Controlled Clinical Trial. Am J Sports Med 2019;47(3):567–77.
66. Hoogeslag RAG, Huis, In't Veld R, et al. Acute Anterior Cruciate Ligament Rupture: Repair or Reconstruction? Five-Year Results of a Randomized Controlled Clinical Trial. Am J Sports Med 2022;50(7):1779–87.
67. Kösters C, Glasbrenner J, Spickermann L, et al. Repair With Dynamic Intraligamentary Stabilization Versus Primary Reconstruction of Acute Anterior Cruciate Ligament Tears: 2-Year Results From a Prospective Randomized Study. Am J Sports Med 2020;48(5):1108–16.
68. Sporsheim AN, Gifstad T, Lundemo TO, et al. Autologous BPTB ACL Reconstruction Results in Lower Failure Rates Than ACL Repair with and without Synthetic Augmentation at 30 Years of Follow-up: A Prospective Randomized Study. Journal of Bone and Joint Surgery - American 2019;101(23):2074–81.
69. van der List JP. Arthroscopic primary repair of the anterior cruciate ligament: rationale, patient selection and early outcomes (PhD Academy Award). Br J Sports Med 2022;56(18):1053–4.
70. van der List JP, Jonkergouw A, van Noort A, et al. Identifying candidates for arthroscopic primary repair of the anterior cruciate ligament: A case-control study. Knee 2019;26(3):619–27.
71. Heusdens CHW. ACL Repair: A Game Changer or Will History Repeat Itself? A Critical Appraisal. J Clin Med 2021;10(5):1–12.
72. Gobbi A, Whyte GP. Long-term Outcomes of Primary Repair of the Anterior Cruciate Ligament Combined With Biologic Healing Augmentation to Treat Incomplete Tears. Am J Sports Med 2018;46(14):3368–77.

Revision Anterior Cruciate Ligament Reconstruction and Associated Procedures

Sahil Dadoo, BS[a,*], Neilen Benvegnu, MD[a], Zachary J. Herman, MD[a], Tetsuya Yamamoto, MD[a,b], Jonathan D. Hughes, MD[a,c], Volker Musahl, MD[a,c]

KEYWORDS

- Revision ACL reconstruction (ACLR) • Graft choice • Staging
- Lateral extra-articular tenodesis (LET) • Osteotomy

KEY POINTS

- Revision anterior cruciate ligament reconstruction (ACLR) is indicated in patients who sustained primary ACLR graft rupture and wish to return to an active lifestyle.
- Several risk factors exist for primary ACLR failure, including demographics, activity level, alignment, and biological factors, and appropriate consideration must be given to these for the optimal, individualized revision ACLR.
- Although 1-stage revision ACLR is preferred to decrease the need for additional surgery and recovery time, a 2-stage revision ACLR may be considered in cases of tunnel malposition or widening that may interfere with the revision procedure.
- In patients with persistent rotatory knee instability and/or coronal and sagittal malalignment, revision ACLR may be performed in combination with lateral extra-articular tenodesis and high tibial osteotomy, respectively.

INTRODUCTION

One of the most common yet devastating complications for patients following primary anterior cruciate ligament (ACL) reconstruction is graft failure or rerupture, occurring in up to 25% of patients.[1] Failure of anterior cruciate ligament reconstruction (ACLR) can lead to persistent knee instability, increased risk of further meniscal or chondral injury, and progression of long-term osteoarthritis (OA).[2] In active patients who wish to return to baseline activity, revision ACLR may be warranted to restore native knee function

[a] Department of Orthopaedic Surgery, UPMC Freddie Fu Sports Medicine Center, University of Pittsburgh, 3200 South Water Street, Pittsburgh, PA 15203, USA; [b] Department of Orthopaedic Surgery, Kobe University Graduate School of Medicine, Kobe, Japan; [c] Department of Orthopaedics, Institute of Clinical Sciences, Sahlgrenska Academy, University of Gothenburg, Gothenburg, Sweden
* Corresponding author.
E-mail address: sahildadoo@gmail.com

Clin Sports Med 43 (2024) 449–464
https://doi.org/10.1016/j.csm.2023.08.012
sportsmed.theclinics.com

and kinematics. However, revision ACLR is a complex and technically challenging procedure associated with inferior clinical outcomes when compared with primary ACLR.[3] As a result, a thorough assessment of the nonmodifiable and modifiable factors contributing to ACLR failure is paramount to reduce the risk of future ACL injury.[4,5]

The purpose of this article is to review the causes of primary ACLR failure and clinical indications for revision ACLR and to explore technical considerations for addressing modifiable risk factors when performing an individualized and patient-centered revision ACLR.

EXPLORING CAUSES OF PRIMARY ANTERIOR CRUCIATE LIGAMENT RECONSTRUCTION FAILURE

Various risk factors for primary ACLR failure have been reported in the literature, and it is crucial during preoperative planning for revision ACLR to identify such factors. These causes can be broadly split into nonmodifiable factors, such as age, sex, and sports participation, and modifiable factors, including tunnel malposition, graft choice during primary ACLR, and lower-limb malalignment.

Nonmodifiable Risk Factors for Anterior Cruciate Ligament Reconstruction Failure

Younger age, female sex, and higher baseline level of activity are well-known risk factors for ACLR failure and subsequent knee surgery following primary ACLR.[6] Although nonmodifiable, understanding of the literature and reported rates of injury is important when synthesizing an appropriate patient-centered plan following ACLR failure. Studies have demonstrated that ipsilateral ACLR failures are nearly 2 times higher in patients aged younger than 21 years compared with patients aged older than 40 years, and the odds of ipsilateral ACLR failure decrease by 0.09 for every yearly increase in patient age.[7,8] Younger female patients in particular are at an increased risk for ACLR failure, with reported rates 2 to 8 times higher than their male counterparts.[1] Higher baseline level of activity and sports participation are associated with a 5-time increase in odds of future ACL injury, with odds of ACLR failure increasing by 0.11 for every increase in baseline Marx activity score.[7] Earlier return to sport (RTS) following primary ACLR has also been identified as a predictor of failure following primary ACLR.[9]

Modifiable Risk Factors for Anterior Cruciate Ligament Reconstruction Failure

Femoral tunnel malposition is often cited as the most common cause of primary ACLR failure. A study by the Multicenter ACL Revision Study (MARS) Group found that technical errors accounted for 60% of primary ACLR failures, of which 80% were attributed to femoral tunnel malposition.[10] Femoral tunnel technique plays a major role in primary ACLR success, with increased ACLR failure rates reported following transtibial versus anteromedial portal drilling, due to the nonanatomic femoral tunnel location following transtibial technique.[11] Additionally, surgeon ACLR volume may play an important role because high-volume surgeons have been shown to place more anatomic (posterior and distal) femoral tunnels compared with low-volume surgeons.[12] Nonanatomic tunnel placement increases the risk of revision ACLR, highlighting the importance of anatomic posterior femoral tunnel placement on the success of primary ACLR.[4]

Graft choice during primary ACLR also plays an important role in failure rates, and understanding of the patient-specific indications for each graft type can reduce the need for future revision ACLR. For younger, higher demand patients (ie, aged <30 years), allograft is generally contraindicated due to the vast literature demonstrating failure rates up to 40% in this age group. Studies have shown a 3-fold increase in failure rates (26.5% vs 8.3%, respectively) and 5.2 times higher odds of ACLR failure following allograft versus autograft use.[7,13] Conversely, autograft choices including bone-patellar tendon-bone (BPTB) and quadriceps tendon (QT) have demonstrated low failure rates and high rates of RTS at short-term and long-term follow-up.[14] Although hamstring tendon (HT) autograft is a popular choice worldwide due to its low failure rates, newer literature may indicate an increased failure rate following HT use compared with BPTB and QT autografts, especially in patients of younger age, female sex, and increased baseline activity.[15,16]

Lower limb malalignment is an important reason for ACLR failure and need for revision ACLR.[17] Varus and valgus malalignment can alter knee biomechanics and increase stress on the native ACL,[18] whereas an increased posterior tibial slope (PTS) greater than 12° has been associated with increased odds of primary ACLR failure, regardless of graft type.[19,20] Due to the increased stress on the ACL, correction of the lower limb malalignment during revision ACLR is crucial to prevent future graft failure.

PREOPERATIVE PLANNING FOR REVISION ANTERIOR CRUCIATE LIGAMENT RECONSTRUCTION

History and Physical Examination

The patient evaluation for suspected failure following primary ACLR should include a thorough history to identify potential risk factors for failure, mechanism of reinjury (ie, traumatic vs nontraumatic), and postoperative course following primary ACLR (ie, successful RTS vs persistent knee instability). Importantly, the patient's desire to return to preinjury level of activity must be elucidated. For older, low-demand patients who are not functionally limited by their knee instability, nonoperative management may be considered. Conversely, for younger, active patients who participate in pivoting sports, revision ACLR may be warranted for successful return to baseline activity level and prevention of further knee damage.

The physical examination for suspected ACLR failure should include maneuvers such as a Lachman test, anterior drawer, and pivot shift examination to evaluate for ACL deficiency. Physical examination may also include instrumented testing, which is available in multiple forms for the Lachman test as well as the pivot shift test.[21,22] Additional testing including valgus, varus, dial, and McMurray tests should be performed to evaluate for concomitant ligamentous and/or meniscus pathologic condition.

Imaging Considerations

Appropriate imaging must be obtained on all patients with suspected ACLR failure, irrespective of if a revision ACLR procedure will be performed. Radiographs of the knee should comprise a full weight-bearing series including a standing anteroposterior (AP) view in extension, 45° flexion weight-bearing postero-anterior (PA), and a Merchant view. Assessment of coronal and sagittal malalignment with full-length standing AP alignment and lateral films are imperative. Earlier implants may additionally be assessed on radiographs to determine the type of fixation used and if hardware removal is needed during the revision surgery.

Careful analysis of tunnel placement and tunnel size are critical for a successful revision procedure. For evaluation of femoral tunnel placement, the total sagittal diameter of the lateral femoral condyle can be divided into 4 equal quadrants along Blumensaat line, and the maximum intercondylar notch height can be divided into 4 equal quadrants as well. The femoral tunnel can be considered in anatomic position when located in the most superoposterior quadrant (**Fig. 1**A).[23] For tibial tunnel evaluation, the tibial plateau can be divided into 4 quadrants on lateral radiographs, and the tibial tunnel

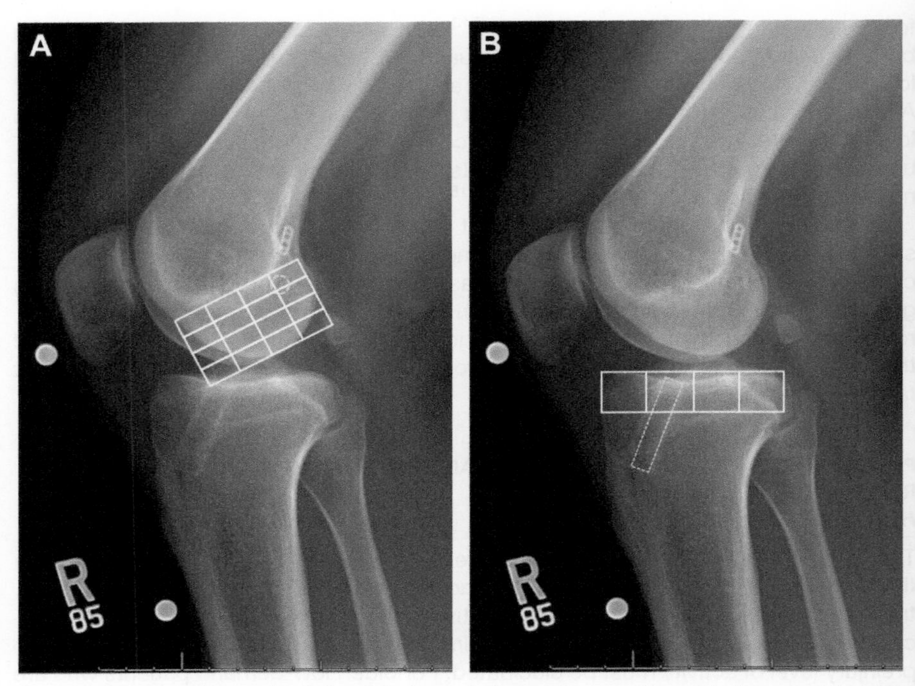

Fig. 1. A lateral radiograph of the right knee is shown. Femoral tunnel placement is determined by dividing Blumensaat line and the maximum intercondylar notch height into 4 equal quadrants each, with appropriate anatomic tunnel placement (*yellow circle*) in the most superoposterior quadrant (*A*). Tibial tunnel placement is determined by dividing the tibial plateau into 4 equal quadrants, with appropriate tunnel placement (*yellow rectangle*) in the posterior third of the second quadrant (*B*).

can be considered in anatomic position if entering the joint in the posterior third of quadrant 2 (**Fig. 1**B).[24] Tunnel obliquity may also be assessed on 45° flexion weight-bearing PA radiographs to determine anatomic versus nonanatomic tunnel placement, with tunnel obliquity less than 32.7° associated with nonanatomic tunnel placement (**Fig. 2**A and B).[25]

Advanced imaging should be obtained on all patients before revision ACLR. MRI is a useful tool for evaluating graft integrity, concomitant meniscal, chondral, and ligamentous injuries, and tunnel position and width.[26] Three-dimensional (3D) computed tomography (CT) imaging is considered the gold standard imaging modality to assess tunnel quality, especially when tunnel malpositioning or widening are suspected based on radiographs or MRI.[27] Tunnel diameter can be measured at the widest point on axial, coronal, and sagittal planes, and measurements greater than 15 mm are consistent with clinically significant tunnel osteolysis that may require bone grafting before, or during, revision ACLR (**Fig. 3**A–C).[28]

CONSIDERATIONS DURING REVISION ANTERIOR CRUCIATE LIGAMENT RECONSTRUCTION

Graft Selection During Revision Anterior Cruciate Ligament Reconstruction

Graft choice for revision ACLR varies significantly across providers despite beliefs that it remains an important factor in the success of the revision procedure.[29] Performing surgeon, prior ACLR graft choice, and patient age are the most influential factors when

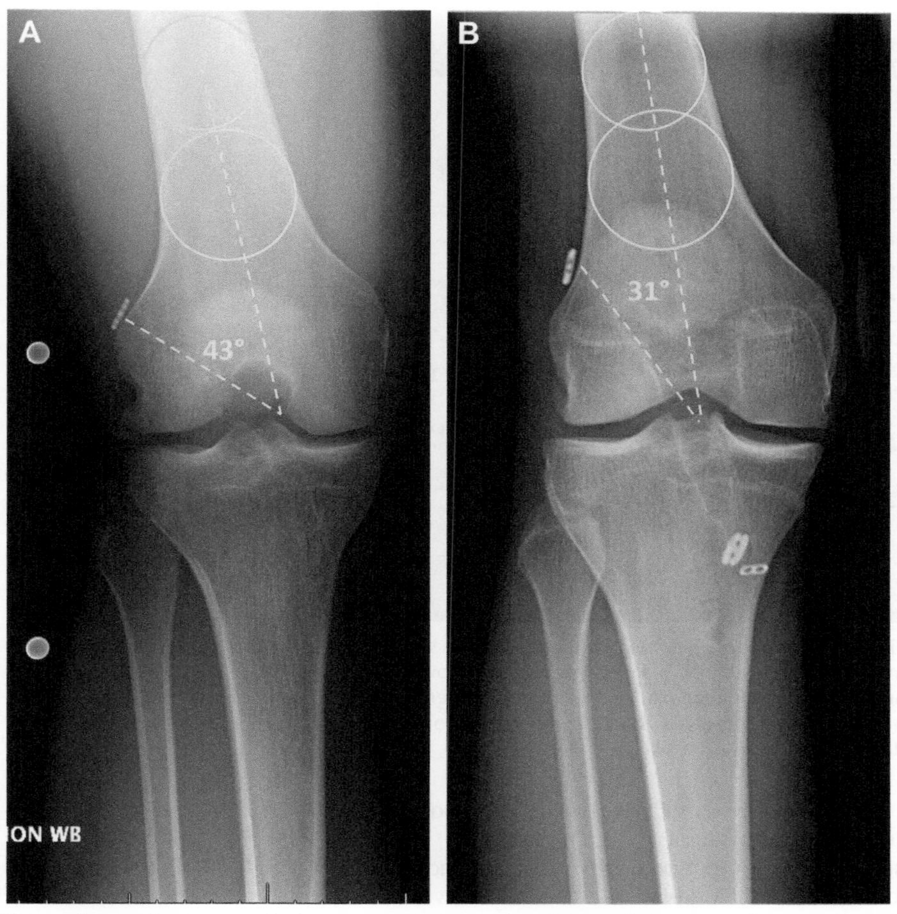

Fig. 2. The 45° flexion weight-bearing PA radiographs of the right knee are shown. Femoral tunnel obliquity can be measured by determining the axis of the femoral shaft, and creating an angle with the direction of the femoral tunnel. An angle greater than 32.7° is consistent with anatomic tunnel placement (*A*), whereas an angle less than 32.7° is consistent with nonanatomic tunnel placement (*B*).

considering the appropriate graft choice for revision ACLR.[30] Graft options for revision ACLR are similar to those for primary ACLR, and include allografts (BPTB, HT, Achilles, tibialis, and peroneal tendons) or autografts (BPTB, QT, and HT).

Allograft is used commonly for revision ACLR due to avoidance of additional donor site morbidity, accounting for 20% to 51% of revision cases.[31] A study by the MARS Group found that allograft was 3.6 times more likely to be chosen for revision ACLR if an autograft was used for primary ACLR.[30] However, there remain questions regarding the risks and benefits of allograft use, as several studies have demonstrated that allograft use is associated with multiple ACL graft failures and leads to a 2.2 times greater rerevision rate following revision ACLR when compared with autograft use.[32,33] In addition, allograft use during ACLR is associated with an increased risk of infection, inferior patient-reported outcomes (PROs) and sports function, and lower cost-effectiveness when compared with autograft choices.[5,34]

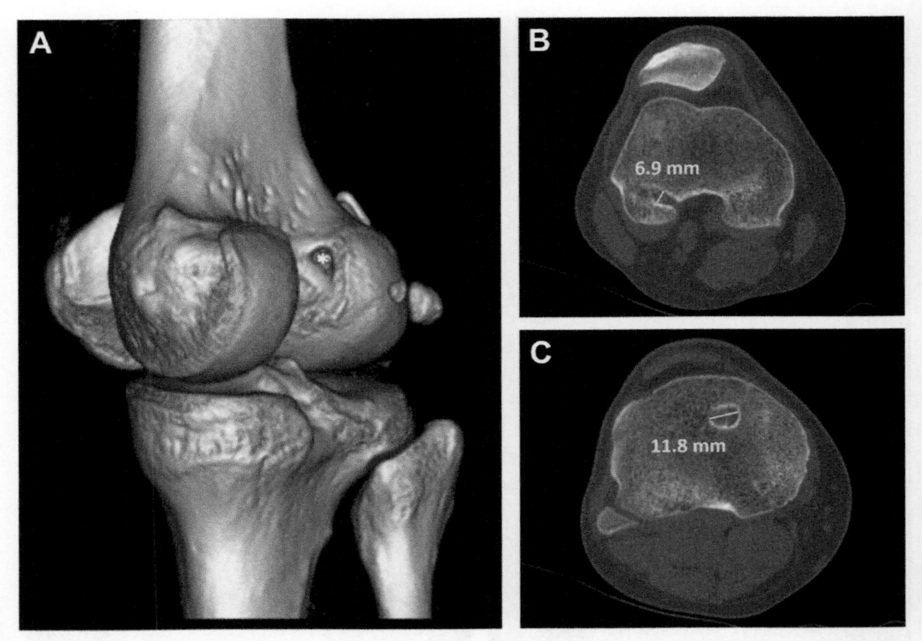

Fig. 3. A 3D CT reconstruction of the knee (*A*) is seen, which can be used to determine placement of earlier tunnels. Axial CT scans of the lower limb can additionally assess femoral (*B*) and tibial (*C*) tunnel width. Tunnel width greater than 15 mm is consistent with clinically significant tunnel osteolysis. 3D CT, three-dimensional computed tomography scan, asterisk indicates femoral tunnel placement.

Autograft choices for revision ACLR include BPTB, QT, and HT, which can be harvested from ipsilateral or contralateral limb, depending on earlier graft use. BPTB is historically the most common autograft choice for revision ACLR procedures, due to the successful long-term outcomes achieved following its use.[35] However, recently, the QT autograft has become increasingly popular for revision ACLR, whereas the HT autograft has declined in use.[36] The emerging evidence demonstrating increased failure rates following HT autograft use and equivalent outcomes between BPTB and QT autografts may contribute to the observed increase in QT autograft use for both primary and revision ACLR. Further, it has been shown that harvesting a second extensor mechanism autograft (BPTB followed by QT, or QT followed by BPTB) results in comparable PROs and RTS to those where only one extensor autograft is used during primary and revision ACLR.[37] Earlier ACLR graft choice plays an important role in graft selection for revision ACLR, and the results of this study encourage the use of QT or BPTB for revision ACLR, which are otherwise favorable graft options.[37]

The authors' recommendation for graft selection during revision ACLR is based on previous graft use and patient age and activity level. In younger, active athletes who desire return to play, QT and BPTB autografts are generally recommended, unless extensor mechanism insufficiency exists following primary ACLR with either graft type. If found, HT autograft is a viable alternative in this population. For patients aged 30 to 40 years, all autografts may be recommended for more active patients, whereas autograft and allograft can both be considered in lower demand patients. For lower demand patients greater than 40 year old, allograft is preferred due to avoidance of further donor site morbidity.

Addressing Concomitant Injuries

Meniscal or chondral injuries have been reported in up to 90% of patients undergoing revision ACLR, with 59% of patients having both types of injuries.[38] These injuries are often overlooked during revision ACLR and are important predictors of poorer PROs up to 6 years following revision ACLR.[39] Additionally, medial meniscus ramp lesions and lateral meniscus root tears are present in up to 52% of primary and revision ACLRs and play an important role in persistent rotatory knee instability following ACLR.[40]

Concomitant ligamentous injury, especially to the MCL, has also been reported in up to 67% of presumed "isolated" ACL tears during primary ACLR.[41] The high incidence of MCL injuries and anteromedial (AM) instability may predispose patients to persistent knee instability following primary ACLR, leading to advanced degenerative changes, further meniscal injury, and failure of ACLR.[41,42] Biomechanical studies have demonstrated that the superficial MCL is the most important restraint to AM instability,[43] and anatomic AM reconstruction of the MCL has been shown to eliminate rotatory instability and reduce failure rates following combined ACL and MCL injuries.[44–46] Further, deficiency of posterolateral corner (PLC) structures has been shown to increase posterolateral laxity and varus load on the ACL graft, leading to an increased risk of failure.[47] A recent systematic review demonstrated that combined ACL and PLC reconstruction is the most effective approach to improve patient outcomes when compared with PLC repair or nonoperative management of these lesions.[48] Therefore, appropriate assessment and management of concomitant meniscus, chondral, and ligamentous injury is crucial for successful outcomes after revision ACLR.

Staging for Revision Anterior Cruciate Ligament Reconstruction

Several factors must be considered by the surgeon when deciding between a single-stage and a 2-stage revision ACLR, including tunnel malposition, tunnel osteolysis, coronal or sagittal malalignment, and concomitant soft-tissue injuries.[49] Patients with appropriately positioned tunnels without excessive osteolysis (<15 mm), or tunnels that do not interfere with anatomic tunnel placement, may be indicated for a single-stage revision.[28] Meniscal and chondral pathologic condition may be addressed and corrective osteotomies performed in a single-stage procedure based on surgeon discretion and thoughtful placement of hardware and tunnels. A 2-stage procedure may primarily be indicated when malpositioned tunnels affect the placement of new tunnels or tunnel osteolysis greater than 15 mm is present. Additionally, the surgeon may decide to perform a first stage to fully evaluate meniscal or chondral injury for subsequent second-stage preoperative planning. Special consideration must be taken when electing for a 2-stage procedure because they typically require a 6-month window between procedures and place the patient at an increased risk for further chondrosis and meniscal injury due to prolonged knee instability.[50] As a result, a 2-stage revision should be reserved for when a 1-stage procedure may not be satisfactorily performed.

During a single-stage revision, earlier tunnels may be avoided but tunnel overlap is not a contraindication to single-stage revision. Earlier tunnels can be filled with bone graft or bone substitute, redrilled, or a divergent tunnel technique may be used. Any retained hardware can be removed, left in place if not interfering with revision tunnel placement (**Fig. 4**), or drilled through (**Fig. 5**A and B). Confirmation should be made that all granulation and foreign material has been removed from the tunnel. It is important to ensure rigid fixation of the graft, and stacked screws should be avoided due to

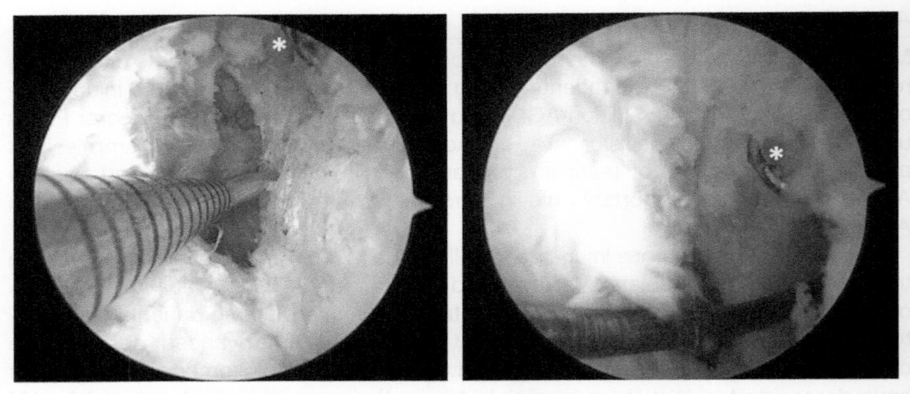

Fig. 4. An anterior arthroscopic view of the lateral femoral notch during revision ACLR is seen. Earlier femoral fixation hardware can be seen left in place while new anatomic femoral tunnels are created because they do not interfere with revision tunnel placement. ACLR, anterior cruciate ligament reconstruction. Asterisk indicates previous ACLR femoral fixation hardware.

risk of graft compromise.[51] If fixation is at all questionable, the revision procedure should be deferred to a second stage.

The goal of a 2-stage procedure is to address tunnel defects that may not allow for a successful single-stage procedure. During the first stage, the tibial and femoral tunnels should be fully debrided and visualized for accurate characterization, all loose hardware should be removed, and bone grafting of tunnels may be achieved using allograft (chips or dowels), autograft, or bone substitutes. Once complete, corrective osteotomies or additional procedures for concomitant meniscal, chondral, or ligamentous injury may be performed. After the initial procedure, the second stage can be performed once CT has confirmed incorporation of bone graft, typically within 3 to 6 months.

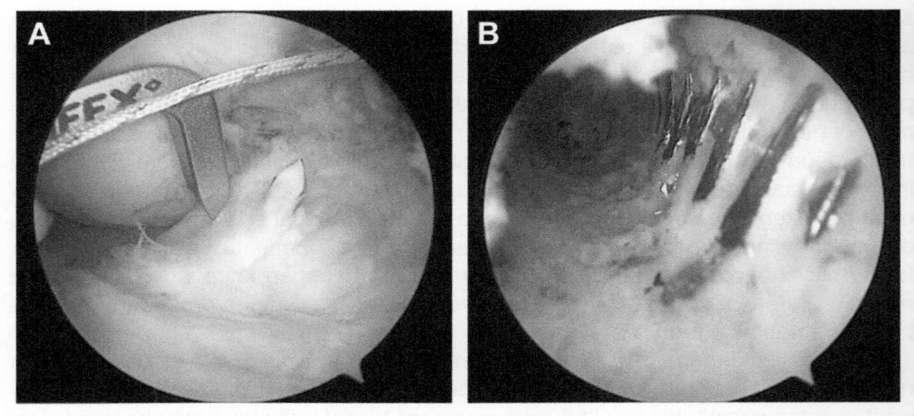

Fig. 5. An anterior arthroscopic view of the tibial stump (*A*) and revision tibial tunnel (*B*) is seen during single-stage revision ACLR. The revision tibial tunnel can be seen drilling through earlier tibial fixation hardware, which is an option during single-stage revision ACLR if new tunnel placement is not interfered with. ACLR, anterior cruciate ligament reconstruction.

Although evidence is limited, the literature suggests equivalent outcomes following single-stage versus 2-stage revision ACLR.[50,52] At 2-year follow-up, no differences in subjective outcomes or failure rates were found between the 2 groups; however, patients undergoing 2-stage revision were predisposed to additional intra-articular lesions and a longer surgical recovery.[50] A systematic analysis comparing outcomes between 1-stage and 2-stage revision ACLR found no significant difference in rate of repeat revision surgery following 1-stage versus 2-stage revision (3.1% vs 6.8%) and equivalent clinical outcomes.[52] As a result, due to the increased time to recovery and need for additional surgery, 2-stage procedures should be performed only when indicated.

Over-the-Top Technique in Revision Anterior Cruciate Ligament Reconstruction

The over-the-top reconstruction (OTT) technique can be used in revision ACLR settings to bypass the need for a multistage procedure, such as when bone grafting of enlarged or malpositioned tunnels may be necessary. The technique involves passing the graft over the superomedial border of the lateral femoral condyle and fixing it to the lateral femoral cortex (**Fig. 6**). Advantages of OTT technique include ease of use, reproducibility, and avoidance of additional femoral tunnel drilling, saving time and cost.[53] Indications for OTT include revision surgery, salvage of intraoperative posterior cortical wall "blowout" of the femoral tunnel, surgery on patients with open physes, and when concomitant anterolateral procedures are being considered.[54]

Although evidence is limited, some studies have reported on the outcomes of the OTT technique in the revision ACLR setting. A 2018 systematic review found comparable PROs, failure rates, and RTS following revision ACLR with OTT technique and traditional revision ACLR methods.[53] Additionally, a 2019 retrospective study found significantly decreased postoperative anterior laxity compared with preoperative states following revision ACLR with OTT technique, and comparable failure rates to

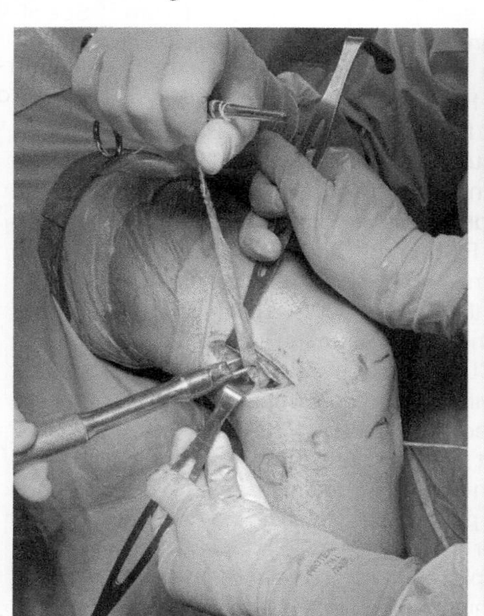

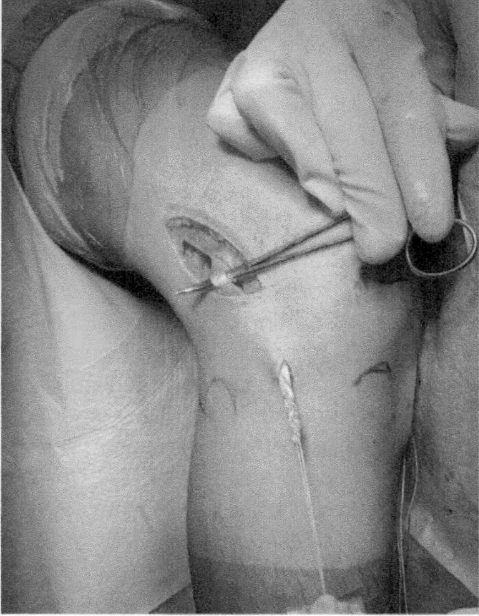

Fig. 6. The OTT technique during revision ACLR is demonstrated here. The technique involves passing the graft over the superomedial border of the lateral femoral condyle and fixing it to the lateral femoral cortex, and provides an alternative approach to bypasses the need for multistage revision ACLR. ACLR, anterior cruciate ligament reconstruction.

traditional revision ACLR.[55] Finally, a recent retrospective study noted no significant differences in clinical outcomes at 2-year follow-up between traditional versus OTT revision ACLR.[56] Although limited, the present literature suggests the technique provides outcomes similar to traditional methods of revision ACLR.

ADDITIONAL PROCEDURES DURING REVISION ANTERIOR CRUCIATE LIGAMENT RECONSTRUCTION

Lateral Extra-Articular Tenodesis

One of the proposed causes of primary ACLR failure is persistent rotatory knee instability, and anterolateral augmentation procedures during ACLR have been shown to control rotatory knee laxity more than isolated ACLR in cadaveric studies.[57,58] Although indications are not well defined, there is consensus that revision ACLR is an indication for lateral extra-articular tenodesis (LET), especially in cases of high-grade pivot shift and persistent rotatory knee instability.[59–61] Although several techniques for LET exist, a common choice is the modified Lemaire procedure, in which a strip of the iliotibial band attached to Gerdy tubercle is passed deep to the lateral collateral ligament (LCL) and fixated proximal to the LCL insertion on the lateral femoral epicondyle.[58] Short-term outcomes of revision ACLR with LET demonstrate improvement in PROs and resolution of pivot shift in most patients postoperatively.[59,60] Importantly, a significant reduction in failure rates and improvement in return to preinjury level of sports have been reported following revision ACLR with LET compared with revision ACLR without LET.[59,61,62]

Role of Osteotomy in Revision Anterior Cruciate Ligament Reconstruction

Lower limb coronal and sagittal malalignment has been shown to increase stress on the native ACL and is associated with an increased risk of primary ACLR failure.[17] Specifically, severe PTS and severe varus malalignment are considered indications for combined osteotomy during revision ACLR. In patients with increased PTS, an anterior closing-wedge high tibial osteotomy (ACW-HTO) can be performed alongside revision ACLR to reduce the tibial slope and prevent future graft failure.[63,64] Relative indications for ACW-HTO include patients who have sustained at least one ACLR failure with an elevated PTS greater than 12°, body mass index (BMI) less than 30 kg/m^2, and without varus malalignment greater than 5°.[65] Studies have reported that combined revision ACLR with ACW-HTO results in improved PROs and clinical outcomes, reduction in anterior tibial translation, and reduction in mean PTS postoperatively (ranging from 4° to 9° of slope reduction).[63–65] Additionally, the role of ACW-HTO is increasingly being reported in the setting of primary ACLR. Although the data are limited, studies suggest that ACW-HTO combined with primary ACLR can effectively reduce tibial slope and anterior laxity of the ACL graft while improving patient outcomes.[66]

Although much attention has been focused on correcting PTS during revision ACLR, correcting varus deformity is also important for preventing future knee instability, revision ACLR failure, and knee OA.[67] In such cases, a medial opening wedge (MOW-HTO) or a lateral closing wedge may be performed. Relative indications for these procedures include patients aged younger than 60 years, BMI less than 30 kg/m^2, intact menisci and cartilage, and unicompartmental mild-to-moderate OA. Biomechanical studies have reported that simultaneous valgus-producing and slope-reducing osteotomy during ACLR further decreased the anterior tibial translation and ACL graft forces in ACL-reconstructed knees, compared with ACLR with only one corrective osteotomy.[68] Further, a systematic review of 18 studies reported that simultaneous HTO and ACLR was effective in correcting varus malalignment (postoperative varus ranging from 0.3° to 7.7°) with low complication and failure rates.[69] Finally, a recent study of 35 patients with combined ACLR and MOW-HTO at 10-year follow-up reported an 80% RTS rate, 31% rate of return to prior activity level, and 10% ACLR failure rate.[70]

Outcomes Following Revision Anterior Cruciate Ligament Reconstruction

In general, outcomes following revision ACLR are inferior when compared with primary ACLR. A 2016 meta-analysis identified significantly higher rates of a grade 2+ pivot shift (7% vs 2%) and radiological evidence of OA (50% vs 25%) after revision ACLR compared with primary ACLR.[3] Patients undergoing revision ACLR also reported significantly inferior International Knee Documentation Committee (IKDC) and Lysholm scores when compared with patients' scores after primary ACLR.[3] Increasingly, lower RTS rates have been reported after revision ACLR compared with primary ACLR, with a recent meta-analysis reporting only 43% of 5365 patients returned to the same level of sport following revision ACLR.[71] An additional systematic review of 13 studies reported rates of RTS at preinjury level as low as 13% after revision ACLR.[72] Finally, subsequent failure rates following revision ACLR have been reported at rates 3 to 4 times higher than failure rates following primary ACLR in both adolescent and adult populations.[73,74] Due to the inferior clinical and functional outcomes reported following revision ACLR, a thorough understanding of the appropriate indications and techniques is paramount to improve patient outcomes in the revision setting.

SUMMARY

Despite improvements in primary ACLR techniques, failure of ACLR remains a common and devastating complication, necessitating the need for a revision ACLR. Identifying the reason for primary ACLR failure is the most important consideration during preoperative planning for revision ACLR. Several patient-related and surgery-related risk factors for ACLR failure exist and must be given the appropriate consideration before revision ACLR. During revision ACLR, special attention must be given to the tunnel size, tunnel position, and concomitant injuries to determine the optimal approach, most commonly 1-stage revision. In patients with persistent rotatory knee instability and/or coronal or sagittal malalignment, LET and HTO may be considered in conjunction with the revision ACLR, respectively. Although outcomes following revision ACLR are generally inferior to those following primary ACLR, it remains an important procedure to improve a patient's quality of life and allow for successful RTS or baseline activity level.

CLINICS CARE POINTS

- Revision ACLR is primarily indicated in patients who sustained failure of primary ACLR and wish to return to an active lifestyle.
- Several risk factors exist for primary ACLR failure, including demographics, activity level, alignment, and biological factors, and appropriate consideration must be given to these for the optimal, individualized revision ACLR.
- Although 1-stage revision ACLR is preferred to decrease the need for additional surgery and recovery time, a 2-stage revision ACLR may be considered in cases of tunnel malposition or widening that may interfere with the revision procedure.
- In patients with persistent rotatory knee instability and/or coronal and sagittal malalignment, revision ACLR can be performed in combination with LET and HTO, respectively.

CONFLICT OF INTEREST

No Disclosure: S. Dadoo, N. Benvegnu, Z.J. Herman, T. Yamamoto, J.D. Hughes. V. Musahl. Education: Smith & Nephew, Arthrex, DePuy Synthes, Conmed. Consulting: Smith & Nephew, Newclip, Ostesys. Royalties: Springer. Shareholder: Ostesys. Board Member: ACL Study Group, AOSSM, ISAKOS, KSSTA (Deputy Editor-in-chief). Codeveloper of iPad app (Serial No. 61/566,761). NIH Grant Support: U01AR076144, W81XWH-16-PRORP-ICTA.

REFERENCES

1. Erickson BJ, Cvetanovich GL, Frank RM, et al. Revision ACL Reconstruction: A Critical Analysis Review. JBJS Rev 2017;5(6):e1.
2. Blaker CL, Zaki S, Little CB, et al. Long-term Effect of a Single Subcritical Knee Injury: Increasing the Risk of Anterior Cruciate Ligament Rupture and Osteoarthritis. Am J Sports Med 2021;49(2):391–403.
3. Grassi A, Ardern CL, Marcheggiani Muccioli GM, et al. Does revision ACL reconstruction measure up to primary surgery? A meta-analysis comparing patient-reported and clinician-reported outcomes, and radiographic results. Br J Sports Med 2016;50(12):716–24.
4. Byrne KJ, Hughes JD, Gibbs C, et al. Non-anatomic tunnel position increases the risk of revision anterior cruciate ligament reconstruction. Knee Surg Sports Traumatol Arthrosc 2022;30(4):1388–95.
5. Group M, Group M. Effect of graft choice on the outcome of revision anterior cruciate ligament reconstruction in the Multicenter ACL Revision Study (MARS) Cohort. Am J Sports Med 2014;42(10):2301–10.
6. Group M, Ding DY, Zhang AL, et al. Subsequent Surgery After Revision Anterior Cruciate Ligament Reconstruction: Rates and Risk Factors From a Multicenter Cohort. Am J Sports Med 2017;45(9):2068–76.
7. Kaeding CC, Pedroza AD, Reinke EK, et al. Risk Factors and Predictors of Subsequent ACL Injury in Either Knee After ACL Reconstruction: Prospective Analysis of 2488 Primary ACL Reconstructions From the MOON Cohort. Am J Sports Med. Jul 2015;43(7):1583–90.
8. Gallo MC, Bolia IK, Jalali O, et al. Risk Factors for Early Subsequent (Revision or Contralateral) ACL Reconstruction: A Retrospective Database Study. Orthop J Sports Med 2020;8(2). 2325967119901173.
9. van Eck CF, Schkrohowsky JG, Working ZM, et al. Prospective analysis of failure rate and predictors of failure after anatomic anterior cruciate ligament reconstruction with allograft. Am J Sports Med 2012;40(4):800–7.
10. Morgan JA, Dahm D, Levy B, et al. Femoral tunnel malposition in ACL revision reconstruction. J Knee Surg 2012;25(5):361–8.
11. Vermeijden HD, Yang XA, van der List JP, et al. Trauma and femoral tunnel position are the most common failure modes of anterior cruciate ligament reconstruction: a systematic review. Knee Surg Sports Traumatol Arthrosc 2020;28(11): 3666–75.
12. Hughes JD, Gibbs CM, Almast A, et al. More anatomic tunnel placement for anterior cruciate ligament reconstruction by surgeons with high volume compared to low volume. Knee Surg Sports Traumatol Arthrosc 2022;30(6):2014–9.
13. Bottoni CR, Smith EL, Shaha J, et al. Autograft versus allograft anterior cruciate ligament reconstruction: a prospective, randomized clinical study with a minimum 10-year follow-up. Am J Sports Med 2015;43(10):2501–9.

14. Sajovic M, Stropnik D, Skaza K. Long-term comparison of semitendinosus and gracilis tendon versus patellar tendon autografts for anterior cruciate ligament reconstruction: a 17-year follow-up of a randomized controlled trial. Am J Sports Med 2018;46(8):1800–8.
15. Mohtadi NG, Chan DS. A Randomized Clinical Trial Comparing Patellar Tendon, Hamstring Tendon, and Double-Bundle ACL Reconstructions: Patient-Reported and Clinical Outcomes at 5-Year Follow-up. J Bone Joint Surg Am 2019; 101(11):949–60.
16. Salem HS, Varzhapetyan V, Patel N, et al. Anterior Cruciate Ligament Reconstruction in Young Female Athletes: Patellar Versus Hamstring Tendon Autografts. Am J Sports Med 2019;47(9):2086–92.
17. Tischer T, Condello V, Menetrey J, et al. Time to focus on ACL revision: ESSKA 2022 consensus. Knee Surg Sports Traumatol Arthrosc 2022. https://doi.org/10.1007/s00167-022-06950-3.
18. van de Pol GJ, Arnold MP, Verdonschot N, et al. Varus alignment leads to increased forces in the anterior cruciate ligament. Am J Sports Med 2009; 37(3):481–7.
19. Webb JM, Salmon LJ, Leclerc E, et al. Posterior tibial slope and further anterior cruciate ligament injuries in the anterior cruciate ligament-reconstructed patient. Am J Sports Med 2013;41(12):2800–4.
20. Christensen JJ, Krych AJ, Engasser WM, et al. Lateral tibial posterior slope is increased in patients with early graft failure after anterior cruciate ligament reconstruction. Am J Sports Med 2015;43(10):2510–4.
21. Hoshino Y, Araujo P, Ahlden M, et al. Quantitative evaluation of the pivot shift by image analysis using the iPad. Knee Surg Sports Traumatol Arthrosc. Apr 2013; 21(4):975–80.
22. Musahl V, Griffith C, Irrgang JJ, et al. Validation of Quantitative Measures of Rotatory Knee Laxity. Am J Sports Med 2016;44(9):2393–8.
23. Bernard M, Hertel P, Hornung H, et al. Femoral insertion of the ACL. Radiographic quadrant method. Am J Knee Surg. Winter 1997;10(1):14–21 [discussion: 21-2].
24. Harner CD, Marks PH, Fu FH, et al. Anterior cruciate ligament reconstruction: endoscopic versus two-incision technique. Arthroscopy 1994;10(5):502–12.
25. Illingworth KD, Hensler D, Working ZM, et al. A simple evaluation of anterior cruciate ligament femoral tunnel position: the inclination angle and femoral tunnel angle. Am J Sports Med. Dec 2011;39(12):2611–8.
26. Rizer M, Foremny GB, Rush A 3rd, et al. Anterior cruciate ligament reconstruction tunnel size: causes of tunnel enlargement and implications for single versus two-stage revision reconstruction. Skeletal Radiol 2017;46(2):161–9.
27. Forsythe B, Kopf S, Wong AK, et al. The location of femoral and tibial tunnels in anatomic double-bundle anterior cruciate ligament reconstruction analyzed by three-dimensional computed tomography models. J Bone Joint Surg Am 2010; 92(6):1418–26.
28. Kamath GV, Redfern JC, Greis PE, et al. Revision anterior cruciate ligament reconstruction. Am J Sports Med 2011;39(1):199–217.
29. Magnussen RA, Trojani C, Granan LP, et al. Patient demographics and surgical characteristics in ACL revision: a comparison of French, Norwegian, and North American cohorts. Knee Surg Sports Traumatol Arthrosc 2015;23(8):2339–48.
30. Group M. Factors influencing graft choice in revision anterior cruciate ligament reconstruction in the mars group. J Knee Surg 2016;29(6):458–63.

31. Condello V, Zdanowicz U, Di Matteo B, et al. Allograft tendons are a safe and effective option for revision ACL reconstruction: a clinical review. Knee Surg Sports Traumatol Arthrosc 2019;27(6):1771–81.
32. Nissen KA, Eysturoy NH, Nielsen TG, et al. Allograft use results in higher re-revision rate for revision anterior cruciate ligament reconstruction. Orthop J Sports Med 2018;6(6). 2325967118775381.
33. Winkler PW, Wagala NN, Hughes JD, et al. A high tibial slope, allograft use, and poor patient-reported outcome scores are associated with multiple ACL graft failures. Knee Surg Sports Traumatol Arthrosc 2022;30(1):139–48.
34. Marom N, Kapadia M, Nguyen JT, et al. Factors associated with an intra-articular infection after anterior cruciate ligament reconstruction: a large single-institution cohort study. Am J Sports Med 2022;50(5):1229–36.
35. Runer A, Csapo R, Hepperger C, et al. Anterior cruciate ligament reconstructions with quadriceps tendon autograft result in lower graft rupture rates but similar patient-reported outcomes as compared with hamstring tendon autograft: a comparison of 875 patients. Am J Sports Med 2020;48(9):2195–204.
36. Winkler PW, Vivacqua T, Thomassen S, et al. Quadriceps tendon autograft is becoming increasingly popular in revision ACL reconstruction. Knee Surg Sports Traumatol Arthrosc 2022;30(1):149–60.
37. Setliff JC, Gibbs CM, Musahl V, et al. Harvesting a second graft from the extensor mechanism for revision ACL reconstruction does not delay return of quadriceps function. Knee Surg Sports Traumatol Arthrosc 2022. https://doi.org/10.1007/s00167-022-07242-6.
38. Group M. Meniscal and Articular Cartilage Predictors of Clinical Outcome After Revision Anterior Cruciate Ligament Reconstruction. Am J Sports Med 2016;44(7):1671–9.
39. Group M, Wright RW, Huston LJ, et al. Meniscal and Articular Cartilage Predictors of Outcome After Revision ACL Reconstruction: A 6-Year Follow-up Cohort Study. Am J Sports Med 2023;51(3):605–14.
40. Magosch A, Mouton C, Nuhrenborger C, et al. Medial meniscus ramp and lateral meniscus posterior root lesions are present in more than a third of primary and revision ACL reconstructions. Knee Surg Sports Traumatol Arthrosc 2021;29(9):3059–67.
41. Willinger L, Balendra G, Pai V, et al. High incidence of superficial and deep medial collateral ligament injuries in 'isolated' anterior cruciate ligament ruptures: a long overlooked injury. Knee Surg Sports Traumatol Arthrosc 2022;30(1):167–75.
42. Alm L, Drenck TC, Frings J, et al. Lower Failure Rates and Improved Patient Outcome Due to Reconstruction of the MCL and Revision ACL Reconstruction in Chronic Medial Knee Instability. Orthop J Sports Med 2021;9(3). 2325967121989312.
43. Wierer G, Milinkovic D, Robinson JR, et al. The superficial medial collateral ligament is the major restraint to anteromedial instability of the knee. Knee Surg Sports Traumatol Arthrosc 2021;29(2):405–16.
44. Behrendt P, Herbst E, Robinson JR, et al. The Control of Anteromedial Rotatory Instability Is Improved With Combined Flat sMCL and Anteromedial Reconstruction. Am J Sports Med 2022;50(8):2093–101.
45. Miyaji N, Holthof SR, Ball SV, et al. Medial Collateral Ligament Reconstruction for Anteromedial Instability of the Knee: A Biomechanical Study In Vitro. Am J Sports Med 2022;50(7):1823–31.

46. Ball S, Stephen JM, El-Daou H, et al. The medial ligaments and the ACL restrain anteromedial laxity of the knee. Knee Surg Sports Traumatol Arthrosc 2020; 28(12):3700–8.
47. Kim SJ, Choi DH, Hwang BY. The influence of posterolateral rotatory instability on ACL reconstruction: comparison between isolated ACL reconstruction and ACL reconstruction combined with posterolateral corner reconstruction. J Bone Joint Surg Am 2012;94(3):253–9.
48. Bonanzinga T, Zaffagnini S, Grassi A, et al. Management of Combined Anterior Cruciate Ligament-Posterolateral Corner Tears: A Systematic Review. Am J Sports Med 2014;42(6):1496–503.
49. Miller MD, Kew ME, Quinn CA. Anterior Cruciate Ligament Revision Reconstruction. J Am Acad Orthop Surg 2021;29(17):723–31.
50. Mitchell JJ, Chahla J, Dean CS, et al. Outcomes After 1-Stage Versus 2-Stage Revision Anterior Cruciate Ligament Reconstruction. Am J Sports Med 2017; 45(8):1790–8.
51. Schliemann B, Treder M, Schulze M, et al. Influence of Different Tibial Fixation Techniques on Initial Stability in Single-Stage Anterior Cruciate Ligament Revision With Confluent Tibial Tunnels: A Biomechanical Laboratory Study. Arthroscopy 2016;32(1):78–89.
52. Mathew C, Palmer JE, Lambert BS, et al. Single-stage versus two-stage revision anterior cruciate ligament reconstruction: a systematic review. Journal of ISAKOS 2018;3(6):345–51.
53. Sarraj M, de Sa D, Shanmugaraj A, et al. Over-the-top ACL reconstruction yields comparable outcomes to traditional ACL reconstruction in primary and revision settings: a systematic review. Knee Surg Sports Traumatol Arthrosc 2019;27(2): 427–44.
54. Melby A, Ewing JW. Arthroscopic Anterior Cruciate Ligament Reconstruction: Over-the-Top Techniques. In: Chow JCY, editor. Advanced arthroscopy. New York: Springer; 2001. p. 435–46.
55. Nagai K, Rothrauff BB, Li RT, et al. Over-the-top ACL reconstruction restores anterior and rotatory knee laxity in skeletally immature individuals and revision settings. Knee Surg Sports Traumatol Arthrosc 2020;28(2):538–43.
56. Kamei G, Nakamae A, Ishikawa M, et al. Equivalent outcomes of ACL revision with over-the-top single and double-bundle reconstruction using hamstring tendon compared to anatomical single and double-bundle reconstruction. Journal of Experimental Orthopaedics 2022;9(1):33.
57. Musahl V, Getgood A, Neyret P, et al. Contributions of the anterolateral complex and the anterolateral ligament to rotatory knee stability in the setting of ACL Injury: a roundtable discussion. Knee Surg Sports Traumatol Arthrosc 2017;25(4): 997–1008.
58. Inderhaug E, Stephen JM, Williams A, et al. Anterolateral Tenodesis or Anterolateral Ligament Complex Reconstruction: Effect of Flexion Angle at Graft Fixation When Combined With ACL Reconstruction. Am J Sports Med 2017;45(13): 3089–97.
59. Alm L, Drenck TC, Frosch KH, et al. Lateral extra-articular tenodesis in patients with revision anterior cruciate ligament (ACL) reconstruction and high-grade anterior knee instability. Knee 2020;27(5):1451–7.
60. Grassi A, Zicaro JP, Costa-Paz M, et al. Good mid-term outcomes and low rates of residual rotatory laxity, complications and failures after revision anterior cruciate ligament reconstruction (ACL) and lateral extra-articular tenodesis (LET). Knee Surg Sports Traumatol Arthrosc 2020;28(2):418–31.

61. Keizer MNJ, Brouwer RW, de Graaff F, et al. Higher return to pre-injury type of sports after revision anterior ligament reconstruction with lateral extra-articular tenodesis compared to without lateral extra-articular tenodesis. Knee Surg Sports Traumatol Arthrosc 2022. https://doi.org/10.1007/s00167-022-07018-y.
62. Saithna A, Monaco E, Carrozzo A, et al. Anterior Cruciate Ligament Revision Plus Lateral Extra-Articular Procedure Results in Superior Stability and Lower Failure Rates Than Does Isolated Anterior Cruciate Ligament Revision but Shows No Difference in Patient-Reported Outcomes or Return to Sports. Arthroscopy 2023; 39(4):1088–98.
63. Dejour D, Saffarini M, Demey G, et al. Tibial slope correction combined with second revision ACL produces good knee stability and prevents graft rupture. Knee Surg Sports Traumatol Arthrosc 2015;23(10):2846–52.
64. Akoto R, Alm L, Drenck TC, et al. Slope-Correction Osteotomy with Lateral Extra-articular Tenodesis and Revision Anterior Cruciate Ligament Reconstruction Is Highly Effective in Treating High-Grade Anterior Knee Laxity. Am J Sports Med 2020;48(14):3478–85.
65. Vivacqua T, Thomassen S, Winkler PW, et al. Closing-Wedge Posterior Tibial Slope-Reducing Osteotomy in Complex Revision ACL Reconstruction. Orthop J Sports Med 2023;11(1). 23259671221144786.
66. Song GY, Ni QK, Zheng T, et al. Slope-Reducing Tibial Osteotomy Combined With Primary Anterior Cruciate Ligament Reconstruction Produces Improved Knee Stability in Patients With Steep Posterior Tibial Slope, Excessive Anterior Tibial Subluxation in Extension, and Chronic Meniscal Posterior Horn Tears. Am J Sports Med 2020;48(14):3486–94.
67. Cantin O, Magnussen RA, Corbi F, et al. The role of high tibial osteotomy in the treatment of knee laxity: a comprehensive review. Knee Surg Sports Traumatol Arthrosc 2015;23(10):3026–37.
68. Imhoff FB, Comer B, Obopilwe E, et al. Effect of Slope and Varus Correction High Tibial Osteotomy in the ACL-Deficient and ACL-Reconstructed Knee on Kinematics and ACL Graft Force: A Biomechanical Analysis. Am J Sports Med 2021;49(2):410–6.
69. Stride D, Wang J, Horner NS, et al. Indications and outcomes of simultaneous high tibial osteotomy and ACL reconstruction. Knee Surg Sports Traumatol Arthrosc 2019;27(4):1320–31.
70. Schneider A, Gaillard R, Gunst S, et al. Combined ACL reconstruction and opening wedge high tibial osteotomy at 10-year follow-up: excellent laxity control but uncertain return to high level sport. Knee Surg Sports Traumatol Arthrosc 2020; 28(3):960–8.
71. Andriolo L, Filardo G, Kon E, et al. Revision anterior cruciate ligament reconstruction: clinical outcome and evidence for return to sport. Knee Surg Sports Traumatol Arthrosc 2015;23(10):2825–45.
72. Glogovac G, Schumaier AP, Grawe BM. Return to Sport Following Revision Anterior Cruciate Ligament Reconstruction in Athletes: A Systematic Review. Arthroscopy 2019;35(7):2222–30.
73. Wright RW, Gill CS, Chen L, et al. Outcome of revision anterior cruciate ligament reconstruction: a systematic review. J Bone Joint Surg Am 2012;94(6):531–6.
74. Ouillette R, Edmonds E, Chambers H, et al. Outcomes of Revision Anterior Cruciate Ligament Surgery in Adolescents. Am J Sports Med 2019;47(6):1346–52.

Complications in Anterior Cruciate Ligament Surgery and How to Avoid Them

Nyaluma N. Wagala, MD, Gabrielle Fatora, MD,
Cortez Brown, MD, Bryson P. Lesniak, MD*

KEYWORDS

• ACL • Complications • ACL reconstruction

KEY POINTS

- Complications following anterior cruciate ligament reconstruction (ACL-R) can include arthrofibrosis, residual instability, graft failure, and infection.
- Thorough physical examinations and accurate diagnosis are key to avoid missing any concomitant injuries which can lead to residual laxity and possible graft failure.
- During ACL-R, surgeons should be aware of techniques for proper graft harvest, tunnel placement, and graft fixation to best restore native knee biomechanics while avoiding impingement and infection.

INTRODUCTION

Successful anterior cruciate ligament (ACL) reconstruction (ACL-R) involves restoring native knee biomechanics that can allow patients to return to desired activities and sport. Beginning at time of initial evaluation, surgeons are responsible for navigating patients throughout the treatment course as complications can occur at any time point. ACL-R has continued to advance over the years leading to improved patient clinical outcomes. Despite this, the risk of complications following ACL-R such as arthrofibrosis, graft failure, and infection persists and can drastically change patient outcomes and need for revision surgery. Therefore, it is important for surgeons to understand how to identify, address, and avoid these complications. The goal of this article is to summarize complications following ACL-R and identify critical steps to reduce the risk of complications during the preoperative, intraoperative, and postoperative stages.

Department of Orthopaedic Surgery, University of Pittsburgh, Pittsburgh, PA, USA
* Corresponding author. University of Pittsburgh, UPMC Freddie Fu Sports Medicine Center, 3200 South Water Street, Pittsburgh, PA 15203.
E-mail address: lesniakbp@upmc.edu

Clin Sports Med 43 (2024) 465–477
https://doi.org/10.1016/j.csm.2023.08.009
sportsmed.theclinics.com
0278-5919/24/

PREOPERATIVE EVALUATION

Avoiding postoperative complications starts during the initial patient evaluation as surgical timing and concomitant injuries can impact clinical outcomes. To minimize risk of complications such as graft failure, recurrent instability, or arthrofibrosis, surgeons must recognize the importance of detailed patient examination, surgical technique, and appropriate rehabilitation.

When evaluating patients with an ACL tear, it is important to complete a thorough examination as concomitant injuries are common and can be missed. Several studies have reported an incidence of concomitant meniscal tears to be as high as 82%.[1–3] Lateral meniscal tears are more commonly associated with acute ACL injuries, while medial meniscus tears tend to be present in chronic ACL injuries.[4,5] Clinical examination may be positive for joint line tenderness and positive McMurray's or Thessaly's testing.[6] Recent studies have shown that posteromedial meniscus lesions, also known as ramp lesions, are common following acute ACL tear with an incidence of roughly 25%.[7] Patients are 3 times more likely to have a ramp lesion if the injury mechanism was due to direct contact.[7] If missed, patients are at risk for persistent and abnormal knee laxity.[7] Although MRI is a useful tool that can identify meniscal pathology, there is a high false-negative rate. Therefore, probing of the menisci during diagnostic arthroscopy is vital to rule out pathology.[8] Using the traditional anteromedial and anterolateral portals may be sufficient for diagnosis; however, the posteromedial portal may be beneficial to successfully identify a ramp lesion.[9–11] Additionally, the modified Gilquist view can be used to visualize the integrity of the posterior meniscocapsular junction and posterior cruciate ligament (PCL) as well as identifying any loose bodies. This typically involves using the anterolateral or anteromedial portal and passing the arthroscope between the medial femoral condyle and PCL to visualize the posterior structures.[12] If a meniscus tear is identified, the surgeon must decide whether it is necessary to address the pathology and choose the appropriate intervention whether that be repair or meniscectomy.

Medial collateral ligament (MCL) tears are also commonly associated with ACL tears occurring in up to 35% of ACL injuries.[1,13] If not diagnosed and addressed, patients can experience persistent knee pain and valgus instability, therefore increasing the risk of ACL-R graft failure.[6] Therefore, a thorough history and a physical examination including valgus stress testing can evaluate for concomitant MCL injuries and subsequently lead to adequate management. Most commonly, treatment involves bracing to allow for the MCL to heal prior to ACL-R with subsequent rehabilitation prior to ACL-R to avoid postoperative arthrofibrosis.[14] Posterolateral corner (PLC) injuries are also associated with ACL tears, can be subtle, and should not be missed on clinical examination.[15,16] The PLC is composed of 3 static stabilizing structures: fibular collateral ligament, popliteus tendon, and the popliteofibular ligament. If not diagnosed initially, patients are at risk for persistent varus or rotational instability and have an increased risk of ACL graft failure.[6] The dial test can help surgeons rule out a PLC injury. This involves externally rotating the patient's lower leg at 30° of knee flexion and if there is a 10° increase in external rotation compared with the uninjured knee then one should be concerned for a possible PLC injury.[17] The pivot shift test is another important examination to perform as it can identify increased rotatory laxity which may suggest the presence of injury to lateral structures such as the lateral meniscus, IT band, and anterolateral capsule.[18] If a high-grade pivot shift is encountered, this may help the surgeon to decide to supplement ACL-R with a lateral extra-articular tenodesis or anterolateral ligament reconstruction as these patients are high risk for postoperative residual laxity.

After a complete assessment of the knee has been made, the next step is to figure out when to proceed with surgical reconstruction. In the past, there has been controversy regarding timing of surgery following an acute ACL tear. Recent studies have shown that delayed surgery may help avoid postoperative stiffness.[19] However, the literature also supports that delayed ACL-R may increase the risk of developing subsequent meniscal injury and osteoarthritis. Various studies have investigated the ideal time for surgical management post-injury; however, there is no consensus. The state of the patient's knee may be the best indicator of when to interventive following an acute injury. If the patient presents with decreased range of motion (ROM) and a tense effusion, then there is a role for preoperative rehabilitation and delaying reconstruction until the acute inflammatory phase has improved.[20] However, studies exist that compare acute (within 48 hours) and delayed (inflammation free phase) ACL-R that demonstrate no significant difference between groups regarding postoperative ROM.[21] There is also literature that concluded that waiting greater than 3 months following injury can increase risk of damage to the articular cartilage and/or menisci. Therefore, surgeons must use their best judgment in regard to surgical timing. It is our practice to address an acute ACL injury within 3 months when possible once the patient has restored ROM and reasonable soft tissues, but this can vary based on both surgeon and patient preference and all treatment should be a shared decision before moving forward.

INTRAOPERATIVE COMPLICATIONS

Graft Harvest

Graft harvest complications vary based on the specific autograft being used. Premature graft amputation or harvesting an insufficient graft can occur with both hamstring and quadriceps autograft harvest; however, this can be avoided by using caution and proper technique. With hamstring autografts, it is essential to release all fascial and soft tissue bands and assess for anomalous tendon insertions prior to harvesting the tendons.[22] Any fold or irregularity in the appearance of the tendon can indicate there are remaining tethers on the hamstring tendon. Further, prior to the surgeon stripping the hamstring tendon, she or he should pull the tendon to be stripped in line with the muscle and watch for any corresponding gastrocnemius movement. The hamstring tendon will cause the gastrocnemius to contract or move if any tethers remain. Typically, the gracilis tendon has 1 large fascial band, whereas the semitendinosus tendon has 2. Identifying and excising these can minimize the risk of premature amputation of the hamstring tendon as the stripper gets caught by the divergent path of the fascial band. Approximately 12 cm of tendon should be free to complete the harvest.[23,24] The hamstring stripper should be applied with constant pressure in line with the tendon while applying countertraction on the tendon.[6]

The most common complication with quadriceps tendon harvest is inadequate graft length. For an all soft-tissue quadriceps graft, it is recommended to harvest from the lateral aspect of the tendon as this side is longer than the medial aspect. The arthroscopic camera can also be used to visualize the proximal extent of the tendon so that an appropriate trajectory can be determined. Similar to hamstring harvest, if a stripping device is used, an inadequate graft can be harvested if the graft is not completely prepared prior to final harvest. Care must be taken to appropriately sharply dissect the quadriceps tendon graft prior to stripping the tendon.

Patella fractures following graft harvest are rare with reported rates ranging up to 2%.[25] This may occur intraoperatively or postoperatively. Despite the rare occurrence, surgeons must pay attention when harvesting a bone-patellar tendon-bone (BPTB) graft or quadriceps tendon graft with bone block. One retrospective study looked at 618 patients who underwent ACL-R with BPTB graft and reported that 8 patients (1.3%) sustained patella fractures. These fractures were identified at a mean of 2 months postoperatively. Of the 8 patients, 5 subsequently underwent surgical fixation of the patella due to fracture displacement. All patients eventually healed their patella fractures and had Lysholm scores ranging from 77 to 98. Despite having good to excellent subjective outcome scores, it is important to note that 4 patients underwent subsequent removal of hardware and 2 patients expressed that the patella fractures had a significant impact on their postoperative progress.[25] Therefore, surgeons must be careful when harvesting the bone block. For BPTB, it is recommended that the bone block should not be more than 10 mm in width and limited to 20 to 30 mm in length or a length that does not pass the middle of the patella height. Additionally, the bone block should not extend more than one-third of the patellar depth.[26] Bone graft can be used based on surgeon preference but should be highly considered in patients with harvest sites wider than 10 mm and deeper than 6 mm.[27] For quad tendon harvest, the bone block should be harvested from the central portion of the patella because a more eccentric position can result in an inadequate remaining bony bridge leading to fracture risk.[23,28]

In regard to neurovascular injuries, the infrapatellar branch of the saphenous nerve (IPBSN) is the most common nerve injured during ACL-R, and is more commonly seen with hamstring autograft harvest. IPBSN injury has been reported in as high as 88% of hamstring autograft cases. Use of an oblique or horizontal incision rather than a vertical incision can minimize the risk of nerve injury.[29] It may also be useful to mark the incision prior to prepping as the pes insertion can be more easily palpated without gloves on.[30] Care should be taken to identify and protect the IPBSN when possible. Additionally, hemarthrosis is an uncommon complication that can lead to joint effusion and arthrofibrosis which may delay a patient's progress in postoperative rehabilitation.[31,32] Adequate hemostasis should be obtained intra-articularly and at the graft donor site prior to closure to help avoid this. Compartment syndrome is another rare complication that may be encountered likely due to extravasation of arthroscopic fluid into the lower leg compartments.[33,34] Although rare, surgeons should be aware of prolonged operative times and should perform immediate postoperative examination of the operative leg to assess the compartments as this is a detrimental complication that would necessitate urgent fasciotomies.

Proper handling of the graft is critical as graft contamination may occur at any point during ACL-R and is a potentially devastating complication. This can involve contact with a nonsterile object during handling or dropping the graft on the floor. Although graft contamination is not a frequent occurrence, one study showed that 25% of surgeons had experienced graft contamination at least once in their career.[35] Implanting a contaminated graft can result in postoperative septic arthritis. To avoid contaminating the graft, careful handling and minimizing handoffs after graft harvest and when transferring between the operating and back table are crucial. Soaking the graft in a vancomycin solution is a technique commonly employed by surgeons, even in cases where obvious contamination has not occurred.[35] Multiple studies have shown promising results in the reduction of rates of postoperative septic arthritis when grafts are soaked in vancomycin by routine.

When a graft is directly contaminated, a decision must be made to sterilize the graft and implant it or discard the graft and either proceed with harvesting of a new autograft or transition to an allograft. If this situation arises, it is recommended that the surgeon should disclose this information and obtain informed consent prior to proceeding with the reconstruction. It is the senior author's practice to obtain consent for possible allograft usage for every ACL-R performed from the patient preoperatively to prevent a pause in the surgery to obtain familial consent once the patient is under anesthesia. Given the morbidity of a second autograft harvest and the preference for autograft over allograft in many cases, it is important to understand effective graft sterilization techniques. Studies have shown that both 2% and 4% chlorhexidine solutions are highly effective with higher success rates than normal saline or povidone-iodine solutions.[36]

Tunnel Placement

Tunnel malposition is the most common technical reason for ACL-R failure and arthrofibrosis. Therefore, it is important to understand the correct placement of both the femoral and tibial tunnels, as well as techniques to avoid improper placement. The femoral tunnel should be centered slightly posterior to the lateral bifurcate ridge, approximately 2.5 mm anterior to the posterior articular cartilage[37] (**Fig. 1**). A tunnel that is too vertical will not restore rotational stability and functional instability may persist. If the femoral tunnel is placed too anteriorly, the knee may be tight in flexion and the graft may impinge in extension and result in stiffness or rupture. To avoid femoral tunnel malposition, it is crucial to have adequate visualization of the medial wall of the lateral femoral condyle, including the posterior wall and resident's ridge. This can be achieved by thorough debridement of the remnant ACL tissue. Notchplasty is also an option to improve visualization, although we find this to never be necessary.[6] Rather, we use visualization of the insertion from the medial and lateral portals or via a 70° arthroscope. Another alternative is to create an accessory medial portal from which to visualize the insertion while drilling through the standard medial portal. Drilling the femoral tunnel via a portal rather than transtibial is thought to allow for creation of a less vertical tunnel.[24] There are a variety of guides that can be used to ensure appropriate femoral tunnel placement and reduce risk of posterior wall blowout; however, tunnel malposition is still possible with use of these guides.[6] To avoid drilling a malpositioned tunnel, the tentative tunnel placement can be marked using a guide or an awl and that position should then be assessed from both anteromedial and anterolateral portals (**Fig. 2**).

Posterior wall blowout is a complication that may be seen when drilling the femoral tunnel. Prior to drilling, the surgeon should clear off the posterior condylar wall of all

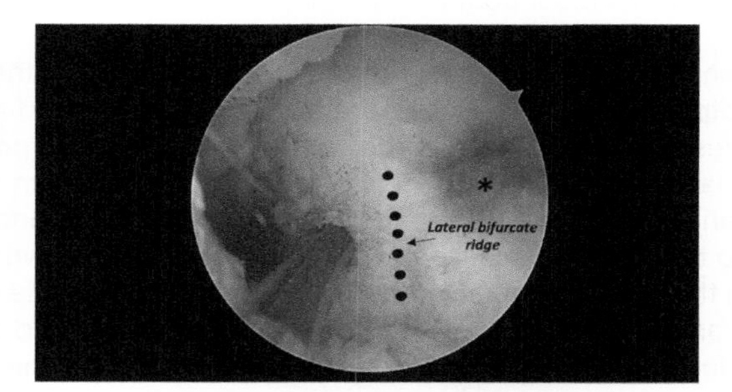

Fig. 1. Femoral tunnel placement is typically just centered slightly posterior to the lateral bifurcate ridge (*dotted line*) and approximately 2.5 mm anterior to the posterior articular cartilage. Anterior to the bifurcate ridge is a previously misplaced anterior femoral tunnel (*asterisk*).

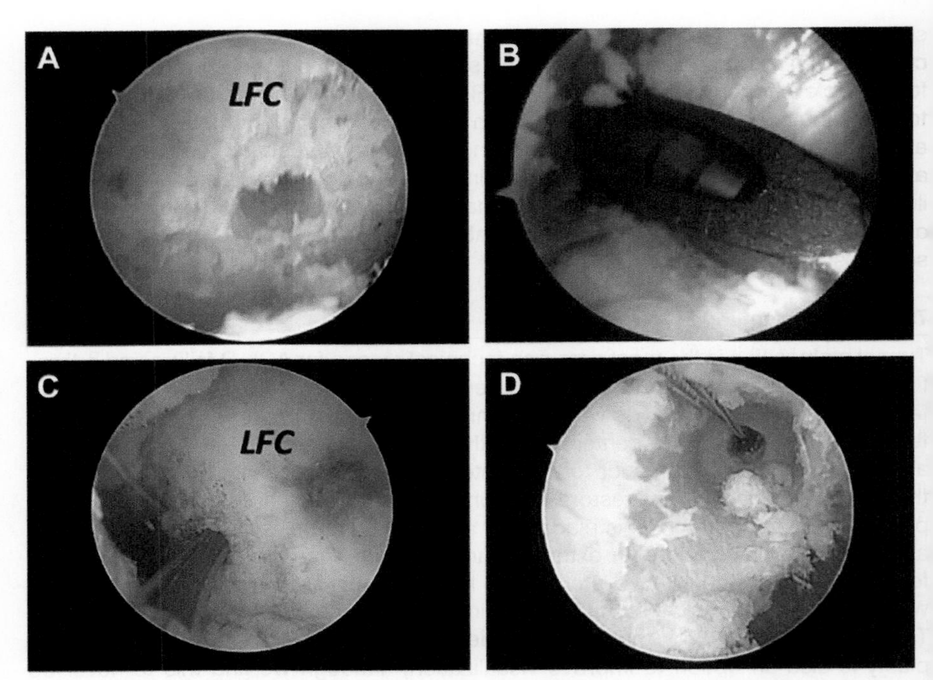

Fig. 2. Anatomic femoral tunnel drilling for ACL reconstruction. (*A*) Arthroscopic view of the lateral femoral condyle with femoral tunnel position marked using a curved awl. (*B*) A flexible guidewire is advanced with the knee in hyperflexion to mark the native footprint of the ACL prior to drilling the tunnel. (*C*) The flexible guidewire is in place slightly posterior to the lateral bifurcate ridge. (*D*) The femoral tunnel with intact posterior wall. ACL, anterior cruciate ligament; LFC, lateral femoral condyle.

soft tissue so that the edge can be easily identified. Placing the knee in greater than 70° of flexion also helps to decrease the risk of compromise of the posterior wall.[24] If the posterior wall is compromised, the ability to secure the graft with aperture fixation is compromised. In this circumstance the graft can be reliably fixed on the femoral side with either a suspensory device on the lateral cortex such as a fixed or adjustable loop button or with a bicortical post and washer placed through a distal and lateral thigh incision.

There have been several studies detailing the optimal position of the tibial tunnel. If the soft tissue footprint remains intact, the tunnel should be centered within that location. If it is not present, tibial tunnel can be in a line even with the posterior edge of anterior horn of lateral meniscus, which is approximately 15 mm anterior to the PCL, and between the intercondylar eminences.[37] A second method is to measure 9 mm posterior to the intermeniscal ligament, which has been shown to be more accurate in locating the anatomic tibial footprint.[38] A tibial tunnel that is too anterior will be tight in flexion and impinge in extension, leading to increased load on the graft and increased risk of failure. If the tibial tunnel is placed too posterior, the graft should be relatively vertical, conferring less rotational stability. There may also be impingement with the PCL. To avoid a malpositioned tibial tunnel, use anatomic landmarks to place the drill guide in the proper position.[6] A high anterolateral portal can aid in visualization of these landmarks.[37]

Graft impingement may be caused by malpositioned tunnels or implantation of a graft larger than the notch. Anterior tibial tunnels may cause roof impingement while a tunnel that is too lateral causes impingement along the intercondylar wall and one that is too medial will cause impingement on the PCL. Preoperatively, the notch can be accurately estimated measured via MRI measurement so that a graft of appropriate width is harvested.[39] If impingement is noted after graft fixation, a notchplasty can be performed to increase the space available for the graft and prevent postoperative complications.

Graft Fixation

Screw-tunnel divergence is another intraoperative complication that can lead to failure after ACL-R. When using a BPTB graft, an interference screw is often placed intra-articularly at the femoral tunnel to secure the graft. Studies have demonstrated that greater than a 15-degree difference between the trajectory of the tunnel and the interference screw results in decreased pullout strength and can ultimately lead to loss of graft fixation.[40] To avoid this complication, a guidewire can be placed in the femoral tunnel with the interference screw placed over this to ensure the proper trajectory and minimize screw-tunnel divergence (**Fig. 3**). Hyperflexion of the knee will make placing the guide wire easier and will also allow advancement of the wire so that the true trajectory of the tunnel is matched by the wire. Another technique to minimize screw-tunnel divergence is to use an inferomedial accessory portal for improved instrument positioning.[24]

Graft-tunnel mismatch is a complication that is seen mainly with BPTB grafts when the length of the graft is longer or shorter than the intra-articular graft distance combined with the femoral and tibial tunnel lengths. If a graft that is too long is passed, there will be protrusion of the bone plug from tibial tunnel that makes tibial fixation more difficult. This may be seen more frequently with anteromedial portal drilling as tunnels tend to be shorter from this approach. To avoid graft-tunnel mismatch, it is crucial to know the length of the harvested BPTB graft prior to drilling femoral or tibial tunnels so that adjustments can be made to tunnel length. For example, a steeper drilling angle for the tibial tunnel will result in a slightly longer tunnel.[41] Alternatively, a technique that can be employed for a long graft involves drilling or burring a deeper trough in the tibia adjacent to the tibial tunnel that the graft can be placed in and then fixed with a staple or screw. Some adjustments can be made to the graft as well. The graft can be effectively shortened by flipping the bone block back onto the adjacent tendon. This method will require larger tunnel diameters to pass the graft.[23] The distal bone plug can also be removed to create a shorter graft and then

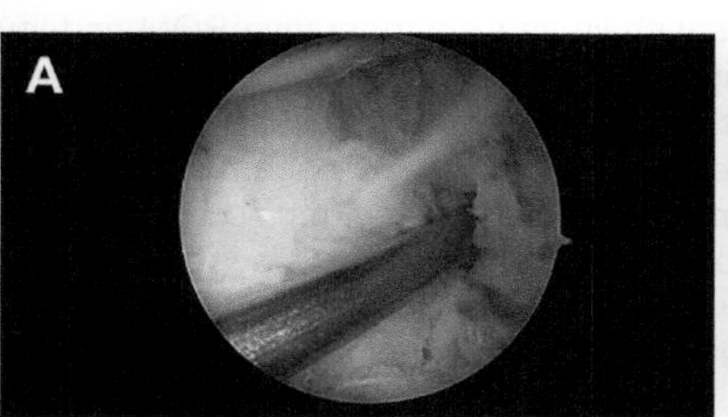

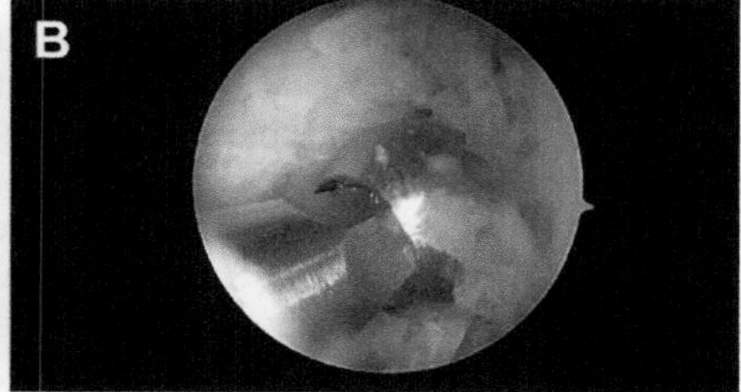

Fig. 3. Fixation of femoral tunnel with interference screw. (*A*) Arthroscopic view of the guidewire in place in femoral tunnel just anterior to ACL graft. (*B*) Interference screw is placed over the guidewire and advanced into the femoral tunnel to fix the ACL graft in place. ACL, anterior cruciate ligament; LFC, lateral femoral condyle.

fixation can be achieved with a soft-tissue interference screw or a bicortical screw and washer.

POSTOPERATIVE COMPLICATIONS

Arthrofibrosis

Arthrofibrosis is one of the more common and impactful postoperative complications following ACL-R. The current literature has reported rates ranging from 2% to 38% following ACL-R.[42–44] A specific definition of arthrofibrosis does not exist; however, it is essentially a significant loss of motion or stiffness of the knee joint. Some studies define it as ROM loss compared with the contralateral knee, presence of a cyclops lesion on MRI with ROM loss, and others use the objective criteria such as more than 5° of extension deficit and less than 90° of flexion.[19,42] Postoperative knee stiffness can lead to limited knee function, delayed return to sport, and can increase the risk of post-traumatic osteoarthritis after ACL-R.[45] Female sex and concomitant ligament or meniscus surgery are known risk factors for arthrofibrosis.[42,43] Additionally, common causes of arthrofibrosis are tunnel malposition, limited preoperative ROM, and an insufficient postoperative rehabilitation program.

Several studies suggested that delayed intervention for an ACL tear may lead to better postoperative ROM.[46,47] One retrospective study looking at 169 patients with acute ACL tears divided patients into groups based on early (0–7 days from injury) or delayed surgery (>7 days) with all patients participating in a conventional or accelerated postoperative rehabilitation program. The accelerated program emphasized early ROM, muscle control, functional exercise, and immediate weight bearing. Patients who underwent delayed surgery had significantly more postoperative ROM compared with the other groups. It is thought this "delayed" period prior to surgery can be used for preoperative physical therapy to regain ROM and improve patient outcomes following surgery. However, there continues to be controversy as recent studies have shown that a combination of modern ACL-R techniques with an accelerated rehabilitation protocol led to no difference in postoperative stiffness when comparing acute versus delayed surgical reconstruction.[48–50] One randomized control trial compared postoperative ROM in acute (within 21 days) versus delayed (>6 weeks) ACL-R. Of the 69 patients, there were no significant differences in postoperative ROM, KT-1000 arthrometer differences, or subjective knee evaluations for the 2 groups. Although there is a lack of consensus on ideal timing, it is recommended for surgeons to wait for acute inflammation and effusion to resolve, as well as, ensuring that patients having adequate preoperative ROM prior to proceeding with ACL-R.

Arthrofibrosis can significantly delay patient recovery and function; therefore, surgeons should keep a close eye on patients with limited postoperative ROM as they are at risk for arthrofibrosis. Close follow-up and early intervention in the initial postoperative period is crucial as adjustments to postoperative rehabilitation can be made with the hope to avoid return to the operating room. Management can vary from physical therapy, corticosteroids, drop out cast application, manipulation under anesthesia (MUA), and arthroscopic lysis of adhesions (LOA). If there is concern for arthrofibrosis within the first 3 postoperative months, it is reasonable to start with an aggressive physical therapy regimen. However, if patients show minimal improvement they should be taken to the operating room. Drop out cast application following arthroscopic LOA is more frequently used for improving extension deficits (**Fig. 4**). Flexion loss is more commonly addressed with MUA with arthroscopic LOA. Surgeons often see more improvement in gaining flexion compared with gaining full extension; therefore, one should consider earlier intervention on patients with extension deficits.

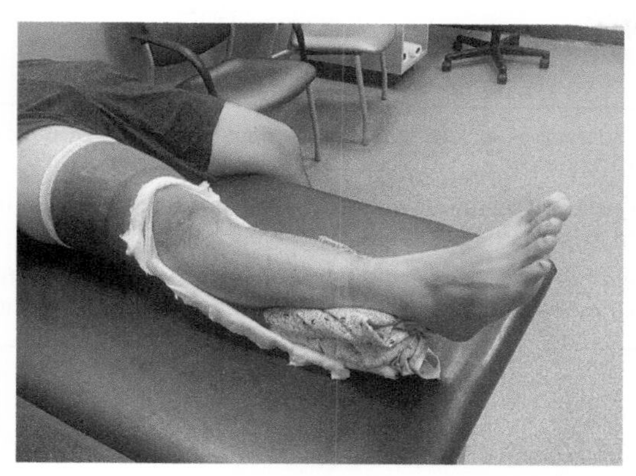

Fig. 4. Drop out cast. The anterior aspect of the cylindrical cast from the knee down is removed and towels are placed underneath the heal to allow for knee to be pushed into full extension.

Infection

Postoperative infection following ACL-R is a rare occurrence with rates ranging up to 2%.[51–53] It has been demonstrated that hamstring autograft has a higher infection rate when compared with other autografts.[54] If concerned for septic arthritis, clinical work-up should include inflammatory labs including white blood cell count, erythrocyte sedimentation rate, C-reactive protein, and joint aspiration. Joint fluid should be sent for cell count and culture. Work-up should be done in a timely manner as septic arthritis warrants urgent surgical intervention to minimize cartilage damage and maintain graft function. The most common pathogen encountered following ACL-R is coagulase-negative Staphylococci.[52,53] The current consensus in the literature is to proceed with either arthroscopic or open irrigation and debridement with graft preservation and antibiotic treatment. If the graft quality is poor at time of surgery or if there is worsening clinical examination following initial debridement, then one should consider graft and hardware removal to help eradicate infection.[52,55] Although infection is rare, it can be detrimental following ACL-R; therefore, surgeons should take care to maintain a sterile field and avoid contamination of instruments and the graft.[6] Additionally, providing patients with strict instructions regarding postoperative wound care management can be beneficial.

SUMMARY

Complications following ACL-R can include arthrofibrosis, residual instability, graft failure, and infection. Although many of these complications are infrequent, they are detrimental to the patient and often lead to inferior clinical outcomes and cause delay in return to baseline function or sport. Surgeons should not only know how to address these complications, but how to avoid them. Thorough physical examination and accurate diagnosis are key to avoid missing any concomitant injuries that can lead to residual laxity and possible graft failure. During ACL-R, surgeons should be aware of techniques for proper graft harvest, tunnel placement, and graft fixation to best restore native knee biomechanics while avoiding impingement and infection. In conclusion, a successful ACL-R without complications requires surgeons to be attentive starting during the clinical evaluation in the office to the last follow-up visit after return to sport.

CLINICS CARE POINTS

- Identifying and addressing concomitant injuries may help improve patient outcomes and reduce risk of graft failure.
- Graft harvest and appropriate tunnel placement are important steps that if done incorrectly can lead to altered joint mechanics and graft failure.
- Decreased preoperative ROM increased the risk for postoperative arthrofibrosis; therefore, surgeons should consider preoperative rehabilitation to avoid this complication.

REFERENCES

1. Borchers JR, Kaeding CC, Pedroza AD, et al. Intra-articular findings in primary and revision anterior cruciate ligament reconstruction surgery: a comparison of the MOON and MARS study groups. Am J Sports Med 2011;39(9):1889–93.
2. Hagino T, Ochiai S, Senga S, et al. Meniscal tears associated with anterior cruciate ligament injury. Arch Orthop Trauma Surg 2015;135(12):1701–6.
3. Musahl V, Karlsson J. Anterior Cruciate Ligament Tear. N Engl J Med 2019;380(24):2341–8.
4. Kilcoyne KG, Dickens JF, Haniuk E, et al. Epidemiology of meniscal injury associated with ACL tears in young athletes. Orthopedics 2012;35(3):208–12.
5. Cipolla M, Scala A, Gianni E, et al. Different patterns of meniscal tears in acute anterior cruciate ligament (ACL) ruptures and in chronic ACL-deficient knees. Classification, staging and timing of treatment. Knee Surg Sports Traumatol Arthrosc 1995;3(3):130–4.
6. Tjoumakaris FP, Herz-Brown AL, Bowers AL, et al. Complications in brief: Anterior cruciate ligament reconstruction. Clin Orthop Relat Res 2012;470(2):630–6.
7. Seil R, Mouton C, Coquay J, et al. Ramp lesions associated with ACL injuries are more likely to be present in contact injuries and complete ACL tears. Knee Surg Sports Traumatol Arthrosc 2018;26(4):1080–5.
8. Rodriguez AN, LaPrade RF, Geeslin AG. Combined Meniscus Repair and Anterior Cruciate Ligament Reconstruction. Arthroscopy 2022;38(3):670–2.
9. Liu X, Feng H, Zhang H, et al. Arthroscopic prevalence of ramp lesion in 868 patients with anterior cruciate ligament injury. Am J Sports Med 2011;39(4):832–7.
10. Ahn JH, Kim SH, Yoo JC, et al. All-inside suture technique using two posteromedial portals in a medial meniscus posterior horn tear. Arthroscopy 2004;20(1):101–8.
11. Bollen SR. Posteromedial meniscocapsular injury associated with rupture of the anterior cruciate ligament: a previously unrecognised association. J Bone Joint Surg Br 2010;92(2):222–3.
12. Lee JY, Chia ZY, Jiang L, et al. A Review of the Gillquist Maneuver: Modifications for a Safer and Easily Reproducible Approach for Knee Transintercondylar Notch Posterior Compartment Arthroscopy. Arthrosc Tech 2020;9(4):e435–8.
13. Ateschrang A, Döbele S, Freude T, et al. Acute MCL and ACL injuries: first results of minimal-invasive MCL ligament bracing with combined ACL single-bundle reconstruction. Arch Orthop Trauma Surg 2016;136(9):1265–72.
14. Petersen W, Laprell H. Combined injuries of the medial collateral ligament and the anterior cruciate ligament. Early ACL reconstruction versus late ACL reconstruction. Arch Orthop Trauma Surg 1999;119(5–6):258–62.

15. Dean RS, LaPrade RF. ACL and Posterolateral Corner Injuries. Curr Rev Musculoskelet Med 2020;13(1):123–32.
16. LaPrade RF, Wentorf FA, Fritts H, et al. A prospective magnetic resonance imaging study of the incidence of posterolateral and multiple ligament injuries in acute knee injuries presenting with a hemarthrosis. Arthroscopy 2007;23(12):1341–7.
17. Krause DA, Levy BA, Shah JP, et al. Reliability of the dial test using a handheld inclinometer. Knee Surg Sports Traumatol Arthrosc 2013;21(5):1011–6.
18. Tanaka M, Vyas D, Moloney G, et al. What does it take to have a high-grade pivot shift? Knee Surg Sports Traumatol Arthrosc 2012;20(4):737–42.
19. Shelbourne KD, Wilckens JH, Mollabashy A, et al. Arthrofibrosis in acute anterior cruciate ligament reconstruction. The effect of timing of reconstruction and rehabilitation. Am J Sports Med 1991;19(4):332–6.
20. Wasilewski SA, Covall DJ, Cohen S. Effect of surgical timing on recovery and associated injuries after anterior cruciate ligament reconstruction. Am J Sports Med 1993;21(3):338–42.
21. Herbst E, Hoser C, Gföller P, et al. Impact of surgical timing on the outcome of anterior cruciate ligament reconstruction. Knee Surg Sports Traumatol Arthrosc 2017;25(2):569–77.
22. Miller MD. PROCEDURE 18 - Single-Bundle Anterior Cruciate Ligament Reconstruction. In: Miller MD, Cole BJ, Cosgarea AJ, et al, editors. Opertaive Techniques: sports knee surgery. Philadelphia: W.B. Saunders; 2008. p. 279–97.
23. Battaglia TC. Management of Intraoperative Graft-related Challenges in Anterior Cruciate Ligament Reconstruction. J Am Acad Orthop Surg 2022;30(10):448–56.
24. Heard WM, Chahal J, Bach BR Jr. Recognizing and managing complications in ACL reconstruction. Sports Med Arthrosc Rev 2013;21(2):106–12.
25. Stein DA, Hunt SA, Rosen JE, et al. The incidence and outcome of patella fractures after anterior cruciate ligament reconstruction. Arthroscopy 2002;18(6):578–83.
26. Malek MM, Kunkle KL, Knable KR. Intraoperative complications of arthroscopically assisted ACL reconstruction using patellar tendon autograft. Instr Course Lect 1996;45:297–302.
27. Benson ER, Barnett PR. A delayed transverse avulsion fracture of the superior pole of the patella after anterior cruciate ligament reconstruction. Arthroscopy 1998;14(1):85–8.
28. Fu FH, Rabuck SJ, West RV, et al. Patellar Fractures After the Harvest of a Quadriceps Tendon Autograft With a Bone Block: A Case Series. Orthop J Sports Med 2019;7(3). 2325967119829051.
29. Grassi A, Perdisa F, Samuelsson K, et al. Association between incision technique for hamstring tendon harvest in anterior cruciate ligament reconstruction and the risk of injury to the infra-patellar branch of the saphenous nerve: a meta-analysis. Knee Surg Sports Traumatol Arthrosc 2018;26(8):2410–23.
30. Frank RM, Hamamoto JT, Bernardoni E, et al. ACL Reconstruction Basics: Quadruple (4-Strand) Hamstring Autograft Harvest. Arthrosc Tech 2017;6(4):e1309–13.
31. Karaaslan F, Karaoğlu S, Yurdakul E. Reducing Intra-articular Hemarthrosis After Arthroscopic Anterior Cruciate Ligament Reconstruction by the Administration of Intravenous Tranexamic Acid:A Prospective, Randomized Controlled Trial. Am J Sports Med 2015;43(11):2720–6.
32. Hooiveld M, Roosendaal G, Vianen M, et al. Blood-induced joint damage: longterm effects in vitro and in vivo. J Rheumatol 2003;30(2):339–44.

33. Jerosch J, Castro WH, Geske B. Intracompartmental pressure in the lower extremity after arthroscopic surgery. Acta Orthop Belg 1991;57(2):97–101.
34. Filho JS, Ramos LA, Sayum J, et al. Leg's compartment syndrome after reconstruction of the anterior cruciate ligament: case report. Revista Brasileira de Ortopedia (English Edition) 2011;46(6):730–2.
35. Izquierdo R Jr, Cadet ER, Bauer R, et al. A survey of sports medicine specialists investigating the preferred management of contaminated anterior cruciate ligament grafts. Arthroscopy 2005;21(11):1348–53.
36. Khan M, Rothrauff BB, Merali F, et al. Management of the contaminated anterior cruciate ligament graft. Arthroscopy 2014;30(2):236–44.
37. Burnham JM, Malempati CS, Carpiaux A, et al. Anatomic Femoral and Tibial Tunnel Placement During Anterior Cruciate Ligament Reconstruction: Anteromedial Portal All-Inside and Outside-In Techniques. Arthrosc Tech 2017;6(2):e275–82.
38. Ferretti M, Doca D, Ingham SM, et al. Bony and soft tissue landmarks of the ACL tibial insertion site: an anatomical study. Knee Surg Sports Traumatol Arthrosc 2012;20(1):62–8.
39. Vaswani R, Meredith SJ, Lian J, et al. Intercondylar Notch Measurement During Arthroscopy and on Preoperative Magnetic Resonance Imaging. Arthrosc Tech 2019;8(10):e1263–7.
40. Rodin D, Levy IM. The use of intraoperative fluoroscopy to reduce femoral interference screw divergence during endoscopic anterior cruciate ligament reconstruction. Arthroscopy 2003;19(3):314–7.
41. Wallace M, Bedi A, Lesniak BP, et al. What effect does anterior cruciate ligament tibial guide orientation have on tibial tunnel length? Arthroscopy 2011;27(6):803–8.
42. Ekhtiari S, Horner NS, de Sa D, et al. Arthrofibrosis after ACL reconstruction is best treated in a step-wise approach with early recognition and intervention: a systematic review. Knee Surg Sports Traumatol Arthrosc 2017;25(12):3929–37.
43. Sanders TL, Kremers HM, Bryan AJ, et al. Procedural intervention for arthrofibrosis after ACL reconstruction: trends over two decades. Knee Surg Sports Traumatol Arthrosc 2017;25(2):532–7.
44. Noyes FR, Berrios-Torres S, Barber-Westin SD, et al. Prevention of permanent arthrofibrosis after anterior cruciate ligament reconstruction alone or combined with associated procedures: a prospective study in 443 knees. Knee Surg Sports Traumatol Arthrosc 2000;8(4):196–206.
45. Shelbourne KD, Benner RW, Gray T. Results of Anterior Cruciate Ligament Reconstruction With Patellar Tendon Autografts: Objective Factors Associated With the Development of Osteoarthritis at 20 to 33 Years After Surgery. Am J Sports Med 2017;45(12):2730–8.
46. Harner CD, Irrgang JJ, Paul J, et al. Loss of motion after anterior cruciate ligament reconstruction. Am J Sports Med 1992;20(5):499–506.
47. Shelbourne KD, Johnson GE. Outpatient surgical management of arthrofibrosis after anterior cruciate ligament surgery. Am J Sports Med 1994;22(2):192–7.
48. Barenius B, Ponzer S, Shalabi A, et al. Increased risk of osteoarthritis after anterior cruciate ligament reconstruction: a 14-year follow-up study of a randomized controlled trial. Am J Sports Med 2014;42(5):1049–57.
49. Raviraj A, Anand A, Kodikal G, et al. A comparison of early and delayed arthroscopically-assisted reconstruction of the anterior cruciate ligament using hamstring autograft. J Bone Joint Surg Br 2010;92(4):521–6.
50. Bottoni CR, Liddell TR, Trainor TJ, et al. Postoperative range of motion following anterior cruciate ligament reconstruction using autograft hamstrings: a prospective

randomized clinical trial of early versus delayed reconstructions. Am J Sports Med 2008;36(4):656–62.
51. Eisenberg MT, Block AM, Vopat ML, et al. Rates of Infection After ACL Reconstruction in Pediatric and Adolescent Patients: A MarketScan Database Study of 44,501 Patients. J Pediatr Orthop 2022;42(4):e362–6.
52. Torres-Claramunt R, Pelfort X, Erquicia J, et al. Knee joint infection after ACL reconstruction: prevalence, management and functional outcomes. Knee Surg Sports Traumatol Arthrosc 2013;21(12):2844–9.
53. Wang C, Ao Y, Wang J, et al. Septic arthritis after arthroscopic anterior cruciate ligament reconstruction: a retrospective analysis of incidence, presentation, treatment, and cause. Arthroscopy 2009;25(3):243–9.
54. Maletis GB, Inacio MC, Reynolds S, et al. Incidence of postoperative anterior cruciate ligament reconstruction infections: graft choice makes a difference. Am J Sports Med 2013;41(8):1780–5.
55. Judd D, Bottoni C, Kim D, et al. Infections following arthroscopic anterior cruciate ligament reconstruction. Arthroscopy 2006;22(4):375–84.

Postoperative

Evaluation of Outcomes After Anterior Cruciate Ligament Reconstruction

What We Know, What We Have, and What to Consider

Hana Marmura, BSc, MPT, PhD (candidate)[a,b,c,d],
Dianne M. Bryant, MSc, PhD[a,b,c,d,e,f,*]

KEYWORDS

• Knee • Anterior cruciate ligament • Orthopedic surgery • Outcome measures
• Clinical outcomes • Patient-reported outcomes

KEY POINTS

- The International Classification of Functioning, Disability and Health (ICF model) can guide decision-making around outcome selection for research or clinical purposes.
- The intent of measurement (diagnosis, prognosis, evaluate change) and demonstrated measurement properties (reliability, validity) are key to instrument selection to assess outcomes following ACLR.
- The feasibility of preferred instruments depends on resources (training, cost, time), patient burden, and in the case of research, influence on sample size.
- The feasibility of making definitive conclusions is influenced by selected outcome measures and their effect on sample size requirements.
- Patient-reported measures help communicate activity- and participation-related outcomes but issues related to response shift may limit their usefulness for long-term outcome measurement.

[a] Faculty of Health Sciences, Western University, 1151 Richmond Street, London, ON N6A 5B9, Canada; [b] Fowler Kennedy Sport Medicine Clinic, 3M Centre, 1151 Richmond Street, London, ON N6A 3K7, Canada; [c] Bone and Joint Institute, Western University, The Dr. Sandy Kirkley Centre for Musculoskeletal Research, University Hospital B6-200, London, ON N6G 2V4, Canada; [d] Lawson Research, London Health Sciences Centre, 800 Commissioners Road East, London, ON N6A 5W9, Canada; [e] Schulich School of Medicine and Dentistry, Western University, 1151 Richmond Street, London, ON N6A 5C1, Canada; [f] Department of Health Research Methods, Evidence and Impact, McMaster University, Health Sciences Centre, 2C1280 Main Street West Hamilton, ON L8S 4L8, Canada
* Corresponding author. Western University, Elborn College, Room 1423, 1201 Western Road, London, ON N6G 1H1.
E-mail address: dianne.bryant@uwo.ca

Clin Sports Med 43 (2024) 479–499
https://doi.org/10.1016/j.csm.2023.08.011 sportsmed.theclinics.com

WHAT WE KNOW

Anterior Cruciate Ligament Reconstruction

Anterior cruciate ligament (ACL) injuries and reconstructions (ACLR) are among the most experienced and widely studied orthopedic injuries and surgeries. Although there has been significant advancement in the field, graft ruptures, subsequent knee injuries, persistent laxity, inability to return to pre-injury sporting levels, and development of post-traumatic osteoarthritis (PTOA) continue to be worrying outcomes following ACLR, and further work is required to optimize patient outcomes.[1] To achieve the universal goal of long-term knee health and quality of life for individuals following ACL injury and reconstruction, it is imperative that interventions are evaluated adequately, and outcomes are reported accurately. Therefore, our definition and understanding of ACLR success hinges on the appropriate use of high-quality and meaningful outcome measures.

Outcome Measures

Outcome measures can be broadly categorized based on who is scoring/assessing them. Patient-reported or subjective outcome measures (PROMs) can be further broken down based on their level of specificity: general health, region specific, joint specific, or condition/injury specific.[2] Observer-reported or objective outcomes can be further broken down into clinical examination, functional performance tests, and imaging.[2] The utility of an outcome can be predictive (ie, limb symmetry index of quadricep strength predicting return to sport), discriminative (ie, international cartilage repair society classification of cartilage injury), or evaluative (ie, improvement in patient-reported quality of life following surgery).[3] Outcome measures can be directly patient-important (ie, pain, return to pre-injury level of sport, perceived knee function), or surrogates assumed to reflect patient-important domains (ie, gait biomechanics, range of motion, graft signal on MRI).[3] Lastly, outcomes may be continuous (ie, scores of 0–100 on a PROM), categorical (ie, pivot shift grades), or dichotomous (ie, graft rupture).

WHAT WE HAVE

Anterior Cruciate Ligament Reconstruction Outcomes

In the wake of evidence-based medicine becoming the gold standard of care, ACLR outcome development and research has exploded over the past few decades. We identified over 100 outcome measures used in the literature to assess ACLR. We then used the International Classification of Functioning, Disability and Health (ICF) model as a system to categorize these outcomes. The ICF model is a framework for the measurement of health and disability approved by the World Health Assembly that can be particularly helpful for organizing and interpreting the multifactorial nature outcomes following ACLR.[4] The ICF model is made up of the following components: body structures and function, activity and function, participation and motivation, and environmental/personal factors, all of which can be applied to ACLR[4,5] (**Fig. 1**). Strengths of this model include its universality, neutrality, acknowledgment of environmental influence, and descriptive profile of functioning rather than a simplistic depiction of a binary good or bad outcome.[4] **Table 1** lists a plethora of possible patient-reported (subjective) outcome measures used with patients undergoing ACLR, organized according to the ICF model.[6–19] **Fig. 2** outlines the observer-reported (objective) outcome measures used for ACLR, which fit mainly into the body structures and function component of the ICF model.[10,11,13–15,17–29,49,50,65,76–97] The large volume of candidate measures can be overwhelming and make comparison across studies and cohorts difficult.

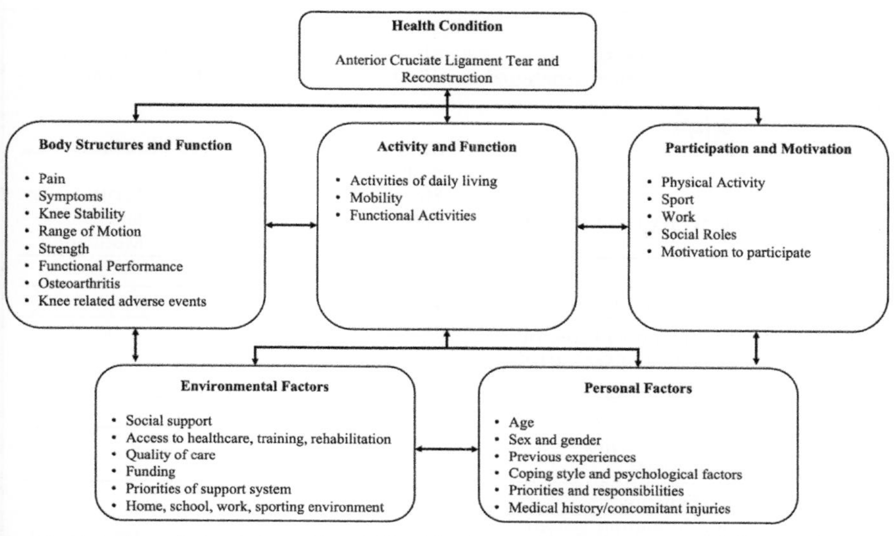

Fig. 1. Domains of the International Classification of Functioning, Disability, and Health Model applied to anterior cruciate ligament injury and reconstruction.

Before new outcome measures are created, work should be directed to validating and/or improving those that exist, unless a clear gap is identified which warrants a novel outcome measure.[6]

WHAT TO CONSIDER

Selecting Outcome Measures

It is important to select outcome measures based on some key considerations to ensure that the results of a study are trustworthy (**Fig. 3**).

Purpose/research question

A study's purpose and research question dictate what outcome(s) are used. The type of study design (diagnostic validity, prognosis/prediction, therapy/harm/intervention) will dictate whether discriminative, predictive, or evaluative outcomes are most appropriate, respectively. Research questions will outline the patient population under investigation. It is important that at least one outcome measure has been specifically developed and validated for the specific study population.[5]

Measurement properties

To have value in clinical decision making, outcome measures must have strong evidence of their measurement properties within the population of interest (in this case, patients undergoing ACLR). **Table 2** briefly outlines measurement properties that should be considered in the selection and interpretation of outcomes, aligning with the Consensus-based Standards for the selection of health Measurement Instruments (COSMIN) and International Society of Quality of Life Research (ISOQOL) reporting standards.[98,99,101–103] These measurement properties fit broadly into the categories of validity, reliability, responsiveness, and practicality (see **Table 2**).

Variety of outcomes and global assessment

Because of the heterogeneity of the ACLR population and in how clinicians, researchers, and patients may define a successful intervention, we recommend including

Table 1
Anterior cruciate ligament reconstruction patient-reported (subjective) outcome measures, categorized according to the international classification of functioning, disability, and health[6–29]

	ICF Model Domain		
Patient-Reported (Subjective) Outcome Measures	**Body Structures and Function**	**Activity and Function**	**Participation and Motivation**
General			
EuroQol 5 Dimension (EQ-5D)[30,a]	✔	✔	✔
Hospital for Special Surgery Pediatric Functional Activity Brief Scale (HSS Pedi-FABS)[31]			✔
Marx Activity Rating Scale (MARS)[32]			✔
International Physical Activity Questionnaire (IPAQ)[33]			✔
Patient-Reported Outcomes Measurement Information System (PROMIS)[34–36]	✔	✔	✔
Quality of Recovery Score (QoR)[37,a]	✔	✔	
Quality of Well-Being Scale (QWB)[38,a]	✔	✔	
Return to participation			✔
Return to performance			✔
Return to sport			✔
Short Form Health Survey (8, 12, 36)[39–41,a]	✔	✔	
Sports Inventory for Pain (SIP)[42]	✔		✔
Subjective Patient Outcome for Return to Sports (SPORTS)[43,44]			✔
Tegner Activity Scale[45]			✔
Tampa Scale for Kinesiophobia 11 (TSK-11)[46,a]		✔	✔
Region Specific: Lower Extremity			
Lower Extremity Functional Scale (LEFS)[47,48]		✔	
Joint Specific: Knee			
Cincinnati Knee Rating System (CKRS)[49,50]: Subjective	✔	✔	✔
Hughston Clinic Questionnaire[51]	✔	✔	✔
International Knee Documentation Committee Subjective Knee Form (IKDC-SKF)[52]	✔	✔	✔
Injury-Psychological Readiness to Return to Sport Scale (I-PPRS)[53,a]			✔
Knee Self Efficacy Scale (K-SES)[54,a]		✔	✔
Knee Injury and Osteoarthritis Outcome Score (KOOS)[55,56]	✔	✔	✔
KOOS-12[57,58]	✔	✔	

(continued on next page)

Table 1
(*continued*)

Patient-Reported (Subjective) Outcome Measures	ICF Model Domain		
	Body Structures and Function	Activity and Function	Participation and Motivation
KOOS-child[59]	✔	✔	✔
KOOS Physical Function Shortform (KOOS-PS)[60]		✔	✔
Knee Outcome Survey (KOS)[61]		✔	✔
Lysholm Score[62]	✔	✔	✔
Pediatric-IKDC (Pedi-IKDC)[63,64]	✔	✔	✔
Test of athletes with knee injuries (TAK)[65]		✔	
Western Ontario and McMaster Universities Osteoarthritis Index (WOMAC)[66,67]	✔	✔	
Condition Specific: ACL Injury			
ACL Quality of Life Questionnaire (ACL-QOL)[68,a]	✔	✔	✔
ACL Return to Sport Index (ACL-RSI)[69,a]	✔		✔
Donor-site-related functional problems following anterior cruciate ligament reconstruction[70]	✔	✔	✔
Japanese ACL Questionnaire 25 (JACL-25)[71]	✔	✔	✔
Knee Numeric Entity Evaluation Score (KNEES-ACL)[72,a]	✔	✔	✔
KOOS-ACL[73,74]		✔	✔
KOOS global[75]	✔	✔	✔
PPLP1 subjective[76,a]	✔		

Abbreviation: ACL, anterior cruciate ligament.
[a] Outcome measure that also assesses quality of life/well-being and/or psychological factors.

multiple outcome measures in a study to reflect different perspectives of health such as those represented using ICF model. The Panther Symposium ACL Injury Clinical Outcomes Consensus Group recommends a comprehensive assessment of ACLR at minimum 2 year follow-up including adverse events, clinical measures of knee function and structure, PROMs, activity level, and recurrent ligament disruption, with measures of PTOA included at 5 years of follow-up.[1] The consensus group also recommends ensuring that this battery includes a knee-related (joint-specific) outcome, an activity scale, and a measure of health-related quality of life.[1] There may also be considerations related to impact and communication of results if different outcome measures are accepted across different regions, or there is a desire to compare new study results with historical results.

Sample size and feasibility

Research involving individuals who have suffered an ACL injury can follow a within-groups design (eg, before-after study) or a between groups design (eg, randomized

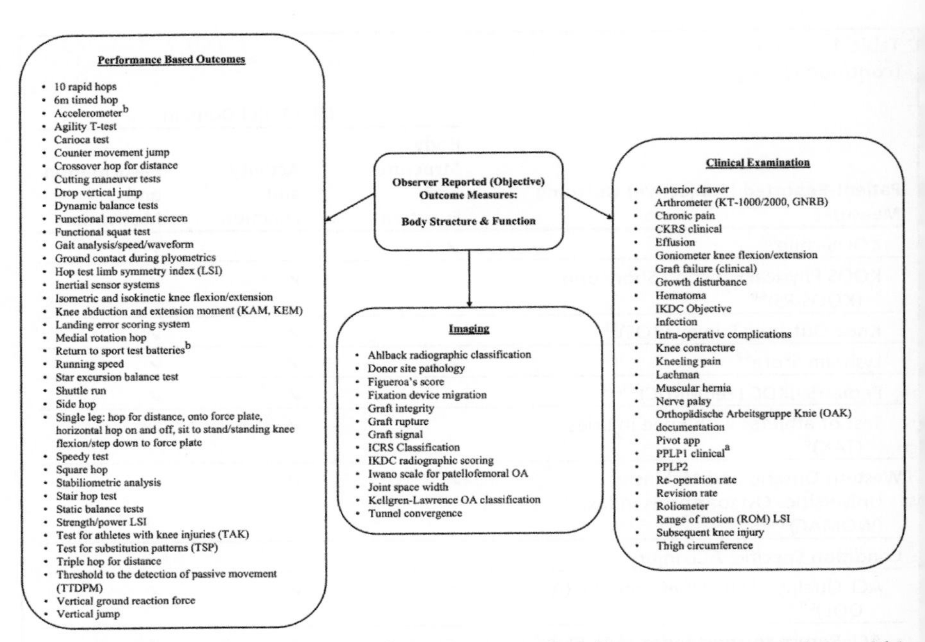

Fig. 2. Objective outcome measures for anterior cruciate ligament reconstruction, within the body structures and function domain of the International Classification of Functioning, Disability and Health (ICF).[a]Also fits within the activities of daily living and functional activities ICF domain [b]Also fits within the participation and motivation ICF domain. CKRS, Cincinnati Knee Rating Scale; ICRS, International Cartilage Regeneration and Joint Preservation Society; IKDC, International Knee Documentation Committee; OA, osteoarthritis.

trial). The sample size for a within-group study will require fewer participants than a between-group study since measuring change in the same group of individuals (within-group) produces less statistical "noise" than differences between individuals who are in separate groups. The greater the "noise," the more difficult it is to see the "signal" and reach statistical significance. Additionally, the change experienced by individuals from before to after an intervention is much larger than differences observed between treatment groups, especially if treatments are similar (eg, ACL reconstruction with single vs double bundle grafts). What we find in most orthopedic studies is a failure to reach statistical significance and more importantly a failure to reach definitive conclusions (ie, statistically significant differences where the confidence interval (CI) includes small, unimportant differences or differences that are not statistically significant where the CIs include clinically important differences).

Why does this happen? A sample size calculation for a between-groups study using a continuous outcome, like a PROM, has 4 main components: Type 1 error rate, Type 2 error rate, standard deviation for the outcome measure in the population (usually derived from pooling results from published studies using the same outcome in the same population or pilot data), and the expected difference between groups. Conventionally, the Type 1 error rate is 5% ($P < .05$) and the Type 2 error rate is 20% (corresponding to 80% power).[3] Very often, the minimally clinically important difference (MCID) is selected to represent the value for the expected difference, which seems logical but is incorrect. Perhaps underappreciated by those performing sample size calculations is that producing an estimate for the MCID for an outcome measure

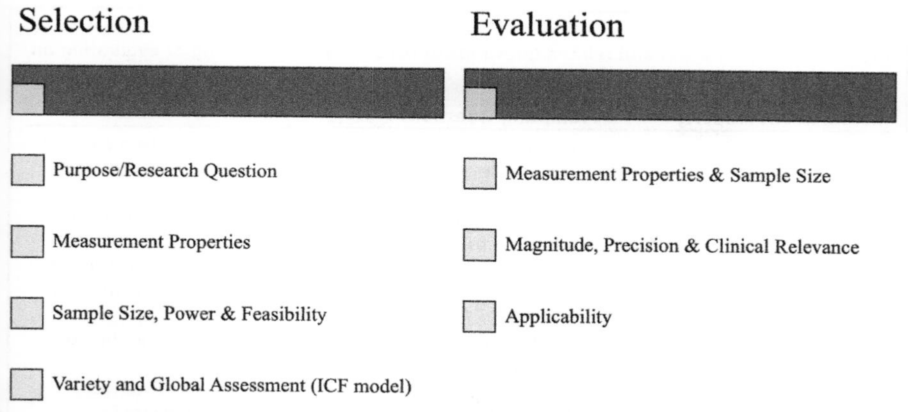

Fig. 3. Checklists for the selection (study design stage) and evaluation/interpretation of outcomes (using the results of the published literature to inform practice or presenting your own results) following anterior cruciate ligament reconstruction.

uses a within-group design. Therefore, the value of the MCID will always overestimate the magnitude of change that one could reasonably expect to observe between 2 groups who are receiving similar treatments. Even if groups are receiving very different treatments (eg, nonoperative vs operative), both usually have a treatment effect such that the amount of change within each group is still likely to be larger than the amount of difference between the 2 groups. In fact, Goldsmith and colleagues[104] found that a reasonable between-group difference was approximately 50% of a within-group change or MCID.

Generally, the larger the sample size of a study, the better its ability to overcome random sampling error and apply to clinical practice[3] with negative effects on feasibility. Collecting outcome data is resource intensive, requiring time, money, and personnel. Strategies to improve feasibility include using a surrogate outcome or including multiple centers (also improves applicability and impact).

Early in the process of evaluating a new intervention, it makes sense to employ a surrogate outcome that is less directly clinically relevant (ie, range of motion vs function), but more easily measured (less expensive, less resource intensive), producing results that are more precise. It is difficult, and more than likely infeasible, to conduct a study with a sufficiently large sample size to detect differences in important proportional outcomes with low event rates, such as graft rupture. However, if there are other published studies that reported surrogate outcomes or less directly important outcomes, the final step to informing the research question may be a very large, multicenter, multicountry effort.[105]

Interpreting Outcome Measures

Effective evidence-based medicine requires the critical evaluation and interpretation of outcomes before results are applied to the real world or added to the rationale for clinical decisions (see **Fig. 3**).

Precision and clinical relevance

Differences in outcome measures may be statistically significant ($P > .05$) but indistinguishable to the individual patient (ie, 3% increase in limb symmetry index for single leg hop tests, or a 4-point improvement on the International Knee Documentation Committee Subjective Knee Form [IKDC-SKF] scored out of 100) and are therefore

Table 2
Measurement properties and related questions to consider when selecting or evaluating an outcome measure[6,98–100]

Measurement Property	Prompting Questions
Validity	Does the outcome measure what it is intended to measure? When assessed a one time point, this is considered cross-sectional validity.
Face validity	Does the outcomes measure appear to measure what it is intended to?
Content validity	Does the outcome measure include a comprehensive set of items that fully assesses the spectrum of the construct of interest?
Construct validity	Does the outcome adequately reflect the construct being measured?
Criterion validity	Does the outcome measure align with the gold standard[a]?
Predictive	Can the outcome measure predict a criterion event?
Convergent	Does the outcome measure have similar results to the gold standard?
Structural validity	Do the outcome scores adequately reflect the dimensionality of the construct being measured?
Longitudinal validity	Does the outcome measure detect change when change has occurred? This property is similar to sensitivity to change, which is the ability of a measure to detect change, given the amount of variability between participants[100]
Hypothesis testing	Do the outcome scores relate to other outcome measures or indicate differences across time/between groups in a way that is consistent with hypotheses?
Cross-cultural validity	Does a translated/cross-culturally adapted outcome measure adequately reflect the intended construct of the original outcome measure?
Reliability	Does the outcome measure produce consistent results when used in the same patients/context when there has been no change in health status?
Internal consistency	Are items measuring a related construct? Or redundant?
Test-retest reliability	Can variance in the outcome scores be attributed to true change/differences?
Measurement error	How much of the variance in outcome scores is attributed to systematic/random error as opposed to true change?
Inter-rater reliability	How much do outcomes vary when carried out by different assessors?
Intra-rater reliability	How much do outcomes vary when carried out by the same assessor at different times or in different contexts?
Responsiveness	Can the outcome detect clinically important change? (ie, changes deemed important by patients and clinicians, worthy of changing practice)
Practicality	Can the outcome measure be reasonably used in a real-world clinical context?
Interpretability	Are the items in the outcome measure clear and easily understood by the average target respondent? Will items likely be interpreted the same way across respondents?
Burden	What is the time and effort required from respondents to complete the measure?

Note: each of these prompting questions must be considered in relation to the target population.
[a] There are no gold standard outcome measurements for constructs such as health-related quality of life or pain. Therefore, outcome measures assessing these constructs can be compared with previously validated and accepted measures assessing the same intended construct.

not clinically relevant. As such, reliance on the *P*-value to make clinical conclusions is insufficient. Relying only on the *P*-value should be saved for early studies where the intention is to evaluate whether a definitive trial is warranted (ie, proof of concept, efficacy studies, cell, or lab-based studies, etc.).[106] MCID, minimal detectable change (MDC), or patient acceptable symptom state (PASS) values can be used to determine if outcome measures have changed by or reached a clinical meaningful threshold. The MCID represents the smallest change in an outcome measure that is considered clinically relevant and would warrant a change in patient care.[107] The MDC represents the smallest change that can be confidently identified as true change beyond measurement error. Change smaller than the MDC would be considered trivial but change beyond the MDC does not necessarily reflect clinical significance.[107] Finally, PASS values indicate the outcome score beyond which patients perceive their current state and well-being as satisfactory.[107] PASS values have been shown to be relatively stable across time and are therefore useful for investigating longitudinal outcomes.[107]

Recall that published MCID values are calculated using within-group change. In an earlier section we suggested that using the MCID as the expected difference in estimations of sample size for between-group comparisons would likely produce an underestimate of the number of participants require to yield a precise result. Along the same lines of reason, if investigators wish to use MCID values to interpret the results of their studies, then robust results are more likely produced when a proportions analysis is used rather than comparing means. In a proportions analysis, each patient is classified as having changed by at least the MCID or not, and the proportion of individuals achieving the MCID within each group is then compared between groups.[11] A significantly larger proportion of patients who have improved by at least the outcome MCID in one group versus the other can be considered clinically relevant. However, if one wishes to compare between-group mean differences, a clinically important difference between groups is likely to be represented by a much smaller value (50% of the MCID), which needs to be taken into consideration when interpreting the 95% CIs around the mean difference between groups.

Precision should be assessed by looking at the lower and upper boundary of 95% confidence intervals. CIs provide a range of plausible results since a single study produces only an estimate of the results influenced by the sample and any number of factors influencing that sample (eg, clinician, institution, health care system, supports, etc.). If a study produces precise results (able to reach a definitive conclusion), each boundary of the 95% CI suggests the same conclusion; either both boundaries imply an important difference in favor of the same intervention or both boundaries exclude the possibility of an important difference between interventions. With imprecise results, each 95% CI boundary suggests a different conclusion is possible (ie, an important difference for the intervention, an important difference for the control, or no important difference).

To illustrate the problem, consider the following: The MCID for the primary outcome is published as 10 points. If the investigator calculates sample size using 10 points as the expected difference, where the standard deviation is 20 points, the 2-sided Type 1 error rate is 5%, and the power to declare a 10-point expected difference as statistically different is 80%, they will require 63 participants per group. If instead, they use 50% of the MCID (ie, 5 points) as the expected difference and recalculate the sample size, they will need 277 participants per group. At first glance, the feasibility of undertaking the study using the second calculation seems a deterrent; but what are the costs of conducting an underpowered study? First, underpowered studies will almost always find the difference not statistically different. Second, because the expected difference is an overestimate of what is truly a reasonable difference between treatment groups, the probability of the nonstatistically significant finding being a Type 2 error (ie, statistically declaring no difference when there is a true difference between groups) is increased, which means the power is less than the 80% planned for in the calculation. Third, the probability increases that a statistically significant finding is a random sampling error and will not be reproducible in future studies or if applied to practice, patients will not experience the benefits predicted by the study. Fourth, underpowered studies will produce wide CIs that lead to imprecise conclusions (ie, lower and upper boundary suggest discrepant findings). Finally, those who do not understand the limitations of *P*-values or how to interpret CIs will be misled and may be influenced or even act on the study's conclusions, especially if the authors have not fully recognized these deficiencies in their limitations and overstated their confidence in the results in their conclusions.

At the end of the trial, in the study that recruited 63 patients per group, if the difference between groups was 8 points (and using a standard deviation of 20 points, as used in the sample size calculation), the result would be 8 (95% CI 1–15). Under the same parameters but with a sample size of 277 patients per group the result would be 8 (95% CI 5–11). In both cases, the results are statistically significant ($P < .05$) but should draw very different conclusions from the authors. Whereas in the study with 63 patients per group, the 95% CI indicates that it is plausible that the difference between groups is as small as one point which is certainly not clinically important, the study with 277 patients per group can confidently conclude that one treatment will offer superior results over the other treatment because even if the difference between the 2 groups is as small as 5 points, it still represents a clinically important difference (ie, >5 points, the between-groups MCID).

Applicability

Lastly, it should be considered whether the context, participants, intervention, and outcomes in a particular study are similar enough to the environment or situation to which the results will be applied. Specific to outcomes, it should be considered whether the outcomes appear relevant to the study participants and whether they will be relevant to other patients.[108]

Current Challenges in Outcome Measurement

It has been discussed here and in other publications that inadequate measurement properties are an issue with outcome measures. Beyond these concerns, we have identified several nuanced issues that warrant discussion and consideration.

Issues with objective outcome measures

As the health care system has shifted toward a shared decision-making model, patient-important outcomes have become emphasized as the optimal choice for evaluating the success of interventions. This inherently highlights the issue with many objective/clinical outcomes that they are not meaningful to patients. It has been shown that patients place greater importance on more functional outcomes that affect their daily life such as returning to sport whereas surgeons place greater importance on clinical outcomes such as knee stability.[109] Both groups emphasize the importance of clinical endpoints such as graft rupture and secondary knee injury.[109] Therefore, patient-reported and patient important outcomes of sport participation or knee function in activities of daily living would be preferred over clinical outcomes like millimeters of anterior tibial translation measured by arthrometers or knee abduction moments during jump landings. Although it could be argued that these outcomes reflect important domains like knee stability and neuromuscular control that will contribute to improved patient function, sport participation, and reduced symptoms, this association is not always borne out in evidence and cannot be assumed.

Issues with subjective outcome measures

Patient-reported outcomes are considered the cornerstone of ACLR evaluation and are often the primary outcome in clinical trials. Patient-reported outcomes drive clinical decision making, health policy, and financial decisions in the health care system (insurance coverage and reimbursement, etc.).

Studies consistently show significant and clinically meaningful improvements in PROMs following ACLR across time. However, a challenge in ACLR research arises when making between-group comparisons in PROMs beyond early post-injury time points when obvious clinical differences between groups exist but between-group comparisons of PROMs yield similar results. For example, in the STABILITY 1 study there was a statistically significant difference in the proportion of graft ruptures at 2 years postoperative between patients who underwent ACLR with or without an additional lateral extra-articular tenodesis (LET) procedure (ACL alone: 11% (34/298) versus ACL + LET: 4% (11/291)) yet the 1 and 2 year between-group mean difference in IKDC scores were 1.7 (95% CI −0.5 to 2.7, P = .14) and −0.7 (95% CI −3.1 to 1.6, P = .54), respectively.[105]

There are a few candidate theories as to why this may occur, and the truth likely lies with unique combinations of reasons in different contexts. First, there may truly be no difference between interventions. It is likely that many ACLR interventions produce a similar effect on patient function and quality of life and are interchangeable.

Second, it is possible that there is a problem with the specific PROMs being used. Perhaps they are outcome measures not intended or evaluated for their fit in ACLR patient populations, or there are ceiling effects that make detection of differences between groups difficult. For example, knee-specific outcome measures only validated for individuals undergoing total knee arthroplasty (typically older, less active patients) may not be appropriate when assessing young active individuals. This has been a consistent argument against the use of the Knee Injury and Osteoarthritis Outcome Score (KOOS) for patients undergoing ACLR[20,110–114] and has led to the development of alternative measures specific to ACLR, such as the KOOS-ACL[73,74] and KOOS global,[75] that used statistical methods to eliminate items deemed irrelevant or problematic for use in the ACL population.

A third explanation could be the general level of success of ACLR. Graft rupture itself is commonly thought of as the most significant endpoint following ACLR, and while rupture rates may remain higher than some clinicians and patients would like, they are still the minority outcome. In the example above, the STABILITY 1 trial investigating ACLR using a hamstring tendon autograft with or without lateral extra-articular tenodesis showed significant improvements in PROMs across time in both groups and a 67% reduction in graft rupture rates at 2 years postoperative in favor of the LET recipients, yet there were no statistically significant differences between groups in any PROM score at the same time point.[105] It is possible that in this 618 patient study, the negative experiences reported by 8% of patients who experienced a graft rupture (45/598) were washed out by the positive outcomes of the remaining 92% (553/598). A greater number of events would mitigate this issue but would require a much larger sample size. Alternatively, choosing a meaningful endpoint with a higher event rate such as return to pre-injury level of sport may mitigate this problem.

Lastly, it is possible that longitudinal assessment of PROMs is muddied by response shift. Response shift is used to describe how patients' perceptions of health-related quality of life is dynamic, changing over time and circumstances.[115] Response shift is defined as the recalibration (change in standards), reprioritization (change in values) and reconceptualization (change in definition) of a target construct in response to a change in health[115] (**Fig. 4**). Evidence of response shift bias has been reported in patients undergoing total knee arthroplasty, knee microfracture for cartilage lesions, and autologous conditioned serum injections for osteoarthritis.[116–121] These shifts are seen across multiple time points (most commonly at 6 and 12 months postoperatively), across multiple PROMs including generic, region-specific and disease-specific measures (patient satisfaction scores, Lysholm, pain visual analog scale (VAS), IKDC, EuroQol 5 Dimension (EQ5D), 36 question Short Form Health Survey (SF-36), Western Ontario and McMaster Univerisities Osteoarthritis Index (WOMAC) KOOS), as well as in qualitative interview responses.[116–121] Although there is some evidence evaluating response shift in patients undergoing knee surgery[116–118,120,122–124] and in the ACLR population,[125–127] more work is required. It seems reasonable to expect a response shift following ACL injury and surgery, especially as the length of time increases between salient, anchoring events like the injury and surgery, and because these patients tend to be younger and at transitional stages of their life, where reconceptualization and reprioritization may be especially prominent.

To illustrate the issue, consider the following: A 24 year old female varsity soccer player, in their final year of eligibility. Her priority and major contributor to her overall health and knee-related quality of life is playing soccer at a highly competitive level. If this athlete ruptures her ACL, the described frame of reference will be reflected in her baseline PROMs. Two years following ACLR, this soccer player has graduated and is entering the workforce. Her priorities have now shifted to work and financial security and her quality of life is maintained at a high level by playing recreational soccer with friends 2 to 3 times per week. This patient has (1) lowered the relative priority of soccer in her life, (2) recalibrated her standards regarding an acceptable level of sport participation, and (3) reconceptualized the construct of return to sport. This new frame of reference will be reflected in her PROMs 2 years after injury which begs the question whether comparison to baseline health-related quality of life is an accurate representation of change over time and/or can be used to qualify success or failure of the operation. Even though this athlete's PROM scores may be similar to pre-injury ratings, this athlete did not achieve return to pre-injury level of sport, which was the primary goal of the patient and surgeon at the time of surgery. However, her quality of life improved by more than the MCID across time for reasons external to the reconstruction.

There are many events and factors that may influence patient perception and outcomes following ACL injury, complicating the assessment of intervention assessment (see **Fig. 4**). Each change or event in a patient's life represents an opportunity for a

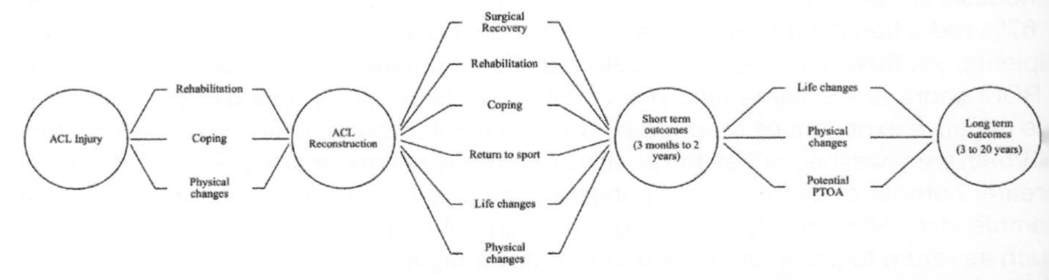

Fig. 4. Timeline of ACL injury recovery, with influential events and factors that can affect outcomes. ACL, anterior cruciate ligament; PTOA, post-traumatic osteoarthritis.

shift in their perceptions (ie, response shift). Again, personal and environmental factors will greatly influence the recovery trajectory.

What is a successful anterior cruciate ligament reconstruction?
Surgeons, physiotherapists, coaches, parents, and patients will likely have different definitions of a successful surgery. Further, individuals within each of these groups may define success differently. Pervasive and reasonable definitions of success for group level analysis appear to be (1) avoidance of graft failure or secondary knee injury, (2) return to pre-injury level of sport, (3) high health-related and/or knee-related quality of life, and (4) freedom from symptoms of PTOA. Critical appraisal of entire bodies of evidence and high-quality research has been important to our understanding of what interventions and predictors may influence this success, including many of the concepts discussed throughout this paper.

Moving to an individual level complicates the concept of ACLR success. Consider how individual definitions (patient, clinician, or researcher) of the previously described "successful outcomes" may differ: What counts as a secondary knee injury? Are graft ruptures counted based on occurrence of revision surgery, clinical assessment, or imaging? At what severity is PTOA problematic (radiographic, symptomatic, interfering with activities)? What is the individual's type and level of pre-injury sport? Do they have the opportunity or desire to return? What is the threshold of acceptable quality of life? Is the surgery successful if a patient is genuinely satisfied years following surgery but did not reach their desired outcome at the time of injury/reconstruction? These nuances emphasize the importance of using a variety of outcome measures and the timing of outcome measurement.

SUMMARY

The ICF model is a useful framework to facilitate decisions about outcome selection and to describe recovery following ACL injury and reconstruction. Study purpose, measurement properties, samples size, clinical relevance, and individuality must be considered when selecting and interpreting outcome measures related to ACLR.

DISCLOSURE

The authors have nothing to disclose.

REFERENCES

1. Svantesson E, Hamrin Senorski E, Webster KE, et al. Clinical Outcomes After Anterior Cruciate Ligament Injury: Panther Symposium ACL Injury Clinical Outcomes Consensus Group. Orthop J Sports Med 2020;8(7):1–19.
2. Vega JF, Spindler KP. Types of Scoring Instruments Available. In: Musahl V, Karlsson J, Hirschmann MT, et al, editors. Basic methods handbook for clinical orthopaedic research. Springer Nature; 2019. p. 97–111.
3. Firth A, Bryant D, Menetrey J, et al. Health Measurement Development and Interpretation. In: Musahl V, Karlsson J, Hirschmann MT, et al, editors. Basic methods handbook for clinical orthopaedic research. Springer Nature; 2019. p. 111–20.
4. Centers for Disease Control and Prevention. The ICF: An Overview.
5. Comins JD, Brodersen J, Siersma V, et al. Choosing the most appropriate PROM for clinical studies in sports medicine. Scand J Med Sci Sports 2021;31(6): 1209–15.

6. Gagnier JJ, Shen Y, Huang H. Psychometric properties of patient-reported outcome measures for use in patients with anterior cruciate ligament injuries: A systematic review. JBJS Rev 2018;6(4):1–15.
7. Meta F, Lizzio VA, Jildeh TR, et al. Which patient reported outcomes to collect after anterior cruciate ligament reconstruction. Ann Jt 2017;2:21.
8. Macri EM, Young JJ, Ingelsrud LH, et al. Meaningful thresholds for patient-reported outcomes following interventions for anterior cruciate ligament tear or traumatic meniscus injury: a systematic review for the OPTIKNEE consensus. Br J Sports Med 2022;56(24):1432–44.
9. Gaal BT, Knapik DM, Gilmore A. Patient-reported outcome measures following surgical intervention for pediatric sports-related injuries to the knee: a systematic review. Curr Rev Musculoskelet Med 2022. https://doi.org/10.1007/s12178-022-09756-5.
10. Kaarre J, Zsidai B, Narup E, et al. Scoping review on ACL surgery and registry data. Curr Rev Musculoskelet Med 2022;15(5):385–93.
11. Almangoush A, Herrington L. Functional performance testing and patient reported outcomes following acl reconstruction: a systematic scoping review. Int Sch Res Notices 2014;2014:1–14.
12. Marinho APR, Nunes GS, Menezes E, et al. Questionnaires for knee instability assessment in people with anterior cruciate ligament injury: a systematic review of original questionnaires and their translated versions. Disabil Rehabil 2020; 42(2):173–82.
13. Ahmad SS, Meyer JC, Krismer AM, et al. Outcome measures in clinical ACL studies: an analysis of highly cited level I trials. Knee Surg Sports Traumatol Arthrosc 2017;25(5):1517–27.
14. Beischer S, Hamrin Senorski E, Thomeé C, et al. How is psychological outcome related to knee function and return to sport among adolescent athletes after anterior cruciate ligament reconstruction? Am J Sports Med 2019;47(7): 1567–75.
15. Everhart JS, Yalcin S, Spindler KP. Twenty-year outcomes after anterior cruciate ligament reconstruction: a systematic review of prospectively collected data. Am J Sports Med 2022;50(10):2842–52.
16. Johnson DS, Smith RB. Outcome measurement in the ACL deficient knee what's the score? Knee 2001;8:5157.
17. Ardern CL, Taylor NF, Feller JA, et al. Fifty-five per cent return to competitive sport following anterior cruciate ligament reconstruction surgery: an updated systematic review and meta-analysis including aspects of physical functioning and contextual factors. Br J Sports Med 2014;48(21):1543–52.
18. Meredith SJ, Rauer T, Chmielewski TL, et al. Return to sport after anterior cruciate ligament injury: panther symposium ACL Injury Return to Sport Consensus Group. Knee Surg Sports Traumatol Arthrosc 2020;28(8):2403–14.
19. Zebis MK, Warming S, Pedersen MB, et al. Outcome Measures After ACL Injury in Pediatric Patients: A Scoping Review. Orthop J Sports Med 2019;7(7). https://doi.org/10.1177/2325967119861803.
20. Svantesson E, Hamrin Senorski E, Webster KE, et al. Clinical outcomes after anterior cruciate ligament injury: Panther Symposium ACL Injury Clinical Outcomes Consensus Group. Journal of ISAKOS 2020;5(5):281–94.
21. Grassi A, Bailey JR, Signorelli C, et al. Magnetic resonance imaging after anterior cruciate ligament reconstruction: A practical guide. World J Orthop 2016; 7(10):638–49.

22. Hanzlíková I, Hébert-Losier K. Is the Landing Error Scoring System Reliable and Valid? A Systematic Review. Sport Health 2020;12(2):181–8.
23. Herbst E, Wierer G, Fischer F, et al. Functional assessments for anterior cruciate ligament reconstruction return to sport. Ann Jt 2017;2:37.
24. Lisee CM, Bjornsen E, Horton WZ, et al. Differences in Gait Biomechanics Between Adolescents and Young Adults With Anterior Cruciate Ligament Reconstruction. J Athl Train 2022;57(9–10):921–8.
25. Marshall DC, Silva FD, Goldenberg BT, et al. Imaging Findings of Complications After Lateral Extra-Articular Tenodesis of the Knee: A Current Concepts Review. Orthop J Sports Med 2022;10(8). https://doi.org/10.1177/23259671221114820.
26. Narducci E, Waltz A, Gorski K, et al. The Clinical Utility of Functional Performance Tests with One-Year Post-ACL Reconstruction: A Systematic Review. International Journal of Sports Physical Therapy 2011;6(4):333–42.
27. Øiestad BE, Engebretsen L, Storheim K, et al. Knee osteoarthritis after anterior cruciate ligament injury: A systematic review. Am J Sports Med 2009;37(7):1434–43.
28. Pedersen M. Long-Term Clinical, Functional, Physical Activity, and Radiographic Outcomes after Anterior Cruciate Ligament Reconstruction or Rehabilitation Alone.; 2022.
29. Strong A, Arumugam A, Tengman E, et al. Properties of knee joint position sense tests for anterior cruciate ligament injury: a systematic review and meta-analysis. Orthop J Sports Med 2021;9(6). https://doi.org/10.1177/23259671211007878.
30. Rabin R, De Charro F. EQ-SD: a measure of health status from the EuroQol Group. Ann Med 2009;33(5):337–43.
31. Fabricant PD, Robles A, Downey-Zayas T, et al. Development and validation of a pediatric sports activity rating scale: the Hospital for Special Surgery Pediatric Functional Activity Brief Scale (HSS Pedi-FABS). Am J Sports Med 2013;41(10):2421–9.
32. Marx RG, Stump TJ, Jones EC, et al. Development and evaluation of an activity rating scale for disorders of the knee. Am J Sports Med 2001;29(2):213–8.
33. Craig CL, Marshall AL, Sjöström M, et al. International physical activity questionnaire: 12-Country reliability and validity. Med Sci Sports Exerc 2003;35(8):1381–95.
34. Fidai MS, Saltzman BM, Meta F, et al. Patient-reported outcomes measurement information system and legacy patient-reported outcome measures in the field of orthopaedics: a systematic review. Arthrosc J Arthrosc Relat Surg 2018;34(2):605–14.
35. Cella D, Yount S, Rothrock N, et al. The patient-reported outcomes measurement information system (PROMIS): progress of an NIH roadmap cooperative group during its first two years. Med Care 2007;45(5 Suppl 1):S3.
36. Reeve BB, Hays RD, Bjorner JB, et al. Psychometric evaluation and calibration of health-related quality of life item banks: plans for the patient-reported outcomes measurement information system (PROMIS). Med Care 2007;45(5 SUPPL. 1):22–31.
37. Stark PA, Myles PS, Burke JA. Development and psychometric evaluation of a postoperative quality of recovery scoreThe QoR-15. Anesthesiology 2013;118(6):1332–40.
38. Kaplan RM, Anderson JP, Ganiats TG. The Quality of Well-being Scale: rationale for a single quality of life index. Quality of life assessment: key issues in the 1990s; 1993. p. 65–94. https://doi.org/10.1007/978-94-011-2988-6_3. Published online.

39. How to score and interpret single-item health status measures: a manual for users of the SF-8TM Health Survey. – ScienceOpen. Available at: https://www.scienceopen.com/document?vid=5c6a3101-a200-45a3-a2dc-f2724767d327. Accessed May 13, 2023.
40. Ware JE, Kosinski M, Keller SD. SF-36 physical and mental health summary scales A user's manual. Boston, MA: The Health Institute, New England Medical Center. - References - Scientific Research Publishing; 1994. Available at: https://www.scirp.org/(S(i43dyn45teexjx455qlt3d2q))/reference/ReferencesPapers.aspx?ReferenceID=1367657. Accessed May 13, 2023.
41. Ware JE, Kosinski M, Keller SD. A 12-Item Short-Form Health Survey: construction of scales and preliminary tests of reliability and validity. Med Care 1996;34(3):220–33.
42. Meyers MC, Bourgeois AE, Stewart S, et al. Predicting Pain Response In Athletes: Development and Assessment of the Sports Inventory for Pain. J Sport Exerc Psychol 1992;14(3):249–61.
43. Bley JA, Master H, Huston LJ, et al. Return to Sports After Anterior Cruciate Ligament Reconstruction: Validity and Reliability of the SPORTS Score at 6 and 12 Months. Orthop J Sports Med 2022;10(6). https://doi.org/10.1177/23259671221098436.
44. Blonna D, Lee G, O'Driscoll SW. Arthroscopic restoration of terminal elbow extension in high-level athletes. Am J Sports Med 2010;38(12):2509–15.
45. Tegner Y, Lysholm J. Rating systems in the evaluation of knee ligament injuries. Clin Orthop Relat Res 1985;198:43–9. Available at: https://pubmed.ncbi.nlm.nih.gov/4028566/. Accessed May 13, 2023.
46. Woby SR, Roach NK, Urmston M, et al. Psychometric properties of the TSK-11: A shortened version of the Tampa Scale for Kinesiophobia. Pain 2005;117(1–2):137–44.
47. Binkley JM, Lott SA. The Lower Extremity Functional Scale (LEFS): Scale Development, Measurement Properties, and Clinical Application. Phys Ther 1999;79(4):371–83.
48. Mehta SP, Fulton A, Quach C, et al. Measurement Properties of the Lower Extremity Functional Scale: A Systematic Review. J Orthop Sports Phys Ther 2016;46(3):200–16.
49. Noyes FR, Moorar PA, Matthews DS, et al. The symptomatic anterior cruciate-deficient knee. Part I: the long-term functional disability in athletically active individuals. J Bone Joint Surg 1983;65(2):154–62.
50. Noyes FR, Matthews DS, Moorar PA, et al. The symptomatic anterior cruciate-deficient knee. Part II: the results of rehabilitation, activity modfication, and counseling on functional disability. J Bone Joint Surg 1983;65(2):163–74.
51. Flandry F, Hunt JP, Terry GC, et al. Analysis of subjective knee complaints using visual analog scales. Am J Sports Med 1991;19(2):112–8.
52. Irrgang JJ, Anderson AF, Boland AL, et al. Development and validation of the International Knee Documentation Committee Subjective Knee Form. Am J Sports Med 2001;29(5):600–13.
53. Glazer DD. Development and Preliminary Validation of the Injury-Psychological Readiness to Return to Sport (I-PRRS) Scale. J Athl Train 2009;44(2):185.
54. Thomeé P, Währborg P, Börjesson M, et al. A new instrument for measuring self-efficacy in patients with an anterior cruciate ligament injury. Scand J Med Sci Sports 2006;16(3):181–7.

55. Roos EM, Lohmander LS. The Knee injury and Osteoarthritis Outcome Score (KOOS): From joint injury to osteoarthritis. Health Qual Life Outcomes 2003; 1:1–8.
56. Roos EM, Roos HP, Lohmander LS, et al. Knee Injury and Osteoarthritis Outcome Score (KOOS) - Development of a self-administered outcome measure. J Orthop Sports Phys Ther 1998;28(2):88–96.
57. Gandek B, Roos EM, Franklin PD, et al. Item selection for 12-item short forms of the Knee injury and Osteoarthritis Outcome Score (KOOS-12) and Hip disability and Osteoarthritis Outcome Score (HOOS-12). Osteoarthritis Cartilage 2019; 27(5):746–53.
58. Gandek B, Roos EM, Franklin PD, et al. A 12-item short form of the Knee injury and Osteoarthritis Outcome Score (KOOS-12): tests of reliability, validity and responsiveness. Osteoarthritis Cartilage 2019;27(5):762–70.
59. Örtqvist M, Roos EM, Broström EW, et al. Development of the Knee Injury and Osteoarthritis Outcome Score for Children (KOOS-Child): Comprehensibility and content validity. Acta Orthop 2012;83(6):666–73.
60. Perruccio AV, Stefan Lohmander L, Canizares M, et al. The development of a short measure of physical function for knee OA KOOS-Physical Function Shortform (KOOS-PS) - an OARSI/OMERACT initiative. Osteoarthritis Cartilage 2008; 16(5):542–50.
61. Irrgang JJ, Snyder-Mackler L, Wainner RS, et al. Development of a patient-reported measure of function of the knee. J Bone Joint Surg Am 1998;80(8): 1132–45.
62. Lysholm J, Gillquist J. Evaluation of knee ligament surgery results with special emphasis on use of a scoring scale. Am J Sports Med 1982;10(3):150–4.
63. Kocher MS, Smith JT, Iversen MD, et al. Reliability, validity, and responsiveness of a modified international knee documentation committee subjective knee form (Pedi-IKDC) in children with knee disorders. Am J Sports Med 2011;39(5): 933–9.
64. Iversen MD, Lee B, Connell P, et al. Validity and comprehensibility of the International Knee Documentation Committee Subjective Knee Evaluation form in Children. Scand J Med Sci Sports 2010;20(1). https://doi.org/10.1111/J.1600-0838.2009.00917.X.
65. Björklund K, Sköld C, Andersson L, et al. Reliability of a criterion-based test of athletes with knee injuries; where the physiotherapist and the patient independently and simultaneously assess the patient's performance. Knee Surg Sports Traumatol Arthrosc 2006;14(2):165–75.
66. McConnell S, Kolopack P, Davis AM. The Western Ontario and McMaster Universities Osteoarthritis Index (WOMAC): a review of its utility and measurement properties. Arthritis Rheum 2001;45(5):453–61.
67. WOMAC 3.1 Index. In WOMAC Osteoarthritis Index. 2021. Available at https://www.womac.com/womac/index.php. Accessed June 13, 2023.
68. Mohtadi N. Development and validation of the quality of life outcome measure (questionnaire) for chronic anterior cruciate ligament deficiency. Am J Sports Med 1998;26(3):350–7.
69. Webster KE, Feller JA. Development and Validation of a Short Version of the Anterior Cruciate Ligament Return to Sport After Injury (ACL-RSI) Scale. Orthop J Sports Med 2018;6(4):1–7.
70. Aufwerber S, Hagströmer M, Heijne A. Donor-site-related functional problems following anterior cruciate ligament reconstruction: development of a self-

administered questionnaire. Knee Surg Sports Traumatol Arthrosc 2012;20(8): 1611–21.

71. Nagao M, Doi T, Saita Y, et al. A novel patient-reported outcome measure for anterior cruciate ligament injury: evaluating the reliability, validity, and responsiveness of Japanese anterior cruciate ligament questionnaire 25. Knee Surg Sports Traumatol Arthrosc 2016;24(9):2973–82.
72. Comins JD, Krogsgaard MR, Brodersen J. Development of the Knee Numeric-Entity Evaluation Score (KNEES - ACL): A condition-specific questionnaire. Scand J Med Sci Sports 2013;23(5). https://doi.org/10.1111/sms.12079.
73. Marmura H, Tremblay PF, Getgood AMJ, et al. Development and Preliminary Validation of the KOOS-ACL: A Short Form Version of the KOOS for Young Active Patients With ACL Tears. Am J Sports Med 2023;51(6):1447–56.
74. Marmura H, Tremblay PF, Bryant DM, et al. External Validation of the KOOS-ACL in the MOON Group Cohort of Young Athletes Followed for 10 Postoperative Years. Am J Sports Med 2023. https://doi.org/10.1177/03635465231160726.
75. Jacobs CA, Peabody MR, Lattermann C, et al. Development of the KOOSglobal patient-reported outcome measurement platform to assess patient-reported outcomes after anterior cruciate ligament reconstruction. Am J Sports Med 2019;46(12):2915–21.
76. Laboute E, Savalli L, Puig PL, et al. Validity and reproducibility of the PPLP scoring scale in the follow-up of athletes after anterior cruciate ligament reconstruction. Ann Phys Rehabil Med 2010;53(3):162–79.
77. Noyes FR, Barber SD, Mangine RE. Abnormal lower limb symmetry determined by function hop tests after anterior cruciate ligament rupture. Am J Sports Med 1991;19(5):513–8.
78. Thomeé R, Kaplan Y, Kvist J, et al. Muscle strength and hop performance criteria prior to return to sports after ACL reconstruction. Knee Surg Sports Traumatol Arthrosc 2011;19(11):1798–805.
79. Reid A, Birmingham TB, Stratford PW, et al. Hop testing provides a reliable and valid outcome measure during rehabilitation after anterior cruciate ligament reconstruction. Phys Ther 2007;87(3):337–49. https://academic.oup.com/ptj/article/87/3/337/2742133.
80. Gustavsson A, Neeter C, Thomeé P, et al. A test battery for evaluating hop performance in patients with an ACL injury and patients who have undergone ACL reconstruction. Knee Surg Sports Traumatol Arthrosc 2006;14(8):778–88.
81. Ebert JR, Preez L, Furzer B, et al. Which hop tests can best identify functional limb asymmetry in patients 9-12 months after anterior cruciate ligament reconstruction employing a hamstrings tendon autograft? Int J Sports Phys Ther 2021;16(2):393–403.
82. Logerstedt D, Grindem H, Lynch A, et al. Single-legged hop tests as predictors of self-reported knee function after anterior cruciate ligament reconstruction: The Delaware-Oslo ACL cohort study. Am J Sports Med 2012;40(10):2348–56.
83. Redler LH, Watling JP, Dennis ER, et al. Reliability of a field-based drop vertical jump screening test for ACL injury risk assessment. Physician Sportsmed 2016; 44(1):46–52.
84. Gray AD, Willis BW, Skubic M, et al. Development and validation of a portable and inexpensive tool to measure the drop vertical jump using the microsoft kinect V2. Sport Health 2017;9(6):537–44.
85. Cook G, Burton L, Hoogenboom BJ, et al. Functional movement screening: the use of fundamental movements as an assessment of function-part 2. Int J Sports

Phys Ther 2014;9(4):549–63. Available at: http://www.ncbi.nlm.nih.gov/pubmed/25133083. Accessed May 18, 2023.
86. Kanko LE, Birmingham TB, Bryant DM, et al. The star excursion balance test is a reliable and valid outcome measure for patients with knee osteoarthritis. Osteoarthritis Cartilage 2019;27(4):580–5.
87. Strong A, Arumugam A, Tengman E, et al. Properties of tests for knee joint threshold to detect passive motion following anterior cruciate ligament injury: a systematic review and meta-analysis. J Orthop Surg Res 2022;17(1). https://doi.org/10.1186/s13018-022-03033-4.
88. Galli M, De Santis V, Tafuro L. Reliability of the Ahlbäck classification of knee osteoarthritis. Osteoarthritis Cartilage 2003;11(8):580–4.
89. Ahlback S. Osteoarthrosis of the knee. A radiographic investigation. Acta Radiol Diagn 1968;277:7–72. Available at: https://cir.nii.ac.jp/crid/1571698599944020608. Accessed May 18, 2023.
90. Logerstedt DS, Scalzitti DA, Bennell KL, et al. Knee Pain and Mobility Impairments: Meniscal and Articular Cartilage Lesions Revision 2018. J Orthop Sports Phys Ther 2018;48(2):A1–50.
91. Iwano T, Kurosawa H, Tokuyama H, et al. Roentgenographic and Clinical Findings of Patellofemoral Ost : Clinical Orthopaedics and Related Research. Clin Orthop Relat Res 1990;252:190–7. Available at: https://journals-lww-com.proxy1.lib.uwo.ca/clinorthop/Abstract/1990/03000/Roentgenographic_and_Clinical_Findings_of.28.aspx?casa_token=3feUjRygT9UAAAAA:3EMLkFGa6BYgutF-Uh5xlkqQUE4yQTZKwcq8tc9IpsdOnteQmIYDYv0NhRH_M3pM-IrFQxaJ2YmBiN4cZz38wQ. Accessed May 18, 2023.
92. Kohn MD, Sassoon AA, Fernando ND. Classifications in Brief: Kellgren-Lawrence Classification of Osteoarthritis. Clin Orthop Relat Res 2016;474(8):1886.
93. Müller W, Biedert R, Hefti F, et al. OAK knee evaluation. A new way to assess knee ligament injuries - PubMed. Clin Orthop Relat Res 1988;232(37):37–50. https://pubmed.ncbi.nlm.nih.gov/3383501/. Accessed May 22, 2023.
94. Mainil-Varlet P, Aigner T, Brittberg M, et al. Histological Assessment of Cartilage Repair : A Report by the Histology Endpoint Committee of the International Cartilage Repair Society (ICRS). J Bone Joint Surg 2003;85(suppl_2):45–57. https://journals.lww.com/jbjsjournal/Citation/2003/00002/Histological_Assessment_of_Cartilage_Repair____A.7.aspx. Accessed May 22, 2023.
95. Kleeman RU, Krocker D, Cedrano A, et al. Altered cartilage mechanics and histology in knee osteoarthritis: relation to clinical assessment (ICRS Grade). Osteoarthritis Cartilage 2005;13(11):958–63.
96. American Orthopaedic Society for Sports Medicine. 2000 IKDC KNEE FORMS. In Resources. 2023. Available at: https://www.sportsmed.org/uploads/main/files/general/IKDC/AOSSM_IKDC_English_US.pdf. Accessed May 14, 2023.
97. Anderson AF, Irrgang JJ, Anderson CN. Development of the IKDC forms. In: Rotatory knee instability: an evidence based approach. Springer International Publishing; 2016. p. 131–46.
98. Mokkink LB, Prinsen CAC, Bouter LM. The COnsensus-based Standards for the selection of health Measurement INstruments (COSMIN) and how to select an outcome measurement instrument. Braz J Phys Ther 2016;20(2):105–13.
99. Brundage M, Blazeby J, Revicki D, et al. Patient-reported outcomes in randomized clinical trials: Development of ISOQOL reporting standards. Qual Life Res 2013;22(6):1161–75.

100. Finch E. Why measurement properties are important. In: Physical rehabilitation outcome measures : a guide to enhanced clinical decision making. 2nd edition. Hamilton, Ont., Baltimore, MD: BC Decker ; Lippincott Williams & Wilkins; ©2002. p. 26–41. Available at: https://www.worldcat.org/title/physical-rehabilitation-outcome-measures-a-guide-to-enhanced-clinical-decision-making/oclc/50638254. Accessed May 15, 2023.
101. Mokkink LB, Terwee CB, Patrick DL, et al. The COSMIN study reached international consensus on taxonomy, terminology, and definitions of measurement properties for health-related patient-reported outcomes. J Clin Epidemiol 2010;63:737–45.
102. Mokkink LB, Terwee CB. The COSMIN checklist for assessing the methodological quality of studies on measurement properties of health status measurement instruments : an international Delphi study. Published online 2010;539–49.
103. Reeve BB, Wyrwich KW, Wu AW, et al. ISOQOL recommends minimum standards for patient-reported outcome measures used in patient-centered outcomes and comparative effectiveness research. Qual Life Res 2013;22(8): 1889–905.
104. Goldsmith CH, Boers M, Bombardier C, et al. Criteria for clinically important changes in outcomes: development, scoring and evaluation of rheumatoid arthritis patient and trial profiles. OMERACT Committee. J Rheumatol 1993; 20(3):561–5. Available at: https://pubmed.ncbi.nlm.nih.gov/8478874/. Accessed May 15, 2023.
105. Getgood AMJ, Bryant DM, Litchfield R, et al. Lateral extra-articular tenodesis reduces failure of hamstring tendon autograft anterior cruciate ligament reconstruction: 2-year outcomes from the STABILITY study randomized clinical trial. Am J Sports Med 2020;48(2):285–97.
106. Docter S, Fathalla Z, Lukacs MJ, et al. Interpreting patient-reported outcome measures in orthopaedic surgery: a systematic review. J Bone Joint Surg Am 2021;103(2):185–90.
107. Popchak A, Lynch AD, Irrgang JJ. Framework for selecting clinical outcomes for clinical trials. In: Volker M, Karlsson J, Hirschmann MR, et al, editors. Basic methods handbook for clinical orthopaedic research. Springer Nature; 2019. p. 133–42.
108. Loudon K, Treweek S, Sullivan F, et al. The PRECIS-2 tool: designing trials that are fit for purpose. BMJ 2015;350.
109. Marmura H, Bryant DM, Birmingham TB, et al. Same knee , different goals : patients and surgeons have different priorities related to ACL reconstruction. Knee Surg Sports Traumatol Arthrosc 2021;29(12):4286–95.
110. Hansen CF, Jensen J, Odgaard A, et al. Four of five frequently used orthopedic PROMs possess inadequate content validity: a COSMIN evaluation of the mHHS, HAGOS, IKDC-SKF, KOOS and KNEES-ACL. Knee Surg Sports Traumatol Arthrosc 2021. https://doi.org/10.1007/s00167-021-06761-y. 0123456789.
111. Marmura H, Tremblay PF, Getgood AMJ, Bryant DM. The Knee Injury and Osteoarthritis Outcome Score Does Not Have Adequate Structural Validity for Use With Young, Active Patients With ACL Tears. Clin Orthop Relat Res 2022; 480(7):1342–50.
112. Polousky J. CORR Insights®: the knee injury and osteoarthritis outcome score does not have adequate structural validity for use with young, active patients with ACL tears. Clin Orthop Relat Res 2022;April:1–3.
113. Terwee CB, Reijman M. Knee injury and osteoarthritis outcome score or international knee documentation committee subjective knee form: which questionnaire

is most useful to monitor patients with an anterior cruciate rupture in the short term? Arthroscopy 2013;29(4):701–15.

114. Zsidai B, Narup E, Senorski EH, et al. The knee injury and osteoarthritis outcome score: shortcomings in evaluating knee function in persons undergoing ACL reconstruction. Knee Surg Sports Traumatol Arthrosc 2022;30(11):3594–8.
115. Vanier A, Oort FJ, Mcclimans L, et al. Response shift in patient - reported outcomes : definition , theory , and a revised model. Qual Life Res 2021;30(12): 3309–22.
116. Razmjou H, Yee A, Ford M, et al. Response shift in outcome assessment in patients undergoing total knee arthroplasty. Journal of Bone and Joint Surgery - Series A 2006;88(12):2590–5.
117. Razmjou H, Schwartz CE, Yee A, et al. Traditional assessment of health outcome following total knee arthroplasty was confounded by response shift phenomenon. J Clin Epidemiol 2009;62(1):91–6.
118. Balain B, Ennis O, Kanes G, et al. Response shift in self-reported functional scores after knee microfracture for full thickness cartilage lesions. Osteoarthritis Cartilage 2009;17(8):1009–13.
119. Howard JS, Mattacola CG, Mullineaux DR, et al. Influence of response shift on early patient-reported outcomes following autologous chondrocyte implanatation. Knee Surg Sports Traumatol Arthrosc 2015;22(9):2163–71.
120. Zhang XH, Li SC, Xie F, et al. An exploratory study of response shift in health-related quality of life and utility assessment among patients with osteoarthritis undergoing total knee replacement surgery in a tertiary hospital in Singapore. Value Health 2012;15(1 SUPPL):72–8.
121. Powden CJ, Hoch MC, Hoch JM. Examination of response shift after rehabilitation for orthopedic conditions : a systematic review. J Sport Rehabil 2018;27(5): 469–79.
122. Felix J, Becker C, Vogl M, et al. Patient characteristics and valuation changes impact quality of life and satisfaction in total knee arthroplasty - Results from a German prospective cohort study. Health Qual Life Outcomes 2019; 17(1):1–10.
123. Rutgers M, Creemers LB, Yang KGA, et al. Osteoarthritis treatment using autologous conditioned serum after placebo: Patient considerations and clinical response in a non-randomized case series. Acta Orthop 2015;86(1):114–8.
124. Woolhead GM, Donovan JL, Dieppe PA. Outcomes of total knee replacement: A qualitative study. Rheumatology 2005;44(8):1032–7.
125. Bryant D, Norman G, Stratford P, et al. Patients undergoing knee surgery provided accurate ratings of preoperative quality of life and function 2 weeks after surgery. J Clin Epidemiol 2006;59(9):984–93.
126. Baez S, Hoch JM, Mattacola C, et al. Use of response shift to improve agreement between patient-reported and performance-based outcomes in knee patients. Clinical Practice in Athletic Training 2021;4(1). https://doi.org/10.31622/2021/0004.1.4.
127. Robling M. Measuring change in patient quality of life over time: an evaluation of scale responsiveness and patient response shift. Dissertation. Cardiff University; 2006. Available at: https://orca.cardiff.ac.uk/54272/1/U584076.pdf. Accessed June 25, 2023.

Biologic Impact of Anterior Cruciate Ligament Injury and Reconstruction

Chilan B.G. Leite, MD, Richard Smith, MD, DPhil, Ophelie Z. Lavoie-Gagne, MD, Simon Görtz, MD, Christian Lattermann, MD*

KEYWORDS

• ACL injury • ACL reconstruction • Inflammation • Graft healing

KEY POINTS

- Inflammatory response plays a critical role in the healing process of anterior cruciate ligament (ACL) injuries.
- The ACL has a limited capacity for spontaneous healing, possibly because of limited scar tissue formation.
- ACL reconstruction triggers a secondary inflammatory response.
- Migration of fibroblasts, production of extracellular matrix, and revascularization contribute to graft integration and maturation after ACL reconstruction.

INTRODUCTION

Anterior cruciate ligament (ACL) tears are common knee injuries that can lead to significant morbidity and functional impairment.[1] ACL tears frequently occur in sports that involve sudden deceleration, jumping, and pivoting, such as soccer, basketball, and football.[2,3] More than 200,000 ACL tears occur per year in the United States, resulting in billions of dollars of annual health care costs.[4,5]

Without appropriate treatment, ACL tears can lead to negative repercussion, such as posttraumatic osteoarthritis (PTOA), knee injuries from chronic instability, reduced mobility and function, and overall decreased quality of life.[6,7] As an intra-articular ligament with limited healing capacity, ACL tears often require surgical intervention to restore knee function.[8] The current gold standard treatment of an ACL tear in moderate-to-high demand individuals is ligament reconstruction using either an autologous or allogenous graft.[9]

Department of Orthopaedic Surgery, Center for Cartilage Repair and Sports Medicine, Brigham and Women's Hospital, Harvard Medical School, 75 Francis Street, Boston, MA 02115, USA
* Corresponding author.
E-mail address: clattermann@bwh.harvard.edu

Clin Sports Med 43 (2024) 501–512
https://doi.org/10.1016/j.csm.2023.07.003

Although ACL reconstructions often have excellent clinical outcomes, it is not without risk. Mechanical factors, such as inappropriate tunnel positioning and graft fixation, can influence the final stability of the knee and in the case of an unstable joint, lead to negative clinical outcomes.[10] Biologic factors can similarly impact the success of ACL reconstruction.[11] The inflammatory response triggered by the injury, surgical intervention, and intra-articular synovial fluid environment may substantially affect the patient's outcome.[8] Hence, understanding the biology of ACL injury and reconstruction is crucial for developing effective treatment strategies and improving patient outcomes. This review outlines some aspects of the biology behind ACL tears, including (1) the inflammatory response of ACL injuries, (2) the lack of spontaneous ACL healing, (3) the second inflammatory "hit" triggered by ACL reconstruction, and (4) the biologic process of graft healing after surgery.

INFLAMMATORY RESPONSE OF ANTERIOR CRUCIATE LIGAMENT INJURY

Inflammation is a complex biologic response to injuries or infections that involves a series of molecular and cellular events. Inflammation plays a critical role in ACL injury biology.[7,12–14] Immediately after an ACL injury, resident immune cells are activated and release proinflammatory molecules, such as cytokines, chemokines, and lipid mediators.[15,16] Preclinical and clinical studies have demonstrated increased synovial fluid levels of tumor necrosis factor-α, interleukin (IL)-1β, IL-6, IL-8, monocyte chemoattractant protein-1 (MCP-1/CCL2), and prostaglandins after ACL injury.[7,17–22] Tissue gene expression analyses have also shown increased expression of matrix-degrading enzymes (eg, metalloproteinase-3) and inducible nitric oxide synthase following an ACL injury.[23] These molecules increase blood supply and attract more immune cells to the site of injury. Neutrophils are the first cells to arrive and phagocytose damaged tissue and release of proinflammatory molecules.[24,25] Following this, recruited monocytes/macrophages phagocytose debris and release cytokines, chemokines, and lipid mediators.[26,27] T cells are also part of the acute immune response to ACL injury and may help facilitate the removal of debris and prompt the healing process to begin.[16]

Although inflammation is crucial for repair, excessive or prolonged inflammation can contribute to tissue degradation and healing impairment. In this regard, the resolution of inflammation needs to occur to ensure the reestablishment of joint homeostasis.[28] Resolution of inflammation is an active process coordinated by specific proresolutive molecules, including the specialized proresolving mediators. Specialized proresolving mediators are omega-3/6 fatty acids–derivatives that resolve inflammation and promote tissue repair by inhibiting proinflammatory mediators, removing immune and apoptotic cells, and ultimately restoring tissue integrity and function.[28] ACL tears trigger a series of cellular and molecular mechanisms aimed at resolving the inflammatory response.[29–31] One critical process involved in the resolution of inflammation is the switch from proinflammatory to anti-inflammatory/proresolutive mediators.[29] This process is driven by changes in macrophage phenotypes from proinflammatory (M1) macrophages, to anti-inflammatory (M2) macrophages.[29,30] During the inflammation resolution phase, the production of proinflammatory molecules switches to anti-inflammatory molecules, such as IL-10, IL-1 receptor antagonist (IL-1Ra), and transforming growth factor-β (TGF-β). Proresolving mediators, including the specialized proresolving mediators (eg, lipoxins, maresins, resolvins, and protectins) eventually conclude the inflammatory response.[32–35] These molecules also stimulate tissue repair and remodeling by secreting cytokines, lipid mediators, and growth factors involved in angiogenesis, modulation of fibroblasts migration and proliferation, and synthesis of extracellular matrix (ECM).[36,37]

Fibroblasts are responsible for the synthesis and deposition of ECM components, such as collagen and proteoglycans, a critical step for healing and remodeling. Indeed, previous studies have demonstrated that, after an ACL injury, fibroblasts migrate to and proliferate within the injured site, where they produce ECM proteins that help to repair the tissue.[38]

Inflammation associated with soft tissue injuries activates the coagulation cascade, leading to the formation of a fibrin clot that normally helps to stabilize the injury site.[39] However, when it comes to the ACL, there usually is a lack of effective clot formation between the two injured ends of the ACL.[8] The absence of clot around the injured ACL may help explain why the inflammatory response after an ACL injury is insufficient to promote healing.

LACK OF SPONTANEOUS HEALING

Unlike extra-articular ligaments, such as the medial collateral ligament (MCL), the ACL is largely intra-articular and cannot heal on its own.[8] Previous research has investigated this peculiarity of the ACL. When comparing ACL fibroblasts with MCL fibroblasts, researchers found that ACL cells are capable of generating a healing response when stimulated in a controlled environment.[40,41] However, the provisional clot found around MCL injuries and other extra-articular ligament tears was missing around ACL tears.[40] This led researchers to hypothesize that lack of significant blood supply may impair the necessary clot formation.[8] Blood vessels play a critical role in tissue healing by delivering nutrients, oxygen, growth factors, and immune cells to the injury site and without this angiogenesis, healing is limited.[8] In addition, the ACL is located within a voluminous joint that is under constant mechanical stress and movement. This joint volume allows for uncontained egress of blood into the synovial joint cavity, whereas mechanical stress causes compressive, tensile, and shear forces that can further disrupt the wound scar eventually formed during the process. Furthermore, the joint is filled with synovial fluid, which is enriched with molecules that limit the formation of scar tissue, such as plasmin and collagenases,[42,43] and the ACL cells themselves produce fewer growth factors (eg, platelet-derived growth factor, TGF-β, and *basic fibroblast growth factor*).[8] Together, these factors explain the absence of spontaneous ACL healing observed.

ANTERIOR CRUCIATE LIGAMENT RECONSTRUCTION AND THE SECOND INFLAMMATORY "HIT"

ACL reconstruction is the preferred treatment because of the ACL's limited healing ability. However, recent advances in ACL repair techniques have been investigated.[44–48] The bridge-enhanced ACL repair (BEAR) uses a scaffold covered by autologous blood that supplies enzymes and growth factors capable of enhancing migration of fibroblasts, nerves, and blood vessels into the torn ACL.[49] These novel strategies have shown promising outcomes and deserve further investigation.

After ACL reconstruction or repair, inflammation can increase because of surgical trauma, response to the foreign material associated with the implanted graft, and mechanical loading during rehabilitation.[50–56] This leads to a second inflammatory response ("second hit") that is, once again, represented by cellular infiltration and release of proinflammatory mediators, which promotes healing. Recent studies have shown that ACL reconstruction triggers an acute inflammatory response with elevated levels of proinflammatory cytokines, such as IL-1β and IL-6.[50] This inflammation can remain present for months to years after ACL reconstruction.[52,57]

Although the inflammatory response is crucial for promoting graft integration, revascularization, and remodeling, excessive or unresolved inflammation is detrimental. It can lead to graft failure, impaired healing, and the development of PTOA.[58,59] Prolonged inflammation can increase the risk of cartilage and bone degeneration leading to PTOA, which is seen in more than 50% of ACL patients, regardless of the ligament reconstruction.[6,60–62]

Nonsteroidal anti-inflammatory drugs are commonly used to manage postoperative pain and inflammation after ACL reconstruction.[63] However, previous evidence suggests that nonsteroidal anti-inflammatory drugs may impair bone, tendon, and ligament healing by inhibiting the necessary inflammatory response and reducing ECM synthesis and the mechanical strength of the repaired tissue.[64–69] Therefore, the use of nonsteroidal anti-inflammatory drugs after ACL reconstruction should be judiciously considered, balancing the benefits of pain relief against the potential adverse effects on healing. With this in mind, several emerging strategies that modulate the inflammatory response after ACL injury and reconstruction have been investigated.[70] These include the use of corticosteroids, anti-inflammatory cytokines, growth factors, and mesenchymal stem cells.[7,70–72] These emerging therapies ultimately aim to promote tissue repair while reducing the detrimental effects of excessive inflammation. Further research is needed to determine the safety and efficacy of these novel therapies.

GRAFT HEALING AFTER ANTERIOR CRUCIATE LIGAMENT RECONSTRUCTION

The biology of graft healing relies on two interrelated stages: midsubstance ligamentization and the osteointegration at the graft-tunnel interface.[70] These stages occur in overlapping phases that include an early healing phase, which involves inflammation, cellular infiltration, and revascularization. This is followed by a proliferative phase and a remodeling phase, where fibroblasts migrate into the healing site and ECM components are produced.[11] Finally, the ligamentization process occurs to restore the native properties of the ACL. At the graft-tunnel interface, Sharpey fibers anchor the graft to the adjacent bone to provide mechanical stability.[73,74]

During the inflammatory phase, the surgical trauma induces the release of cytokines and chemokines that recruit additional inflammatory cells to the site of injury.[50,57] In this phase, the graft is initially populated by host immune cells that secrete cytokines, chemokines, reactive oxygen species, and growth factors that cause cell migration, cell proliferation, revascularization, and synthesis of ECM molecules.[75,76] This response is critical for clearing away cellular debris and creating a permissive environment for subsequent stages of healing and graft maturation. Neutrophils and macrophages invade the periphery of the graft and initiate tissue remodeling.[75] The hypoxia that occurs after reconstruction also plays a crucial role by releasing vascular endothelial growth factor, which induces revascularization that provides a source of nutrients and oxygen.[76,77] Particularly in the first month after surgery, the number of cells in the graft decreases and central areas of the graft suffer necrosis.[77]

As the inflammation subsides, cells derived from synovial tissue, remnant ACL, and host bone marrow infiltrate the graft. This marks the proliferative phase of healing.[11,78] During this phase between the sixth to eighth week postoperatively, the graft is weak because of the grafts' initial hypocellularity.[38] This corresponds to the vulnerable phase for graft rupturing observed clinically around this timeframe.[79] Following this period, the cellularity progressively increases from the periphery to the center of the graft until there are more cells in the graft than in a native ACL.[80] These cells, mainly formed by mesenchymal stem cells and fibroblasts, secrete various growth factors

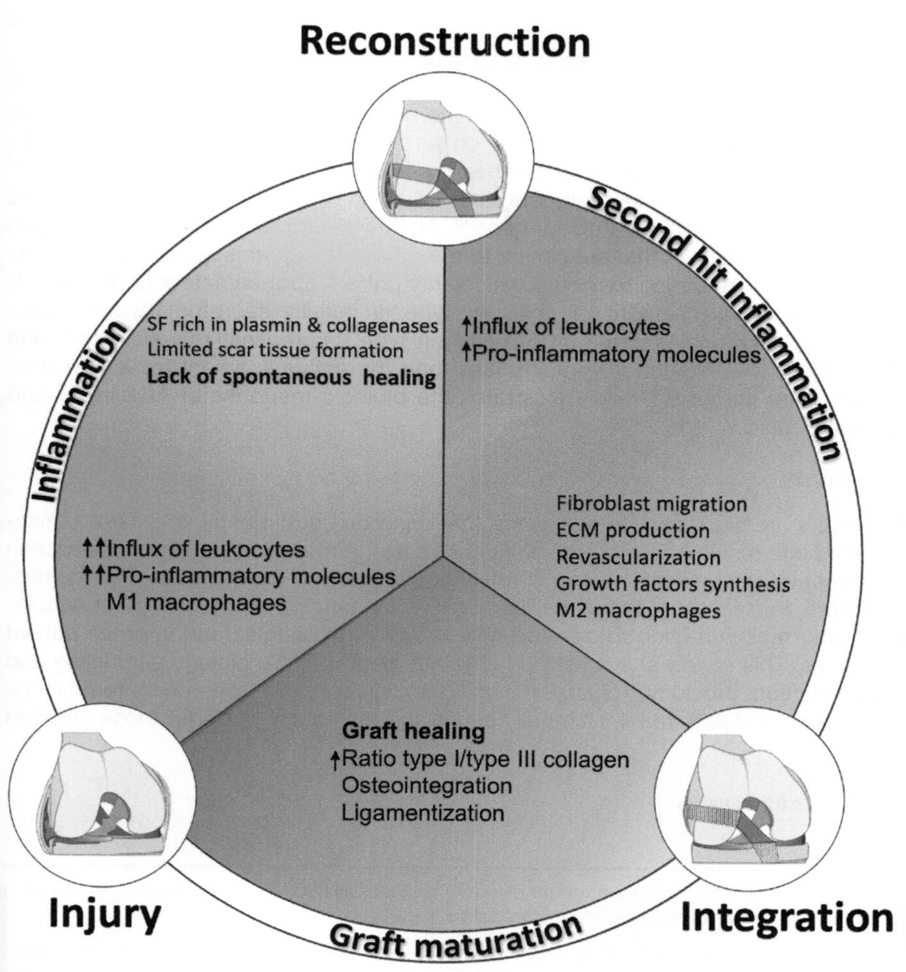

Fig. 1. The biologic response of ACL injury and reconstruction. ACL injury leads to an initial inflammation characterized by the influx of leukocytes and release of proinflammatory molecules. However, spontaneous healing of the ACL does not usually occur, mainly because of the presence of plasmin and collagenases in the synovial fluid (SF) that limit scar formation. After ACL reconstruction, a second hit of inflammation is triggered, leading to another influx of leukocyte and release of proinflammatory molecules. This process is followed by fibroblast migration, extracellular matrix (ECM) production, and revascularization, eventually culminating in graft osteointegration and maturation.

that stimulates tissue repair including *basic fibroblast growth factor*, TGF-β, and platelet-derived growth factor.[81] The number of myofibroblasts also increases, which are responsible for the tensioning structure necessary for the ligamentization process.[82] Mesenchymal stem cells have also been shown to be crucial for graft osteointegration by differentiating into osteoblasts and osteoclasts, which contribute to new bone formation.[83] Osteoblasts are responsible for producing the ECM that forms the bone matrix, whereas osteoclasts are responsible for removing old bone tissue. In addition, the ECM deposited mainly by fibroblasts during graft integration is composed of a variety of proteins, including collagen and glycosaminoglycans.[38] These proteins provide the scaffold for new bone growth in the graft-tunnel interface and are regulated by a variety of molecular signals, including bone morphogenetic proteins and TGF-β.[84–86] The bone maturation at the graft-tunnel interface gradually evolves, and seems to be dependent on an adequate resolution of inflammation response, as shown by the enhanced healing when M2 macrophages take over.[30,87]

At the midsubstance portion, the intra-articular ligamentization process starts approximately 3 months after surgery.[38] At this point, the graft has developed several characteristics that are similar to the native ACL. In this phase, vascularization decreases, returning to normal vascularity pattern approximately 12 months after surgery.[38] The amount of collagen type III initially secreted by fibroblasts decreases, whereas the amount of collagen type I increases. However, the ratio of collagen I to collagen III remains less than the native ligament for longer than 3 years after surgery.[88] **Fig. 1** illustrates the biologic response of ACL injury and reconstruction.

SUMMARY

ACL tears are significant knee injuries that can have detrimental long-term consequences and result in significant health care costs. Although ligament reconstruction is currently the standard treatment, biologic factors can impact patient outcomes. Therefore, it is essential to have a thorough understanding of the biology of ACL injuries and reconstruction to develop new treatment strategies and improve patient outcomes. This review sheds light on critical aspects of ACL biology after injury and reconstruction, providing valuable insights for clinicians and researchers to advance the treatment of ACL tears, ultimately enhancing the quality of life for those affected by this injury.

CLINICS CARE POINTS

- ACL injuries lead to an inflammatory response that is crucial for healing. However, sustained or unresolved inflammation is detrimental to tissue repair.
- The ACL has a limited healing capacity. This may be caused by the inability to form an effective clot between the injured ends of the ligament.
- ACL reconstruction leads to a second inflammatory "hit" that decreases over time, although signs of inflammation remain present for an extended period after surgery.
- Strategies that modulate the biologic response after ACL injury and its reconstruction could help improve patient outcomes.

DISCLOSURE OF FUNDING SOURCE

None.

FINANCIAL DISCLOSURE

Authors have no financial relationships relevant to this study to disclose.

CONFLICT OF INTEREST

Authors have no conflict of interest to disclose.

REFERENCES

1. Lyman S, Koulouvaris P, Sherman S, et al. Epidemiology of anterior cruciate ligament reconstruction. J Bone Joint Surg Am 2009;91(10):2321–8.
2. Waldén M, Krosshaug T, Bjørneboe J, et al. Three distinct mechanisms predominate in non-contact anterior cruciate ligament injuries in male professional football players: a systematic video analysis of 39 cases. Br J Sports Med 2015; 49(22):1452–60.
3. Krosshaug T, Nakamae A, Boden BP, et al. Mechanisms of anterior cruciate ligament injury in basketball: video analysis of 39 cases. Am J Sports Med 2007; 35(3):359–67.
4. Mall NA, Chalmers PN, Moric M, et al. Incidence and trends of anterior cruciate ligament reconstruction in the United States. Am J Sports Med 2014;42(10): 2363–70.
5. Mather RC 3rd, Koenig L, Kocher MS, et al. Societal and economic impact of anterior cruciate ligament tears. J Bone Joint Surg Am 2013;95(19):1751–9.
6. Øiestad BE, Engebretsen L, Storheim K, et al. Knee osteoarthritis after anterior cruciate ligament injury: a systematic review. Am J Sports Med 2009;37(7): 1434–43.
7. Lattermann C, Jacobs CA, Proffitt Bunnell M, et al. A multicenter study of early anti-inflammatory treatment in patients with acute anterior cruciate ligament tear. Am J Sports Med 2017;45(2):325–33.
8. Murray MM, Fleming BC. Biology of anterior cruciate ligament injury and repair: Kappa Delta Ann Doner Vaughn award paper 2013. J Orthop Res 2013;31(10): 1501–6.
9. Chambat P, Guier C, Sonnery-Cottet B, et al. The evolution of ACL reconstruction over the last fifty years. Int Orthop 2013;37(2):181–6.
10. Celiktas M, Kose O, Sarpel Y, et al. Can we use intraoperative femoral tunnel length measurement as a clue for proper femoral tunnel placement on coronal plane during ACL reconstruction? Arch Orthop Trauma Surg 2015;135(4):523–8.
11. Leite CBG, Demange MK. Biological enhancements for anterior cruciate ligament reconstruction. Acta Ortop Bras 2019;27(6):325–30.
12. Bigoni M, Sacerdote P, Turati M, et al. Acute and late changes in intraarticular cytokine levels following anterior cruciate ligament injury. J Orthop Res 2013; 31(2):315–21.
13. Dare D, Rodeo S. Mechanisms of post-traumatic osteoarthritis after ACL injury. Curr Rheumatol Rep 2014;16(10):448.
14. Swärd P, Frobell R, Englund M, et al. Cartilage and bone markers and inflammatory cytokines are increased in synovial fluid in the acute phase of knee injury (hemarthrosis): a cross-sectional analysis. Osteoarthritis Cartilage 2012;20(11): 1302–8.
15. Amano K, Huebner JL, Stabler TV, et al. Synovial fluid profile at the time of anterior cruciate ligament reconstruction and its association with cartilage matrix composition 3 years after surgery. Am J Sports Med 2018;46(4):890–9.
16. Kim-Wang SY, Holt AG, McGowan AM, et al. Immune cell profiles in synovial fluid after anterior cruciate ligament and meniscus injuries. Arthritis Res Ther 2021; 23(1):280.
17. Catterall JB, Stabler TV, Flannery CR, et al. Changes in serum and synovial fluid biomarkers after acute injury (NCT00332254). Arthritis Res Ther 2010;12(6):R229.

18. King JD, Rowland G, Villasante Tezanos AG, et al. Joint fluid proteome after anterior cruciate ligament rupture reflects an acute posttraumatic inflammatory and chondrodegenerative state. Cartilage 2018. 1947603518790009.
19. Braza-Boïls A, Alcaraz MJ, Ferrándiz ML. Regulation of the inflammatory response by tin protoporphyrin IX in the rat anterior cruciate ligament transection model of osteoarthritis. J Orthop Res 2011;29(9):1375–82.
20. Irie K, Uchiyama E, Iwaso H. Intraarticular inflammatory cytokines in acute anterior cruciate ligament injured knee. Knee 2003;10(1):93–6.
21. Keil LG, Onuscheck DS, Pratson LF 2nd, et al. Bone bruising severity after anterior cruciate ligament rupture predicts elevation of chemokine MCP-1 associated with osteoarthritis. J Exp Orthop 2022;9(1):37.
22. Bigoni M, Turati M, Zatti G, et al. Intra-articular cytokine levels in adolescent patients after anterior cruciate ligament tear. Mediators Inflamm 2018;2018: 4210593.
23. Gilbert SJ, Bonnet CS, Stadnik P, et al. Inflammatory and degenerative phases resulting from anterior cruciate rupture in a non-invasive murine model of post-traumatic osteoarthritis. J Orthop Res 2018;17. https://doi.org/10.1002/jor.23872.
24. Haslauer CM, Proffen BL, Johnson VM, et al. Gene expression of catabolic inflammatory cytokines peak before anabolic inflammatory cytokines after ACL injury in a preclinical model. J Inflamm 2014;11(1):34.
25. Wilgus TA, Roy S, McDaniel JC. Neutrophils and wound repair: positive actions and negative reactions. Adv Wound Care 2013;2(7):379–88.
26. Fujii T, Wada S, Carballo CB, et al. Distinct inflammatory macrophage populations sequentially infiltrate bone-to-tendon interface tissue after anterior cruciate ligament (ACL) reconstruction surgery in mice. JBMR Plus 2022;6(7):e10635.
27. Butterfield TA, Best TM, Merrick MA. The dual roles of neutrophils and macrophages in inflammation: a critical balance between tissue damage and repair. J Athl Train 2006;41(4):457–65.
28. Serhan CN, Savill J. Resolution of inflammation: the beginning programs the end. Nat Immunol 2005;6(12):1191–7.
29. Fadok VA, Bratton DL, Konowal A, et al. Macrophages that have ingested apoptotic cells in vitro inhibit proinflammatory cytokine production through autocrine/paracrine mechanisms involving TGF-beta, PGE2, and PAF. J Clin Invest 1998;101(4):890–8.
30. Liu S, Lin J, Luo Z, et al. Changes in macrophage polarization during tendon-to-bone healing after ACL reconstruction with insertion-preserved hamstring tendon: results in a rabbit model. Orthop J Sports Med 2022;10(5). 23259671221090896.
31. Turati M, Franchi S, Leone G, et al. Resolvin E1 and cytokines environment in skeletally immature and adult ACL tears. Front Med 2021;8:610866.
32. Liu T, Xiang A, Peng T, et al. HMGB1-C1q complexes regulate macrophage function by switching between leukotriene and specialized proresolving mediator biosynthesis. Proc Natl Acad Sci U S A 2019;116(46):23254–63.
33. Ortega-Gómez A, Perretti M, Soehnlein O. Resolution of inflammation: an integrated view. EMBO Mol Med 2013;5(5):661–74.
34. Chandrasekharan JA, Sharma-Walia N. Lipoxins: nature's way to resolve inflammation. J Inflamm Res 2015;8:181–92.
35. Arnardottir HH, Dalli J, Norling LV, et al. Resolvin D3 is dysregulated in arthritis and reduces arthritic inflammation. J Immunol 2016;197(6):2362–8.
36. Pils V, Terlecki-Zaniewicz L, Schosserer M, et al. The role of lipid-based signalling in wound healing and senescence. Mech Ageing Dev 2021;198(111527):111527.

37. Wang R, Xu B, Xu HG. Up-regulation of TGF-β promotes tendon-to-bone healing after anterior cruciate ligament reconstruction using bone marrow-derived mesenchymal stem cells through the TGF-β/MAPK signaling pathway in a New Zealand white rabbit model. Cell Physiol Biochem 2017;41(1):213–26.
38. Scheffler SU, Unterhauser FN, Weiler A. Graft remodeling and ligamentization after cruciate ligament reconstruction. Knee Surg Sports Traumatol Arthrosc 2008; 16(9):834–42.
39. Levi M, van der Poll T. Inflammation and coagulation. Crit Care Med 2010;38(2 Suppl):S26–34.
40. Murray MM, Spindler KP, Ballard P, et al. Enhanced histologic repair in a central wound in the anterior cruciate ligament with a collagen-platelet-rich plasma scaffold. J Orthop Res 2007;25(8):1007–17.
41. Murray MM, Spector M. The migration of cells from the ruptured human anterior cruciate ligament into collagen-glycosaminoglycan regeneration templates in vitro. Biomaterials 2001;22(17):2393–402.
42. Rość D, Powierza W, Zastawna E, et al. Post-traumatic plasminogenesis in intraarticular exudate in the knee joint. Med Sci Monit 2002;8(5):CR371–8.
43. Tang Z, Yang L, Wang Y, et al. Contributions of different intraarticular tissues to the acute phase elevation of synovial fluid MMP-2 following rat ACL rupture. J Orthop Res 2009;27(2):243–8.
44. Murray MM, Spindler KP, Abreu E, et al. Collagen-platelet rich plasma hydrogel enhances primary repair of the porcine anterior cruciate ligament. J Orthop Res 2007;25(1):81–91.
45. DiFelice GS, Villegas C, Taylor S. Anterior cruciate ligament preservation: early results of a novel arthroscopic technique for suture anchor primary anterior cruciate ligament repair. Arthroscopy 2015;31(11):2162–71.
46. Heusdens CHW, Hopper GP, Dossche L, et al. Anterior cruciate ligament repair with independent suture tape reinforcement: a case series with 2-year follow-up. Knee Surg Sports Traumatol Arthrosc 2019;27(1):60–7.
47. DiFelice GS, van der List JP. Clinical outcomes of arthroscopic primary repair of proximal anterior cruciate ligament tears are maintained at mid-term follow-up. Arthroscopy 2018;34(4):1085–93.
48. Kohl S, Evangelopoulos DS, Ahmad SS, et al. A novel technique, dynamic intraligamentary stabilization creates optimal conditions for primary ACL healing: a preliminary biomechanical study. Knee 2014;21(2):477–80.
49. Murray MM, Fleming BC, Badger GJ, et al. Bridge-enhanced anterior cruciate ligament repair is not inferior to autograft anterior cruciate ligament reconstruction at 2 years: results of a prospective randomized clinical trial. Am J Sports Med 2020; 48(6):1305–15.
50. Hunt ER, Jacobs CA, Conley CEW, et al. Anterior cruciate ligament reconstruction reinitiates an inflammatory and chondrodegenerative process in the knee joint. J Orthop Res 2021;39(6):1281–8.
51. Eriksson K, von Essen C, Jönhagen S, et al. No risk of arthrofibrosis after acute anterior cruciate ligament reconstruction. Knee Surg Sports Traumatol Arthrosc 2018;26(10):2875–82.
52. Bigoni M, Turati M, Gandolla M, et al. Effects of ACL reconstructive surgery on temporal variations of cytokine levels in synovial fluid. Mediators Inflamm 2016; 2016:8243601.
53. Hayward AL, Deehan DJ, Aspden RM, et al. Analysis of sequential cytokine release after ACL reconstruction. Knee Surg Sports Traumatol Arthrosc 2011; 19(10):1709–15.

54. Yang R, Zhang Z, Song B, et al. Ratio of T helper to regulatory T cells in synovial fluid and postoperative joint laxity after allograft anterior cruciate ligament reconstruction. Transplantation 2012;94(11):1160–6.
55. Nishikawa Y, Kokubun T, Kanemura N, et al. Effects of controlled abnormal joint movement on the molecular biological response in intra-articular tissues during the acute phase of anterior cruciate ligament injury in a rat model. BMC Musculoskelet Disord 2018;19(1). https://doi.org/10.1186/s12891-018-2107-6.
56. Brophy RH, Kovacevic D, Imhauser CW, et al. Effect of short-duration low-magnitude cyclic loading versus immobilization on tendon-bone healing after ACL reconstruction in a rat model. J Bone Joint Surg Am 2011;93(4):381–93.
57. Larsson S, Struglics A, Lohmander LS, et al. Surgical reconstruction of ruptured anterior cruciate ligament prolongs trauma-induced increase of inflammatory cytokines in synovial fluid: an exploratory analysis in the KANON trial. Osteoarthritis Cartilage 2017;25(9):1443–51.
58. Habouri L, El Mansouri FE, Ouhaddi Y, et al. Deletion of 12/15-lipoxygenase accelerates the development of aging-associated and instability-induced osteoarthritis. Osteoarthritis Cartilage 2017;25(10):1719–28.
59. Song B, Jiang C, Luo H, et al. Macrophage M1 plays a positive role in aseptic inflammation-related graft loosening after anterior cruciate ligament reconstruction surgery. Inflammation 2017;40(6):1815–24.
60. Buller LT, Best MJ, Baraga MG, et al. Trends in anterior cruciate ligament reconstruction in the United States. Orthop J Sports Med 2015;3(1). 2325967114563664.
61. Ayral X, Pickering EH, Woodworth TG, et al. Synovitis: a potential predictive factor of structural progression of medial tibiofemoral knee osteoarthritis: results of a 1 year longitudinal arthroscopic study in 422 patients. Osteoarthritis Cartilage 2005;13(5):361–7.
62. Attur M, Belitskaya-Lévy I, Oh C, et al. Increased interleukin-1β gene expression in peripheral blood leukocytes is associated with increased pain and predicts risk for progression of symptomatic knee osteoarthritis. Arthritis Rheum 2011;63(7): 1908–17.
63. Ge H, Liu C, Shrestha A, et al. Do nonsteroidal anti-inflammatory drugs affect tissue healing after arthroscopic anterior cruciate ligament reconstruction? Med Sc Monit 2018;24:6038–43.
64. Schug SA. Do NSAIDs really interfere with healing after surgery? J Clin Med 2021 10(11):2359.
65. Lisowska B, Kosson D, Domaracka K. Positives and negatives of nonsteroida anti-inflammatory drugs in bone healing: the effects of these drugs on bone repair. Drug Des Devel Ther 2018;12:1809–14.
66. Wheatley BM, Nappo KE, Christensen DL, et al. Effect of NSAIDs on bone healing rates: a meta-analysis. J Am Acad Orthop Surg 2019;27(7):e330–6.
67. Ghosh N, Kolade OO, Shontz E, et al. Nonsteroidal anti-inflammatory drugs (NSAIDs) and their effect on musculoskeletal soft-tissue healing: a scoping review. JBJS Rev 2019;7(12):e4.
68. Riley GP, Cox M, Harrall RL, et al. Inhibition of tendon cell proliferation and matrix glycosaminoglycan synthesis by non-steroidal anti-inflammatory drugs in vitro J Hand Surg Br 2001;26(3):224–8.
69. Carroll CC, Dickinson JM, LeMoine JK, et al. Influence of acetaminophen and ibuprofen on in vivo patellar tendon adaptations to knee extensor resistance exercise in older adults. J Appl Physiol 2011;111(2):508–15.

70. Hexter AT, Thangarajah T, Blunn G, et al. Biological augmentation of graft healing in anterior cruciate ligament reconstruction: a systematic review. Bone Joint Lett J 2018;100-B(3):271–84.
71. Khella CM, Horvath JM, Asgarian R, et al. Anti-inflammatory therapeutic approaches to prevent or delay post-traumatic osteoarthritis (PTOA) of the knee joint with a focus on sustained delivery approaches. Int J Mol Sci 2021;22(15): 8005.
72. Jacobs CA, Conley CEW, Kraus VB, et al. MOntelukast as a potential CHondroprotective treatment following Anterior cruciate ligament reconstruction (MOCHA Trial): study protocol for a double-blind, randomized, placebo-controlled clinical trial. Trials 2022;23(1):98.
73. Liu SH, Panossian V, al-Shaikh R, et al. Morphology and matrix composition during early tendon to bone healing. Clin Orthop Relat Res 1997;339(339):253–60.
74. Chen CH, Lee CH. Biological fixation in anterior cruciate ligament surgery. Asia-Pacific Journal of Sports Medicine, Arthroscopy, Rehabilitation and Technology 2014;1(2):48–53.
75. Ekdahl M, Wang JHC, Ronga M, et al. Graft healing in anterior cruciate ligament reconstruction. Knee Surg Sports Traumatol Arthrosc 2008;16(10):935–47.
76. Leite CBG, Tavares LP, Leite MS, et al. Revisiting the role of hyperbaric oxygen therapy in knee injuries: potential benefits and mechanisms. J Cell Physiol 2023;17. https://doi.org/10.1002/jcp.30947.
77. Janssen RPA, Scheffler SU. Intra-articular remodelling of hamstring tendon grafts after anterior cruciate ligament reconstruction. Knee Surg Sports Traumatol Arthrosc 2014;22(9):2102–8.
78. Ménétrey J, Duthon VB, Laumonier T, et al. "Biological failure" of the anterior cruciate ligament graft. Knee Surg Sports Traumatol Arthrosc 2008;16(3):224–31.
79. Zaffagnini S, De Pasquale V, Marchesini Reggiani L, et al. Neoligamentization process of BTPB used for ACL graft: histological evaluation from 6 months to 10 years. Knee 2007;14(2):87–93.
80. Scheffler S, Becker R. Graft Remodeling and Bony Ingrowth After ACL Reconstruction. In: Doral M., Karlsson J. (eds), Sports Injuries. Springer, Berlin, Heidelberg. 2013, Available at: https://doi.org/10.1007/978-3-642-36801-1_98-1.
81. Kuroda R, Kurosaka M, Yoshiya S, et al. Localization of growth factors in the reconstructed anterior cruciate ligament: immunohistological study in dogs. Knee Surg Sports Traumatol Arthrosc 2000;8(2):120–6.
82. Unterhauser FN, Bosch U, Zeichen J, et al. Alpha-smooth muscle actin containing contractile fibroblastic cells in human knee arthrofibrosis tissue. Winner of the AGA-DonJoy Award 2003. Arch Orthop Trauma Surg 2004;124(9):585–91.
83. Steinert AF, Kunz M, Prager P, et al. Mesenchymal stem cell characteristics of human anterior cruciate ligament outgrowth cells. Tissue Eng Part A 2011;17(9–10): 1375–88.
84. Gulotta LV, Rodeo SA. Biology of autograft and allograft healing in anterior cruciate ligament reconstruction. Clin Sports Med 2007;26(4):509–24.
85. Martinek V, Latterman C, Usas A, et al. Enhancement of tendon-bone integration of anterior cruciate ligament grafts with bone morphogenetic protein-2 gene transfer. J Bone Joint Surg Am 2002;84(7):1123–31.
86. Yasuda K, Tomita F, Yamazaki S, et al. The effect of growth factors on biomechanical properties of the bone-patellar tendon-bone graft after anterior cruciate ligament reconstruction: a canine model study. Am J Sports Med 2004;32(4):870–80.

87. Li Z, Li Q, Tong K, et al. BMSC-derived exosomes promote tendon-bone healing after anterior cruciate ligament reconstruction by regulating M1/M2 macrophage polarization in rats. Stem Cell Res Ther 2022;13(1):295.
88. Ng GY, Oakes BW, Deacon OW, et al. Long-term study of the biochemistry and biomechanics of anterior cruciate ligament-patellar tendon autografts in goats. J Orthop Res 1996;14(6):851–6.

Rehabilitation and Return to Sport After Anterior Cruciate Ligament Reconstruction

Rebecca Simonsson, PT, MSc[a,b,c], Ramana Piussi, PT, MSc[a,b,c], Johan Högberg, PT, MSc[a,b,c], Axel Sundberg, PT, MSc[b,c,d], Eric Hamrin Senorski, PT, PhD[a,b,c,e,*]

KEYWORDS

• ACL • Physical activity • Physical therapy • ACL injury • Prevention

KEY POINTS

- Rehabilitation is performed in phases with specific goals to guide progression within each phase and progression to the following phase.
- Before return to sport, patients should be both physically and psychologically ready for the demands that their sport imply.
- Physical and psychological readiness is determined by muscle function testing, psychological outcome scores, and on field testing involving change of direction tests but also by consultation between patient, physical therapist, surgeon, and coach.
- To minimize the risk for second ACL injury or subsequent injury, patients are advised to maintain strength and neuromuscular training as a form of prevention after having returned to sport.

BACKGROUND

Anterior cruciate ligament (ACL) injuries are severe traumatic knee injuries that are commonly sustained while particpating in sports, especially within cutting and pivoting sports, with an incidence of 68.6 injuries per 100,000 person-years.[1] The most frequently reported maneuvers for the occurrence of an ACL injury are a rapid deceleration, change of direction (COD), or landing after a jump during competitive sport.[2] Patients who aim to return to sport (RTS) after suffering an ACL injury are usually

[a] Sportrehab Sports Medicine Clinic, Stampgatan 14, Gothenburg SE-411 01, Sweden; [b] Sahlgrenska Sports Medicine Center, Gothenburg, Sweden; [c] Unit of Physiotherapy, Department of Health and Rehabilitation, Institute of Neuroscience and Physiology, Sahlgrenska Academy, University of Gothenburg, Box 455, Gothenburg SE-405 30, Sweden; [d] Capio Ortho Center, Arvid Wallgrens Backe 4a, Gothenburg SE-413 13, Sweden; [e] Swedish Olympic Committee, Olympiastadion 114 33, Stockholm, Sweden
* Corresponding author. Sportrehab Sports Medicine Clinic, Stampgatan 14, Gothenburg SE-411 01, Sweden.
E-mail address: eric.hamrin.senorski@gu.se

Clin Sports Med 43 (2024) 513–533
https://doi.org/10.1016/j.csm.2023.07.004
0278-5919/24/

recommended treatment consisting of rehabilitation with additional ACL reconstructive surgery.[3–5] Alternatively, patients can be offered treatment consisting of rehabilitation alone. Several factors, such as the degree of knee laxity, perceived knee instability, level of physical activity, age, and concomitant injuries are considered when chosing treatment because these factors can affect treatment outcomes.[3] Patients who are especially thought to benefit from ACL reconstruction, are patients who aim to RTS, are younger, and have greater knee laxity or greater perceived knee instability.[6,7] Reconstructive surgery can be performed with a bodily tendon (autograft) or a donated tendon (allograft). Among autografts, the use of the hamstring tendon (HT) autograft has increased during the past 3 decades compared with the bone-patellar tendon-bone (BPTB) autograft which, until 1992, was the dominant autograft for primary ACL reconstruction.[8] In the last decade, the quadriceps tendon (QT) autograft has also become a more common option as a reconstructive autograft after ACL injury.[8] The QT, HT, and BPTB tendons show comparable functional outcomes and, compared with the BPTB, the QT shows less harvesting donor-site pain, with survival rates similar to those of the HT and BPTB.[9] Despite an increase in the use of QT tendon autografts, the HT is still the most frequently used tendon, with 50% of primary reconstruction cases, followed by the BPTB (40%) and others (including the QT) in 10% of cases.[8]

After an ACL reconstruction, the subsequent rehabilitation lasts for a considerable period, that is, typically 9 to 12 months,[10] with some recommendations suggesting up to 2 years.[11] Rehabilitation aims to regain muscle strength, hop performance, and movement quality of the body and the knee and to restore knee-related quality of life, with a safe RTS as the ultimate goal, that is, without sustaining a second ACL injury.[3] Nevertheless, 1 in 4 young patients who return to pivoting sport sustains a second ACL injury.[12] Similar rates of second ACL injury are observed for men in professional elite soccer, with 1 in 5 sustaining a second ACL injury after RTS.[13] In addition, other subsequent knee injuries apart from a second ACL injury, such as meniscal or osteochondral injuries, are also common.[14] Worryingly, the rate of ACL injuries seems to be increasing, with increasing rates reported from Australia, especially in the young population.[15,16] The increasing rates of primary ACL injuries and the relatively high risk of a subsequent knee injury upon RTS after ACL reconstruction highlight the need for improvements in the care of patients treated with ACL reconstruction.

REHABILITATION

Preoperative Rehabilitation

The timing of ACL reconstruction is a subject of debate but in the absence of extensive symptoms of instability, surgery is often recommended to be scheduled in 4 to 12 weeks to reduce the inflammatory process related to the trauma, eliminate knee-joint effusion and improve range of motion and muscle function.[17] Despite the 4 to 12-week recommendation, there is great variability in the time between injury and reconstruction, due to regional differences in the health-care system. If ACL reconstruction is delayed for more than 8 weeks, it is important to maintain/increase quadriceps strength in particular because deficits in the injured leg of greater than 20% of the uninjured leg may result in a persistent quadriceps deficit up to 2 years after ACL reconstruction.[18] In line with previous findings, symmetric knee strength preoperatively has been shown to increase the likelihood of restoring strength earlier in the postoperative period.[19] Consequently, improving strength preoperatively is an important step in a successful rehabilitation after ACL reconstruction.

Goals

The goal is to prepare the patient for surgery physically by restoring knee-joint range of motion and improving muscle function.

Procedure

Restoring range of motion and muscle function while the knee recovers from the initial trauma of the injury situation. This is followed by strength training as tolerated by the affected knee.

Psychological Aspects

A central part of the preoperative preparations includes psychological groundwork for the patient to accept the postoperative rehabilitation process, especially the time requirement. Before ACL reconstruction, 84% of patients report that they expect full sports participation at the same level as preinjury, whereas unfortunately only 1 in 4 patients actually achieves this aim.[20]

The phases of ACL rehabilitation are presented in **Fig. 1**, and a schematic view of phases, goals, and evaluations is presented in **Table 1**. It is important to note that the phases merge into one another and never have a definite ending or beginning.

EARLY POSTOPERATIVE REHABILITATION—SETTLE THE KNEE AND CREATE A SOLID PLATFORM

An ACL reconstruction is a trauma to the knee, which ultimately leads to symptoms similar to those at the time of the ACL injury, such as hematoma, pain, joint effusion, arthrogenic muscle inhibition (AMI) and reduced range of motion.[21] Consequently, the different type of graft selection implies different types of donor-site morbidity and pain, where PT and QT autografts infer an increased risk of more prominent AMI, which negatively affects the voluntary activation of the quadriceps muscle, active knee extension at normal gait pattern and can contribute to pronounced muscle atrophy with a negative long-term impact on the extensor mechanism.[22–24] The magnitude of muscle atrophy is a significant part of the following rehabilitation process and, for individuals who suffer from AMI, neuromuscular electrostimulation or cryotherapy might be useful as supplements in early rehabilitation.[25] Reconstruction with the HT seems to produce milder early short-term effects but it can instead have a negative long-term impact on hamstring architecture and knee flexor strength potential.[26]

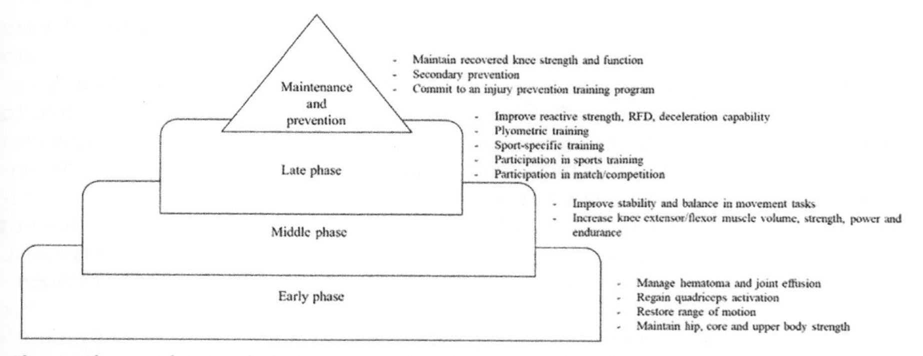

Fig. 1. Phases of ACL rehabilitation. RFD, rate of force development.

Table 1
Phases of rehabilitation, goals, and recommended evaluation

Phase of Rehabilitation	Goals	Evaluation
Early	Reduce swelling and pain; increase range of motion and muscle function	PROs; Stroke test Range of motion Numerical rating scale
Middle	Regain muscle strength	Muscle function tests and PROs
Late	Increase athletic performance and prepare the patient for a safe RTS and for the demands of the respective sport	Muscle function test; power, endurance, eccentric strength, hop performance, and PROs
Maintenance and prevention	Maintain physical fitness and perform an injury prevention program regularly	No evaluation recommended

PROs, patient reported outcomes; RTS, return to sport.

Goals

To reduce swelling and pain, minimize AMI and increase muscle function. At the end of the early postoperative rehabilitation phase, the aim is to have full range of motion and active terminal knee extension similar to the contralateral knee and to have initiated strength training and aerobic conditioning without any increase in swelling and pain following the rehabilitation session.

Procedure

For the standard procedure of ACL reconstruction, the current recommendations for early postoperative rehabilitation (<6 weeks) include full weight-bearing and range of motion immediately, but concomitant surgical treatments, such as meniscal sutures or cartilage procedures, may affect this approach.[25] Strength training includes both open kinetic chain (OKC) and closed kinetic chain (CKC) exercises (**Fig. 2**),[25] which can be initiated during the first weeks. At this stage, the training regimen should involve low stress on the ACL-reconstructed knee and its surrounding structures, and it is recommended to be performed several times a day with regard to pain and eventual joint effusion, to achieve the desired adaptations. Exercises start with no weight to light weight and this can then be increased depending on knee function and tolerance. Using OKC exercises can facilitate increased quadriceps strength, which is superior to CKC exercises alone,[27,28] without compromising graft integrity, regardless of the choice of autograft.[29–31] Both OKC and CKC exercises should be performed in the early stages of rehabilitation because the risk of increased anterior tibial laxity is very small for OKC compared with CKC exercises.[29] As a complement to weighted training, aquatic training is considered helpful to reduce pain and swelling, maintain cardiovascular fitness, and optimize motor patterns, which facilitates the recovery of gait and also improve recovery between weighted training sessions.[32]

In addition, a newly highlighted complement in rehabilitation is blood flow restriction (BFR) training, which has been proven to facilitate muscle growth and improve strength with lighter weights to the same extent as heavier weights in the early stages of rehabilitation.[33]

In order to maintain general conditioning, strength training for the upper body, core and lower body beyond knee-joint muscles should be implemented without

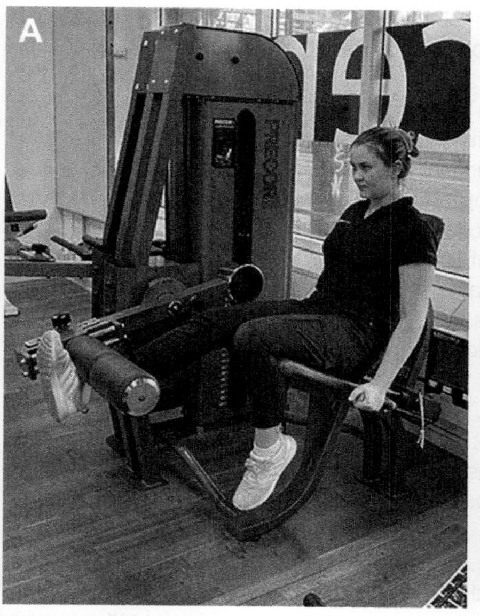

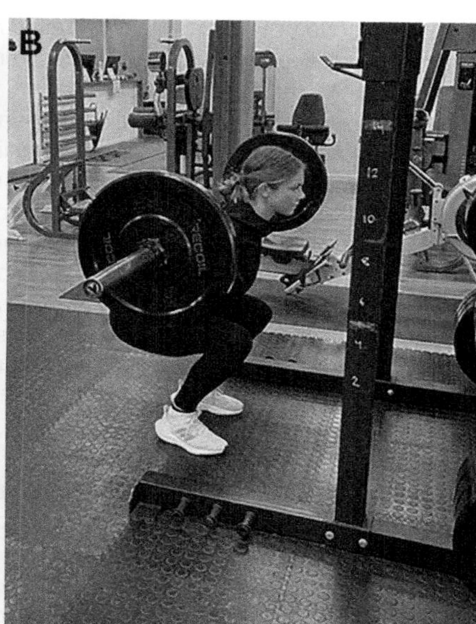

ig. 2. (*A*) Open chain and (*B*) closed chain.

estrictions. Aerobic conditioning on a stationary bike can be performed as tolerated. ntense strength training for the healthy limb is recommended, as strength improvenents in the reconstructed limb can be attained through the cross-education henomenon.[34]

sychological Aspects

n the weeks just before and just after surgery, patients can report high levels of sympoms of depression and anxiety.[35] This is especially important because early negative sychological reactions can affect rehabilitation outcomes up to 12 months after recontruction.[36] Consequently, therapists should be aware that the early phase after econstruction is a psychologically challenging period for patients. Having open ommunication and searching for eventual psychological problems is very important n this phase. Whenever there is a clinical suspicion that eventual symptoms of depression might result in a clinical diagnosis, referral to a sport psychologist is warranted.

valuation

he early use of patient-reported outcomes (PROs) can facilitate screening for evenual psychological distress, which might influence long-term outcomes.[37] The stroke est can be used objectively to assess knee joint swelling[38] and a numerical rating cale can be used for subjective measurements of perceived pain. Full active knee xtension should be achieved and knee flexion is recommended to be at least 90% f that in the contralateral knee.[39,40]

IDDLE PHASE—IMPROVE LOAD TOLERANCE AND STRENGTH AND START TO IOVE LIKE AN ATHLETE

nce the objectives of the initial phase have been achieved, the aim of rehabilitation hifts toward regaining muscle strength, with the uninjured limb commonly used as a proxy for recovery. Patients who undergo ACL reconstruction have been reported to struggle to achieve both symmetry and preoperative knee function in a battery of tests up to 12 months after reconstruction.[41,42]

The recovery of strength depends on an interaction between neural and muscular adaptations. Neural effects involve the ability to increase voluntary muscle activation, increase firing rate and intramuscular and intermuscular coordination such as the inhibition of antagonists.[43] Muscular hypertrophy occurs preferentially through 3 mechanisms: (1) muscular tension, (2) metabolic stress, and (3) training-induced cell damage and repair, all of which are relevant to consider when planning the rehabilitation process.[44] The structure of strength training and volume is based on the individual's previous training level, receptiveness, and training response but it follows the general guidelines for strength training, such as principles of overload, progression, and variation.[45]

Goals

The goal of rehabilitation in the middle phase is to regain muscle strength, both symmetric and preoperative strength (when possible to compare).

Procedure

Load, volume, and intensity should be modified throughout rehabilitation for different purposes, for example, muscular endurance, maximum strength, or explosive capacity, with both OKC and CKC exercises, such as squats (with possible variations, eg, back squats and front squats), leg press, or leg extension.[46] In addition, exercises should be performed both bilaterally and unilaterally to ensure that the uninjured limb does not compensate by taking an additional load, thereby increasing muscular gain in the injured limb.[46] By overloading the eccentric phase of repetitions, high-threshold motor units can be activated more efficiently, which is a prerequisite for optimal power and strength development.[47] Even in this phase of rehabilitation, BFR can help to optimize motor neuron recruitment and increase muscle strength. The focus during the rehabilitation should differ, depending on the choice of autograft for surgical reconstruction. For patients with an HT autograft, knee flexion strength exercises should be carried out in various positions and in a wide spectrum of knee flexion angles to optimize the contribution from both the medial and lateral knee flexors.[48–50] These exercises can include the Nordic hamstring, the seated leg curl, and hip extension exercises. However, PT and QT autografts need a clear approach to restore strength in knee extension moments within a deeper knee flexion range of motion, which means the simultaneous tension of the extensor complex.[51]

Parallel to strength improvements, the patient is gradually introduced to athletic movements, such as running. One milestone in this process for many athletes is to return to running. The functional criteria that should be met before running have not yet been determined. The most widely used criterion is postoperative time, where 12 weeks is the usual time-point to allow patients to start running.[52] At about this time-point, hop training and plyometrics are also introduced at an appropriate intensity level. The purpose is to recreate the ability of the knee joint and the lower kinetic chain effectively to use the stretch-shortening effect and improve the ability for rapid power development in multiplanar directions, as well as the reactive strength and stability during landing moments.[53]

Psychological Aspects

The middle phase can be challenging psychologically because it is difficult to maintain a high level of motivation and a large volume of training needs to be performed to achieve physical milestones. Achieving preset goals (eg, squat a certain weight) has been reported by both patients and physical therapists as a great source of motivation.[54,55] As more athletic movements such as jumps are introduced, patients might experience fear of reinjury,[56] and they should be guided with tasks of successively increasing difficulty, starting with simple, safe tasks. It is important to recognize that psychological and physical aspects during the middle phase do not necessarily correlate[57] and, despite improving physical capabilities, the patient might still not perceive the knee as better. For this reason, the respective aspects should be considered independently.

Evaluation

Patients should be continuously evaluated with muscle function tests and PROs in order to follow their progression and assist caregivers in load management and focus areas of rehabilitation. Strength tests with an isokinetic dynamometer are regarded as the "gold standard" for evaluating muscle strength.[58] Several different velocities and contraction modes have been investigated and the most frequently used angular velocities for tests are 60° to 180° per second. In addition to strength tests, a battery of hop performance tests is recommended to evaluate the ability for explosiveness, dynamic stability, and functional performance.[59] An asymmetry of greater than 20% between the ACL-reconstructed and uninjured limb has been suggested as reduced knee function.[60] For this reason, strength symmetry is suggested to range between 80% and 90%, based predominantly on consensus statements and expert opinions.[46] However, symmetry might not be trustworthy as the sole evaluation of knee function for the future. Instead, strength in relation to bodyweight (Newton meters/kilograms) has been proposed as an alternative to present adequate references for strength.[61] Several different PROs of varying methodological quality are used for patients who suffer an ACL injury.[62] Cut-offs for commonly used PROs for passing muscle function tests have shown no ability to discriminate between patients who sustain a second ACL injury and patients who do not.[63] Consequently, PROs should be used to evaluate self-reported symptoms at the specific time of evaluation but should not be regarded as having a prognostic value for sustaining a second ACL injury.

LATE PHASE—GET EXPLOSIVE AND PHYSICALLY ROBUST

On having regained symmetric muscle strength, patients enter the last part of rehabilitation before the process of RTS. Returning to sport after an ACL reconstruction entails increased exposure to the risk of suffering a second ACL injury,[12] where factors such as female sex,[64] younger age,[12] concomitant injuries, and surgical outcomes interplay[65,66] in the second ACL injury risk. Having symmetric knee strength represents a reduction in second ACL injury rates[67] and this can consequently be regarded as important during rehabilitation. A strength evaluation usually consists of tests of maximum strength, that is, with limited regard to rapid force production. The rapid stabilization of the knee joint when changing direction and landing is regarded as a key aspect in the prevention of knee injury and this function may be more dependent on the ability to increase force quickly from onset, the so-called rate of force development (RFD), rather than maximum strength.[68] The RFD can be categorized into different time frames where the later part of RFD, greater than 150 milliseconds from force onset, has a strong correlation to changes in maximum muscle strength. However, early RFD (0–100 milliseconds) is more closely associated with factors affecting relative RFD, such as the level of agonist muscle activation at activation onset, the contractile properties of the muscle, muscle fiber type, and the architectural characteristics of the muscle.[69] After ACL reconstruction, early RFD can be significantly reduced compared with the uninvolved limb, despite symmetric maximum strength.[70] In addition to improving explosive muscular function, approaching RTS means that rehabilitation needs to prepare sport-specific movement tasks. This involves the physically demanding training of deceleration capacity, the ability to perform multiplanar movements and improving both muscular endurance and aerobic capacity to cope with the demands of sport.[71]

Goals

The last part of rehabilitation aims to increase athletic performance and prepare the patient for a safe RTS, that is, without sustaining a second ACL injury.

Procedure

In addition to strength training, more intense plyometric training in combination with agility, endurance, and power should be used to restore explosiveness and physical robustness. Plyometric training is constituted by the peak external load of the task at hand, joint-specific internal moments, reactivity, muscle forces and control challenges, all of which are important for participation in sports.[53] In order to improve neuromuscular control in sports, strength training itself is not enough and plyometric exercises can be more transferable to athletic movements.[53] Due to the complexity of plyometric training, rehabilitation should include linear and multiplanar tasks, strength, and movement quality. The intensity of exercise performance should be adjusted based on purpose, where sessions focused on high explosiveness can be alternated with high-volume sessions focusing on improving aerobic capacity to match competitive levels. For example, Almeida and colleagues[72] reported that professional soccer players at 6 months after ACL reconstruction have a markedly reduced aerobic capacity compared with uninjured controls.

Psychological Aspects

Patients have reported that, when approaching RTS, psychological barriers, such as fear of reinjury, are perceived as greater compared with physical barriers.[73] Importantly, patients who suffered a second ACL injury after ACL reconstruction have reported not feeling ready to RTS, despite physical tests showing satisfactory outcomes,[55] and physical and psychological measurements of training intensity do not generally correlate.[74] Consequently, clinicians working with patients who rehabilitate after ACL reconstruction should apply clear and concise communication, in order to support patients, in case psychological impairments are experienced. Importantly, clinicians should check how patients would like to receive support before providing it. With regard to psychological impairments and second ACL injury, previous research has shown that patients who have both a strong or a weak psychological profile run a higher risk of sustaining a second ACL injury.[75,76] As the psychological spectra are broad, ranging from fear to confidence in the reconstructed knee, it is likely that the psychological response curve is U-shaped (**Fig. 3**), implying that extremes in both a positive and a negative direction can increase the risk of a second ACL injury.[77] A close observation of psychological factors during rehabilitation might therefore be just as important as the physical factors.

Evaluation

Before RTS, the continuous and meticulous evaluation of patients with muscle function tests and patient-reported results is central. When possible, measurements of RFD, muscular endurance and aerobic capacity are encouraged. PROs that are

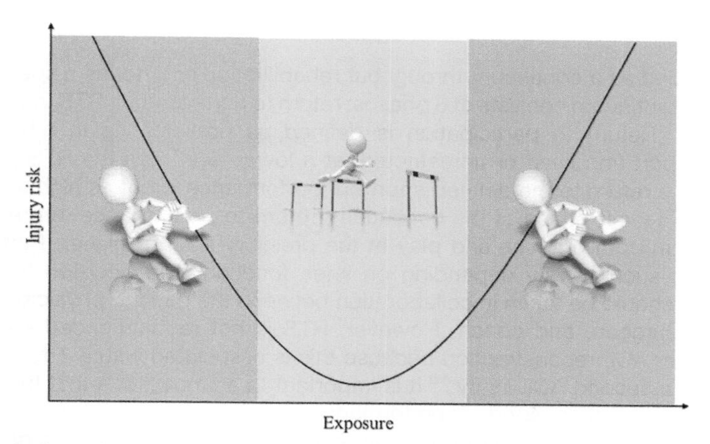

Fig. 3. Psychological response. Red zones indicate an increased risk of injury; the green zone indicates a reduced risk of injury.

designed for later stage rehabilitation, such as the ACL Return to Sport after Injury Scale, can be paid more attention compared with less sensitive scales, such as the Knee injury and Osteoarthritis Outcome Score subscales of symptoms or activities of daily living.

MAINTENANCE AND PREVENTION PHASE

After a successful RTS and performance, patients are encouraged to maintain knee function through regular gym sessions and, ideally, to perform a knee-specific secondary prevention program in parallel with sports training.

Goals

The goal in the maintenance phase is to maintain knee-load tolerance and the strength and stability attained during rehabilitation and to minimize the risk of a second ACL injury via secondary prevention programs. Recommended preventive training programs include a combination of neuromuscular training, strengthening, balance, and proximal control exercises[78] but the optimal combination of exercises to include in a secondary prevention program is still unclear.[37]

Procedure

Knee-specific prevention training can be performed on a weekly basis but it should be adapted to every specific patient, taking account of the specific patient's training schedule, volume, and perceived exertion.[74]

Psychological Aspects

A history of stressors, that is, having had several stressful events, and stress response, that is, how a certain patient reacts to stress, has been shown to have the strongest association with sport injury risks.[79] Consequently, when a patient has returned to performance, screening for stressful events and considering how a patient reacts to stress might be helpful in minimizing the risk of a second ACL injury.

Evaluation

No specific evaluation is recommended during this phase.

RETURN TO SPORT

RTS is regarded as a continuum throughout rehabilitation and not as a specific time-point.[80] The continuum consists of 3 phases: return to participation, RTS, and return to performance. Return to participation is defined as participating in rehabilitation, training, or sport (modified or unrestricted) at a lower level than the RTS goal. RTS is defined as a return to the defined sport but performance is not as high as the pre-injury level. The last phase of the continuum, return to performance, represents full participation in both practice and play at the preinjury level or higher. Participation can increase successively depending on knee function. The decision to increase participation should be taken in collaboration between the patient, physical therapist, responsible surgeon, and coach. However, RTS is not recommended earlier than 9 months after ACL reconstruction because this is associated with a 7-fold increase in the risk of a second ACL injury.[10] It is important to acknowledge that the decision to return to participation, sport, or performance is multifactorial and is not dependent on only muscle strength or psychological readiness and should not be determined based on one variable, such as time. To ascertain that patients are ready to RTS, objective tests of muscle strength and functional skills that demonstrate the appropriate quality of movement, as well as some test of psychological readiness, are paramount but the results need to be interpreted in each specific case.[81] The results of muscle function tests are usually presented as the limb symmetry index (LSI), where 90% or greater LSI is regarded as meeting the RTS criteria. Evidence of whether meeting the RTS criteria comprising muscle function tests infers a reduced risk of second ACL injuries on RTS is conflicting.[82–85] The conflicting evidence may reflect the nature of sports, with a "chaos" of unpredictable and reactive movements often with multiple stimuli occurring simultaneously. Although the tests used in the RTS process may vary, they are often predictable; that is, patients are aware of the task at hand and the tests that are used may not be sufficient to ascertain whether patients are ready to return to their specific sport.

In many cases, the ACL injury occurs at the time of a sudden COD. Accordingly, the deceleration phase in high-speed runs before a COD is a crucial movement strategy for reducing body momentum and the following knee load at the final ground contact when performing a COD maneuver. An improved deceleration performance during COD maneuvers can, therefore, be regarded as a modifiable risk factor for ACL injury.[86] There is, however, limited research on COD as a part of the test procedure before RTS and COD is therefore seldom integrated in the discharge criteria for RTS.[87] Despite symmetric strength, laboratory studies have identified compensatory strategies such as knee abduction and adduction in ACL-injured patients compared with uninjured patients.[88] As a result, on-field tests might be recommended in an attempt to screen for compensatory strategies before RTS. Unfortunately, many COD tests are not particularly similar to the athlete's movement in sport-specific situations and are therefore not transferable to sports participation and performance.[89] Furthermore, several COD tests are difficult to perform in clinical settings and have a long duration, which means less focus on the COD performance and more on linear sprinting and anaerobic power capacity.[84,90,91] The 505-agility test (**Fig. 4**) is one of several COD tests described in the literature.[92] Because the 505-agility test is performed with a short total test time (2.0–3.0 seconds), it can provide a more accurate measurement of COD performance. However, the COD tests analyzed in the literature (505-agility test, triangle test, square test, Gewandtheitslauf test, T-agility test, and Illinois agility test) all measure task-specific performances.[93] The test should therefore be chosen depending on the requirement of the athlete.

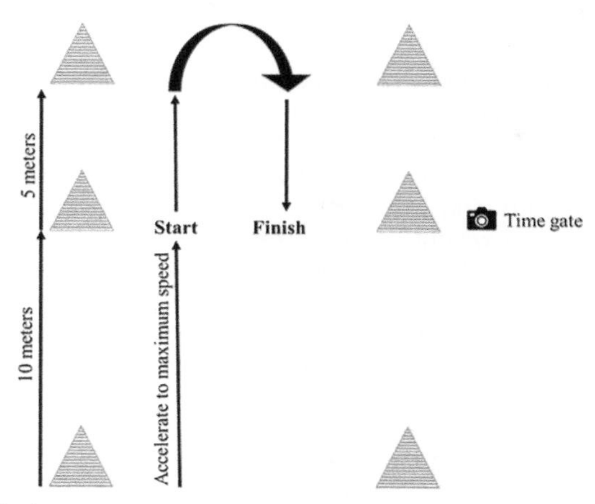

Fig. 4. 505-agility test.

In order to bridge the gap between predictable assessments in rehabilitation and the sport-specific "chaos" at RTS, the BEAST (BEtter And Safer return to sporT) protocol was established by Moksnes and colleagues.[94] The BEAST protocol includes continuous assessments of knee stability, effusion, quadriceps power-and-hop ability, followed by a sport-specific return to training protocol dependent on the knee assessment results at each follow-up. The sport-specific return to a training protocol is divided into 6 levels, where levels 1 to 3 consist of sport-specific movements in a controlled environment, for example, technique and passing drills, whereas levels 4 to 6 consist of participation in team practice, initially with restrictions before full participation. To advance to the next level, patients should perform at least 4 sessions during 2 weeks without experiencing effusion, pain, or insecurity. In addition, every 8 weeks, patients return to the clinic to perform the knee assessment and to ascertain that their knee function is maintained. Ideally, communication among the health caregiver, the patient, and the coach should be maintained throughout the increasing demands during the RTS continuum.

In the RTS continuum, patients who have low self-efficacy beliefs,[95] avoidance tendencies toward movements and fear of reinjury, lack clear expectations and have less social support report inferior perceived knee function, as well as inferior confidence and emotions in relation to returning to sport.[96] Considering that patients who RTS and sustained a second ACL injury did not feel psychologically ready and were unsure of what the knee was able to withstand, the monitoring of psychological outcomes is important even during the latter phases of the RTS continuum. With this in mind, close communication with the patient with regard to the psychological attitude toward RTS should be as important as the results of muscle function tests. Consequently, the recovery of muscle function and psychological readiness should be of equal importance before RTS.

Currently, RTS testing, which comprises muscle function (strength and hop) tests, some subjective patient-reported outcome, and some measurement of movement quality, is recommended.[97,98] How to interpret the test results and which cut-offs should be used to define whether or not a patient has passed the test vary in the literature.[83] Accordingly, an evaluation of test results should be carried out together with the patient and the results should be considered in the light of the specific patient and the sport to which the patient wishes to return. The RTS tests can be performed continuously until the patient has returned to performance.

DISCUSSION

The great influence an ACL injury has on a patient, both physically and psychologically, and the relatively high risk of a subsequent knee injury on RTS highlights the need to improve the care of ACL-reconstructed patients.

Immediate knee mobilization and strength/neuromuscular training should be used both preoperatively and during ACL postoperative rehabilitation. In order to restore quadriceps activation, full weight-bearing exercises and early OKC and CKC exercises should be used according to individual circumstances. One important aspect to consider is that the progression of rehabilitation exercises with increases in load/volume and difficulty needs to be tolerated by the knee. Eventual increments in the training programs should take place when the current training program does not cause pain, swelling, or major joint discomfort. Although the initial phase of rehabilitation does not have a decisive influence on the patient's ability to RTS, this phase is important to provide a solid foundation for the further rehabilitation process, matching the patient's expectations of progress and allowing sufficient time for the more physically challenging phases of rehabilitation.

A rationale for the relatively high risk of a subsequent knee injury on RTS might be that patients are not sufficiently prepared physically or mentally. Many patients fail to meet RTS passing criteria (≥90% LSI) in all the tests included in a test battery before RTS (muscle strength, hop performance, and PROs), indicating that they have not fully recovered.[99] However, patients who meet RTS criteria do not necessarily run a lower risk of a subsequent knee injury such as a meniscal, cartilage, or ligament injury.[83,100,101] Furthermore, the interpretation of the results of strength tests and hop performance is made in relation to the uninjured leg, that is, the LSI. The LSI can be regarded as a *proxy* for estimates of the recovery of the reconstructed limb and should not be considered solely when patients have recovered muscle function because deconditioning of the uninjured limb can occur during rehabilitation, causing symmetric values due to bilateral weakness.[42,102] On this topic, the Aspetar group[103] suggested that the LSI cut-off values to define that a patient has passed a test should be higher than 90%, suggesting 100% in quadriceps and hamstring strength measured isokinetically before RTS. In addition, the achievement of preoperative strength values or normative strength values is recommended, depending on sport and activity level.[103] Even though isokinetic assessments of muscle strength are regarded as the "gold standard," this is not easily accessible to clinicians. According to a survey of more than 1000 physical therapists working with rehabilitation after ACL reconstruction, manual muscle testing using a handheld dynamometer was more frequently used to assess muscle strength.[104] In addition to assessing muscle strength, single-leg-hop testing was the most frequently used measurement to permit a return to modified sports activity, according to the survey.[104] Nevertheless, it has been suggested that hop tests, such as the hop for distance, mask lower limb biomechanics, with less contribution from the knee, compensated by the hip and ankle, and, as a result, using hop performance in the knee evaluation after ACL injury, can be questioned.[105] However, the vertical hop seems to be more promising as knee deficits of the injured limb may be apparent despite achieving symmetric (≥90% LSI) values in the hop for distance and in the quadriceps strength test.[106] Collectively, currently used test batteries should not be regarded as an RTS criterion but more as an indicator of knee function throughout rehabilitation to obtain information on whether the patient is ready for the next phase of rehabilitation. The LSI should be interpreted in conjunction with preoperative or normative values and the movement quality of the hop test in order to be aware of compensatory movements that can be masked by high LSI values.

The fact that that the majority of ACL injuries occur as noncontact injuries[2] during the first 50 milliseconds of initial ground contact accompanied by an external focus[107] highlights the discrepancy between the injury mechanism and current tests used before RTS. The current test batteries thus lack explosive, reactive, and neurocognitive components more specific to sports. In support of this notion, deficits of explosive strength in the hamstring and quadriceps have been reported, despite the recovery of symmetric and preoperative strength values.[108–110] Furthermore, greater deficits between the reconstructed and the uninjured limb have been reported when a reactive phase was added to hop performance, for example, a vertical drop hop compared with a vertical hop, indicating that the reactive phase may unmask deficits not previously observed in hop performance from the commonly used test battery.[106] During sports participation, athletes must divide their attention between different stimuli, for example, performing a defensive cutting maneuver while reacting to the opponents' movement.[111] Adding a cognitive challenge may worsen biomechanical movements, such as reducing the knee flexion angle and increasing the knee abduction angle at initial contact, or increasing peak vertical ground forces, factors all associated with ACL injuries.[112] Consequently, integrating cognitive performance with a functional RTS test may add information on whether the patients are ready for the "chaos" of sports before RTS. However, more research is needed when it comes to the validation and reliability of tests included in the battery and the determination of the tests that are missing in terms of optimizing RTS testing.

SUMMARY

The current RTS test batteries that are used after ACL injury need to develop and evolve with the emerging evidence. Rehabilitation specialists need to look beyond maximum strength, distance, and time in hop performance and consider the ability to produce force in a short period of time, as well as movement quality and reactive ability. In addition, the integration of neurocognitive aspects to prepare patients before RTS should be considered and the patient's perspective and feeling of readiness must be acknowledged in the complicated RTS after an ACL reconstruction equation.

CLINICS CARE POINTS

- Rehabilitation is performed in phases with specific goals
- Patients should be physically and psychologically ready before return to sport
- Readiness should be determined with tests and consultation between patient, physical therapist, surgeon and coach
- Patients should continue knee specific training for maintenance and prevention even after return to sport

DISCLOSURE

The authors have nothing to disclose.

REFERENCES

1. Sanders TL, Maradit Kremers H, Bryan AJ, et al. Incidence of Anterior Cruciate Ligament Tears and Reconstruction: A 21-Year Population-Based Study. Am J Sports Med 2016;44(6):1502–7.

2. Della Villa F, Buckthorpe M, Grassi A, et al. Systematic video analysis of ACL injuries in professional male football (soccer): injury mechanisms, situational patterns and biomechanics study on 134 consecutive cases. Br J Sports Med 2020;54(23):1423–32.
3. Diermeier T, Rothrauff BB, Engebretsen L, et al. Treatment after anterior cruciate ligament injury: Panther Symposium ACL Treatment Consensus Group. Knee Surg Sports Traumatol Arthrosc 2020;28(8):2390–402.
4. Chalmers PN, Mall NA, Moric M, et al. Does ACL reconstruction alter natural history?: A systematic literature review of long-term outcomes. J Bone Joint Surg Am 2014;96(4):292–300.
5. Snoeker BA, Roemer FW, Turkiewicz A, et al. Does early anterior cruciate ligament reconstruction prevent development of meniscal damage? Results from a secondary analysis of a randomised controlled trial. Br J Sports Med 2020;54(10):612–7.
6. Beard DJ, Davies L, Cook JA, et al. Rehabilitation versus surgical reconstruction for non-acute anterior cruciate ligament injury (ACL SNNAP): a pragmatic randomised controlled trial. Lancet 2022;400(10352):605–15.
7. Kim SJ, Choi CH, Kim SH, et al. Bone-patellar tendon-bone autograft could be recommended as a superior graft to hamstring autograft for ACL reconstruction in patients with generalized joint laxity: 2- and 5-year follow-up study. Knee Surg Sports Traumatol Arthrosc 2018;26(9):2568–79.
8. Arnold MP, Calcei JG, Vogel N, et al. ACL Study Group survey reveals the evolution of anterior cruciate ligament reconstruction graft choice over the past three decades. Knee Surg Sports Traumatol Arthrosc 2021;29(11):3871–6.
9. Mouarbes D, Menetrey J, Marot V, et al. Anterior Cruciate Ligament Reconstruction: A Systematic Review and Meta-analysis of Outcomes for Quadriceps Tendon Autograft Versus Bone-Patellar Tendon-Bone and Hamstring-Tendon Autografts. Am J Sports Med 2019;47(14):3531–40.
10. Beischer S, Gustavsson L, Senorski EH, et al. Young Athletes Who Return to Sport Before 9 Months After Anterior Cruciate Ligament Reconstruction Have a Rate of New Injury 7 Times That of Those Who Delay Return. J Orthop Sports Phys Ther 2020;50(2):83–90.
11. Nagelli CV, Hewett TE. Should Return to Sport be Delayed Until 2 Years After Anterior Cruciate Ligament Reconstruction? Biological and Functional Considerations. Sports Med 2017;47(2):221–32.
12. Wiggins AJ, Grandhi RK, Schneider DK, et al. Risk of Secondary Injury in Younger Athletes After Anterior Cruciate Ligament Reconstruction: A Systematic Review and Meta-analysis. Am J Sports Med 2016;44(7):1861–76.
13. Della Villa F, Hägglund M, Della Villa S, et al. High rate of second ACL injury following ACL reconstruction in male professional footballers: an updated longitudinal analysis from 118 players in the UEFA Elite Club Injury Study. Br J Sports Med 2021;55(23):1350–6.
14. Fältström A, Kvist J, Hägglund M. High Risk of New Knee Injuries in Female Soccer Players After Primary Anterior Cruciate Ligament Reconstruction at 5- to 10-Year Follow-up. Am J Sports Med 2021;49(13):3479–87.
15. Zbrojkiewicz D, Vertullo C, Grayson JE. Increasing rates of anterior cruciate ligament reconstruction in young Australians, 2000-2015. Med J Aust 2018;208(8):354–8.
16. Maniar N, Verhagen E, Bryant AL, et al. Trends in Australian knee injury rates: An epidemiological analysis of 228,344 knee injuries over 20 years. Lancet Reg Health West Pac 2022;21:100409.

17. Musahl V, Diermeier T, de Sa D, et al. ACL surgery: when to do it? Knee Surg Sports Traumatol Arthrosc 2020;28(7):2023–6.
18. Eitzen I, Holm I, Risberg MA. Preoperative quadriceps strength is a significant predictor of knee function two years after anterior cruciate ligament reconstruction. Br J Sports Med 2009;43(5):371–6.
19. Grindem H, Granan LP, Risberg MA, et al. How does a combined preoperative and postoperative rehabilitation programme influence the outcome of ACL reconstruction 2 years after surgery? A comparison between patients in the Delaware-Oslo ACL Cohort and the Norwegian National Knee Ligament Registry. Br J Sports Med 2015;49(6):385–9.
20. Webster KE, Feller JA. Expectations for Return to Preinjury Sport Before and After Anterior Cruciate Ligament Reconstruction. Am J Sports Med 2019;47(3): 578–83.
21. Paterno MV. Non-operative Care of the Patient with an ACL-Deficient Knee. Curr Rev Musculoskelet Med 2017;10(3):322–7.
22. Sonnery-Cottet B, Saithna A, Quelard B, et al. Arthrogenic muscle inhibition after ACL reconstruction: a scoping review of the efficacy of interventions. Br J Sports Med 2019;53(5):289–98.
23. Kennedy JC, Alexander IJ, Hayes KC. Nerve supply of the human knee and its functional importance. Am J Sports Med 1982;10(6):329–35.
24. Mayr HO, Hochrein A, Hein W, et al. Rehabilitation results following anterior cruciate ligament reconstruction using a hard brace compared to a fluid-filled soft brace. Knee 2010;17(2):119–26.
25. Andrade R, Pereira R, van Cingel R, et al. How should clinicians rehabilitate patients after ACL reconstruction? A systematic review of clinical practice guidelines (CPGs) with a focus on quality appraisal (AGREE II). Br J Sports Med 2020;54(9):512–9.
26. Konrath JM, Vertullo CJ, Kennedy BA, et al. Morphologic Characteristics and Strength of the Hamstring Muscles Remain Altered at 2 Years After Use of a Hamstring Tendon Graft in Anterior Cruciate Ligament Reconstruction. Am J Sports Med 2016;44(10):2589–98.
27. Mikkelsen C, Werner S, Eriksson E. Closed kinetic chain alone compared to combined open and closed kinetic chain exercises for quadriceps strengthening after anterior cruciate ligament reconstruction with respect to return to sports: a prospective matched follow-up study. Knee Surg Sports Traumatol Arthrosc 2000;8(6):337–42.
28. Tagesson S, Oberg B, Good L, et al. A comprehensive rehabilitation program with quadriceps strengthening in closed versus open kinetic chain exercise in patients with anterior cruciate ligament deficiency: a randomized clinical trial evaluating dynamic tibial translation and muscle function. Am J Sports Med 2008;36(2):298–307.
29. Perriman A, Leahy E, Semciw AI. The Effect of Open- Versus Closed-Kinetic-Chain Exercises on Anterior Tibial Laxity, Strength, and Function Following Anterior Cruciate Ligament Reconstruction: A Systematic Review and Meta-analysis. J Orthop Sports Phys Ther 2018;48(7):552–66.
30. Jewiss D, Ostman C, Smart N. Open versus Closed Kinetic Chain Exercises following an Anterior Cruciate Ligament Reconstruction: A Systematic Review and Meta-Analysis. J Sports Med 2017;2017:4721548.
31. Ebert JR, Edwards P, Joss B, et al. A structured accelerated versus control rehabilitation pathway after anterior cruciate ligament reconstruction using autologous hamstrings demonstrates earlier improvement in physical outcomes

without increasing graft laxity: A randomized controlled trial. Phys Ther Sport 2022;55:271–81.

32. Buckthorpe M, Pirotti E, Villa FD. Benefits and use of aquatic therapy during rehabilitation after acl reconstruction -a clinical commentary. Int J Sports Phys Ther 2019;14(6):978–93.
33. Hughes L, Rosenblatt B, Haddad F, et al. Comparing the Effectiveness of Blood Flow Restriction and Traditional Heavy Load Resistance Training in the Post-Surgery Rehabilitation of Anterior Cruciate Ligament Reconstruction Patients: A UK National Health Service Randomised Controlled Trial. Sports Med 2019; 49(11):1787–805.
34. Harput G, Ulusoy B, Yildiz TI, et al. Cross-education improves quadriceps strength recovery after ACL reconstruction: a randomized controlled trial. Knee Surg Sports Traumatol Arthrosc 2019;27(1):68–75.
35. Piussi R, Berghdal T, Sundemo D, et al. Self-Reported Symptoms of Depression and Anxiety After ACL Injury: A Systematic Review. Orthop J Sports Med 2022; 10(1). 23259671211066493.
36. Piussi R, Beischer S, Thomeé R, et al. Superior knee self-efficacy and quality of life throughout the first year in patients who recover symmetrical muscle function after ACL reconstruction. Knee Surg Sports Traumatol Arthrosc 2020;28(2): 555–67.
37. Johnson JL, Capin JJ, Arundale AJH, et al. A Secondary Injury Prevention Program May Decrease Contralateral Anterior Cruciate Ligament Injuries in Female Athletes: 2-Year Injury Rates in the ACL-SPORTS Randomized Controlled Trial. J Orthop Sports Phys Ther 2020;50(9):523–30.
38. Sturgill LP, Snyder-Mackler L, Manal TJ, et al. Interrater reliability of a clinical scale to assess knee joint effusion. J Orthop Sports Phys Ther 2009;39(12): 845–9.
39. Pinto FG, Thaunat M, Daggett M, et al. Hamstring Contracture After ACL Reconstruction Is Associated With an Increased Risk of Cyclops Syndrome. Orthop J Sports Med 2017;5(1). 2325967116684121.
40. Noll S, Garrison JC, Bothwell J, et al. Knee Extension Range of Motion at 4 Weeks Is Related to Knee Extension Loss at 12 Weeks After Anterior Cruciate Ligament Reconstruction. Orthop J Sports Med 2015;3(5). 2325967115583632.
41. Broman D, Piussi R, Thomeé R, et al. A clinician-friendly test battery with a passing rate similar to a 'gold standard' return-to-sport test battery 1 year after ACL reconstruction: Results from a rehabilitation outcome registry. Phys Ther Sport 2023;59:144–50.
42. Piussi R, Broman D, Musslinder E, et al. Recovery of preoperative absolute knee extension and flexion strength after ACL reconstruction. BMC Sports Sci Med Rehabil 2020;12(1):77.
43. Buckthorpe M, La Rosa G, Villa FD. Restoring knee extensor strength after anterior cruciate ligament reconstruction: a clinical commentary. Int J Sports Phys Ther 2019;14(1):159–72.
44. Schoenfeld BJ. The mechanisms of muscle hypertrophy and their application to resistance training. J Strength Condit Res 2010;24(10):2857–72.
45. American College of Sports Medicine position stand. Progression models in resistance training for healthy adults. Med Sci Sports Exerc 2009;41(3): 687–708.
46. Buckthorpe M, Della Villa F. Optimising the 'Mid-Stage' Training and Testing Process After ACL Reconstruction. Sports Med 2020;50(4):657–78.

47. Lepley LK, Palmieri-Smith R. Effect of eccentric strengthening after anterior cruciate ligament reconstruction on quadriceps strength. J Sport Rehabil 2013; 22(2):150–6.
48. Bourne MN, Duhig SJ, Timmins RG, et al. Impact of the Nordic hamstring and hip extension exercises on hamstring architecture and morphology: implications for injury prevention. Br J Sports Med 2017;51(5):469–77.
49. Bourne MN, Williams MD, Opar DA, et al. Impact of exercise selection on hamstring muscle activation. Br J Sports Med 2017;51(13):1021–8.
50. Högberg J, Bergentoft E, Piussi R, et al. Persistent knee flexor strength deficits identified through the NordBord eccentric test not seen with "gold standard" isokinetic concentric testing during the first year after anterior cruciate ligament reconstruction with a hamstring tendon autograft. Phys Ther Sport 2022;55: 119–24.
51. Solie B, Monson J, Larson C. Graft-Specific Surgical and Rehabilitation Considerations for Anterior Cruciate Ligament Reconstruction with the Quadriceps Tendon Autograft. Int J Sports Phys Ther 2023;18(2):493–512.
52. Van Cant J, Pairot de Fontenay B, Douaihy C, et al. Characteristics of return to running programs following an anterior cruciate ligament reconstruction: A scoping review of 64 studies with clinical perspectives. Phys Ther Sport 2022; 57:61–70.
53. Buckthorpe M, Della Villa F. Recommendations for Plyometric Training after ACL Reconstruction - A Clinical Commentary. Int J Sports Phys Ther 2021;16(3): 879–95.
54. Alexanders J, Perry J, Douglas C. Goal setting practices used within anterior cruciate ligament rehabilitation: An exploration of physiotherapists understanding, training and experiences. Muscoskel Care 2021;19(3):293–305.
55. Piussi R, Krupic F, Sundemo D, et al. 'I was young, I wanted to return to sport, and re-ruptured my ACL' - young active female patients' voices on the experience of sustaining an ACL re-rupture, a qualitative study. BMC Muscoskel Disord 2022;23(1):760.
56. Filbay S, Kvist J. Fear of Reinjury Following Surgical and Nonsurgical Management of Anterior Cruciate Ligament Injury: An Exploratory Analysis of the NACOX Multicenter Longitudinal Cohort Study. Phys Ther 2022;102(2).
57. Högberg J, Piussi R, Simonson R, et al. Is absolute or relative knee flexor strength related to patient-reported outcomes in patients treated with ACL reconstruction with a hamstring tendon autograft? An analysis of eccentric Nordic hamstring strength and seated concentric isokinetic strength. Knee 2023;41:161–70.
58. van der Horst N, Denderen RV. Isokinetic hamstring and quadriceps strength interpretation guideline for football (soccer) players with ACL reconstruction: a Delphi consensus study in the Netherlands. Sci Med Footb 2022;6(4):434–45.
59. Gustavsson A, Neeter C, Thomeé P, et al. A test battery for evaluating hop performance in patients with an ACL injury and patients who have undergone ACL reconstruction. Knee Surg Sports Traumatol Arthrosc 2006;14(8):778–88.
60. Palmieri-Smith RM, Lepley LK. Quadriceps Strength Asymmetry After Anterior Cruciate Ligament Reconstruction Alters Knee Joint Biomechanics and Functional Performance at Time of Return to Activity. Am J Sports Med 2015;43(7): 1662–9.
61. Simonson R, Piussi R, Högberg J, et al. Effect of Quadriceps and Hamstring Strength Relative to Body Weight on Risk of a Second ACL Injury: A Cohort

Study of 835 Patients Who Returned to Sport After ACL Reconstruction. Orthop J Sports Med 2023;11(4). 23259671231157386.
62. Gagnier JJ, Shen Y, Huang H. Psychometric Properties of Patient-Reported Outcome Measures for Use in Patients with Anterior Cruciate Ligament Injuries: A Systematic Review. JBJS Rev 2018;6(4):e5.
63. Piussi R, Simonson R, Högberg J, et al. Psychological Patient-reported Outcomes Cannot Predict a Second Anterior Cruciate Ligament Injury in Patients who Return to Sports after an Anterior Cruciate Ligament Reconstruction. Int J Sports Phys Ther 2022;17(7):1340–50.
64. Patel AD, Bullock GS, Wrigley J, et al. Does sex affect second ACL injury risk? A systematic review with meta-analysis. Br J Sports Med 2021;55(15):873–82.
65. Snaebjörnsson T, Hamrin Senorski E, Svantesson E, et al. Graft Fixation and Timing of Surgery Are Predictors of Early Anterior Cruciate Ligament Revision: A Cohort Study from the Swedish and Norwegian Knee Ligament Registries Based on 18,425 Patients. JB JS Open Access 2019;4(4):e0037.
66. Rahardja R, Zhu M, Love H, et al. Effect of Graft Choice on Revision and Contralateral Anterior Cruciate Ligament Reconstruction: Results From the New Zealand ACL Registry. Am J Sports Med 2020;48(1):63–9.
67. Grindem H, Snyder-Mackler L, Moksnes H, et al. Simple decision rules can reduce reinjury risk by 84% after ACL reconstruction: the Delaware-Oslo ACL cohort study. Br J Sports Med 2016;50(13):804–8.
68. Buckthorpe M. Optimising the Late-Stage Rehabilitation and Return-to-Sport Training and Testing Process After ACL Reconstruction. Sports Med 2019; 49(7):1043–58.
69. Andersen LL, Aagaard P. Influence of maximal muscle strength and intrinsic muscle contractile properties on contractile rate of force development. Eur J Appl Physiol 2006;96(1):46–52.
70. Turpeinen JT, Freitas TT, Rubio-Arias J, et al. Contractile rate of force development after anterior cruciate ligament reconstruction-a comprehensive review and meta-analysis. Scand J Med Sci Sports 2020;30(9):1572–85.
71. Harper DJ, Kiely J. Damaging nature of decelerations: Do we adequately prepare players? BMJ Open Sport & Exercise Medicine 2018;4(1):e000379.
72. Almeida AM, Santos Silva PR, Pedrinelli A, et al. Aerobic fitness in professional soccer players after anterior cruciate ligament reconstruction. PLoS One 2018; 13(3):e0194432.
73. Burland JP, Toonstra JL, Howard JS. Psychosocial Barriers After Anterior Cruciate Ligament Reconstruction: A Clinical Review of Factors Influencing Postoperative Success. Sport Health 2019;11(6):528–34.
74. Saw AE, Main LC, Gastin PB. Monitoring the athlete training response: subjective self-reported measures trump commonly used objective measures: a systematic review. Br J Sports Med 2016;50(5):281–91.
75. Piussi R, Beischer S, Thomeé R, et al. Greater Psychological Readiness to Return to Sport, as Well as Greater Present and Future Knee-Related Self-Efficacy, Can Increase the Risk for an Anterior Cruciate Ligament Re-Rupture: A Matched Cohort Study. Arthroscopy 2022;38(4):1267–76.e1261.
76. McPherson AL, Feller JA, Hewett TE, et al. Psychological Readiness to Return to Sport Is Associated With Second Anterior Cruciate Ligament Injuries. Am J Sports Med 2019;47(4):857–62.
77. Fältström A, Kvist J, Bittencourt NFN, et al. Clinical Risk Profile for a Second Anterior Cruciate Ligament Injury in Female Soccer Players After Anterior Cruciate Ligament Reconstruction. Am J Sports Med 2021;49(6):1421–30.

78. Sugimoto D, Myer GD, Foss KD, et al. Specific exercise effects of preventive neuromuscular training intervention on anterior cruciate ligament injury risk reduction in young females: meta-analysis and subgroup analysis. Br J Sports Med 2015;49(5):282–9.
79. Ivarsson A, Johnson U, Andersen MB, et al. Psychosocial Factors and Sport Injuries: Meta-analyses for Prediction and Prevention. Sports Med 2017;47(2):353–65.
80. Ardern CL, Glasgow P, Schneiders A, et al. Consensus statement on return to sport from the First World Congress in Sports Physical Therapy, Bern. Br J Sports Med 2016;50(14):853.
81. Meredith SJ, Rauer T, Chmielewski TL, et al. Return to Sport After Anterior Cruciate Ligament Injury: Panther Symposium ACL Injury Return to Sport Consensus Group. Orthop J Sports Med 2020;8(6). 2325967120930829.
82. Turk R, Shah S, Chilton M, et al. Return to Sport After Anterior Cruciate Ligament Reconstruction Requires Evaluation of >2 Functional Tests, Psychological Readiness, Quadriceps/Hamstring Strength, and Time After Surgery of 8 Months. Arthroscopy 2023;39(3):790–801.e796.
83. Webster KE, Hewett TE. What is the Evidence for and Validity of Return-to-Sport Testing after Anterior Cruciate Ligament Reconstruction Surgery? A Systematic Review and Meta-Analysis. Sports Med 2019;49(6):917–29.
84. Kyritsis P, Bahr R, Landreau P, et al. Likelihood of ACL graft rupture: not meeting six clinical discharge criteria before return to sport is associated with a four times greater risk of rupture. Br J Sports Med 2016;50(15):946–51.
85. Welling W, Benjaminse A, Lemmink K, et al. Passing return to sports tests after ACL reconstruction is associated with greater likelihood for return to sport but fail to identify second injury risk. Knee 2020;27(3):949–57.
86. McBurnie AJ, Harper DJ, Jones PA, et al. Deceleration Training in Team Sports: Another Potential 'Vaccine' for Sports-Related Injury? Sports Med 2022;52(1):1–12.
87. Gokeler A, Dingenen B, Hewett TE. Rehabilitation and Return to Sport Testing After Anterior Cruciate Ligament Reconstruction: Where Are We in 2022? Arthrosc Sports Med Rehabil 2022;4(1):e77–82.
88. Pollard CD, Stearns KM, Hayes AT, et al. Altered lower extremity movement variability in female soccer players during side-step cutting after anterior cruciate ligament reconstruction. Am J Sports Med 2015;43(2):460–5.
89. Jang SH, Kim JG, Ha JK, et al. Functional performance tests as indicators of returning to sports after anterior cruciate ligament reconstruction. Knee 2014;21(1):95–101.
90. Myer GD, Schmitt LC, Brent JL, et al. Utilization of modified NFL combine testing to identify functional deficits in athletes following ACL reconstruction. J Orthop Sports Phys Ther 2011;41(6):377–87.
91. Nimphius S, Callaghan SJ, Spiteri T, et al. Change of Direction Deficit: A More Isolated Measure of Change of Direction Performance Than Total 505 Time. J Strength Condit Res 2016;30(11):3024–32.
92. Emmonds S, Nicholson G, Begg C, et al. Importance of Physical Qualities for Speed and Change of Direction Ability in Elite Female Soccer Players. J Strength Condit Res 2019;33(6):1669–77.
93. Kadlubowski B, Keiner M, Hartmann H, et al. The Relationship between Change of Direction Tests in Elite Youth Soccer Players. Sports (Basel) 2019;7(5).
94. Moksnes H, Ardern CL, Kvist J, et al. Assessing implementation, limited efficacy, and acceptability of the BEAST tool: A rehabilitation and return-to-sport decision

tool for nonprofessional athletes with anterior cruciate ligament reconstruction. Phys Ther Sport 2021;52:147–54.
95. Thomeé P, Währborg P, Börjesson M, et al. Self-efficacy, symptoms and physical activity in patients with an anterior cruciate ligament injury: a prospective study. Scand J Med Sci Sports 2007;17(3):238–45.
96. Burland JP, Howard JS, Lepley AS, et al. What Are Our Patients Really Telling Us? Psychological Constructs Associated With Patient-Reported Outcomes After Anterior Cruciate Ligament Reconstruction. J Athl Train 2020;55(7):707–16.
97. Svantesson E, Hamrin Senorski E, Webster KE, et al. Clinical Outcomes After Anterior Cruciate Ligament Injury: Panther Symposium ACL Injury Clinical Outcomes Consensus Group. Orthop J Sports Med 2020;8(7). 2325967120934751.
98. Di Paolo S, Zaffagnini S, Tosarelli F, et al. Beyond Distance: A Simple Qualitative Assessment of the Single-Leg Hop Test in Return-to-Play Testing. Sport Health 2022;14(6):906–11.
99. Lynch AD, Logerstedt DS, Grindem H, et al. Consensus criteria for defining 'successful outcome' after ACL injury and reconstruction: a Delaware-Oslo ACL cohort investigation. Br J Sports Med 2015;49(5):335–42.
100. Turk R, Shah S, Chilton M, et al. Return to Sport After Anterior Cruciate Ligament Reconstruction Requires Evaluation of >2 Functional Tests, Psychological Readiness, Quadriceps/Hamstring Strength, and Time After. Surgery of 8 Months. Arthroscopy. 2023;39(3):790–801.e6.
101. Jauhiainen S, Kauppi JP, Krosshaug T, et al. Predicting ACL Injury Using Machine Learning on Data From an Extensive Screening Test Battery of 880 Female Elite Athletes. Am J Sports Med 2022;50(11):2917–24.
102. Wellsandt E, Failla MJ, Snyder-Mackler L. Limb Symmetry Indexes Can Overestimate Knee Function After Anterior Cruciate Ligament Injury. J Orthop Sports Phys Ther 2017;47(5):334–8.
103. Kotsifaki R, Korakakis V, King E, et al. Aspetar clinical practice guideline on rehabilitation after anterior cruciate ligament reconstruction. Br J Sports Med 2023;57(9):500–14.
104. Greenberg EM, Greenberg ET, Albaugh J, et al. Rehabilitation Practice Patterns Following Anterior Cruciate Ligament Reconstruction: A Survey of Physical Therapists. J Orthop Sports Phys Ther 2018;48(10):801–11.
105. Kotsifaki A, Whiteley R, Van Rossom S, et al. Single leg hop for distance symmetry masks lower limb biomechanics: time to discuss hop distance as decision criterion for return to sport after ACL reconstruction? Br J Sports Med 2022; 56(5):249–56.
106. Kotsifaki A, Van Rossom S, Whiteley R, et al. Single leg vertical jump performance identifies knee function deficits at return to sport after ACL reconstruction in male athletes. Br J Sports Med 2022;56(9):490–8.
107. Krosshaug T, Nakamae A, Boden BP, et al. Mechanisms of anterior cruciate ligament injury in basketball: video analysis of 39 cases. Am J Sports Med 2007; 35(3):359–67.
108. San Jose AT, Maniar N, Timmins RG, et al. Explosive hamstrings strength asymmetry persists despite maximal hamstring strength recovery following anterior cruciate ligament reconstruction using hamstring tendon autografts. Knee Surg Sports Traumatol Arthrosc : official journal of the ESSKA 2022. https://doi.org/10.1007/s00167-022-07096-y.
109. Knezevic OM, Mirkov DM, Kadija M, et al. Asymmetries in explosive strength following anterior cruciate ligament reconstruction. Knee 2014;21(6):1039–45.

110. Maestroni L, Read P, Turner A, et al. Strength, rate of force development, power and reactive strength in adult male athletic populations post anterior cruciate ligament reconstruction - A systematic review and meta-analysis. Phys Ther Sport 2021;47:91–104.
111. Waldén M, Krosshaug T, Bjørneboe J, et al. Three distinct mechanisms predominate in non-contact anterior cruciate ligament injuries in male professional football players: a systematic video analysis of 39 cases. Br J Sports Med 2015; 49(22):1452–60.
112. McCarren G, Chaput M, Grooms DR, et al. Cognitive Load Influences Drop Jump Landing Mechanics During Cognitive-Motor-Simulated Shooting. Mil Med 2023. https://doi.org/10.1093/milmed/usad003.

Precision Anterior Cruciate Ligament Reconstruction

Zachary J. Herman, MD[a,*], Janina Kaarre, MD, MSc[a,b],
Alan M.J. Getgood, MPhil, MD, FRCS(Tr&Orth)[c,d,e], Volker Musahl, MD[a]

KEYWORDS

- Precision • ACLR • Individualized • Anterior cruciate ligament

KEY POINTS

- Precision anterior cruciate ligament reconstruction (ACLR) refers to the individualized approach to prerehabilitation, surgery (including anatomy, bony morphology, and repair/reconstruction of concomitant injuries), postrehabilitation, and functional recovery.
- The future of precision ACLR is likely to involve the incorporation of artificial intelligence and machine learning algorithms, along with innovations in robotic-assisted surgery as well as regenerative medicine.
- As the new technologies continue to improve, orthopedic sports medicine is likely to experience a new era, marked by a paradigm shift toward more individualized and precise patient care.

INTRODUCTION

Anterior cruciate ligament reconstruction (ACLR) is a comprehensive, precise process involving an accurate diagnosis of the ACL rupture and numerous concomitant injuries, an individualized assessment and treatment plan, proper postoperative management and rehabilitation, and patient education. Precision ACLR refers to the individualized approach to prerehabilitation, surgery (including anatomy, bony morphology, and repair/reconstruction of concomitant injuries), postrehabilitation, and functional recovery. The purpose of this article is to provide an explanatory summary framework for precision ACLR, from the time of diagnosis to that of returning to play, with additional insight into what is to come for the future of ACLR.

[a] Department of Orthopaedic Surgery, UPMC Freddie Fu Sports Medicine Center, University of Pittsburgh, Pittsburgh, USA; [b] Department of Orthopaedics, Institute of Clinical Sciences, Sahlgrenska Academy, University of Gothenburg, Gothenburg, Sweden; [c] Department of Orthopaedic Surgery, London Health Sciences Centre, University Hospital, London, Ontario N6A 5A5, Canada; [d] Department of Surgery, Fowler-Kennedy Sports Medicine Clinic 3M Centre, Western University, London, Ontario N6A 3K7, Canada; [e] Western's Bone and Joint Institute, University Hospital, London, Ontario N6G 2V4, Canada
* Corresponding author. 3200 South Water Street, Pittsburgh, PA 15203.
E-mail address: hermanz@upmc.edu

Clin Sports Med 43 (2024) 535–546
https://doi.org/10.1016/j.csm.2023.08.010 **sportsmed.theclinics.com**

INDIVIDUALIZED ANTERIOR CRUCIATE LIGAMENT RECONSTRUCTION

The ACL is a dynamic structure, rich in neurovascular supply and composed of 2 distinct bundles, which function synergistically to facilitate normal knee kinematics in concert with bony morphology.[1] Because there is considerable variation across individuals regarding ACL width and orientation, footprint size, and notch morphology, individualized ACLR must meet patient needs as the functional restoration of the ACL to its native dimensions, collagen orientation, and insertion sites according to unique anatomy.[2] By adapting the surgery to the anatomy of each individual patient, the surgeon creates an appropriately sized and positioned graft for superior restoration of knee kinematics, in turn improving clinical outcomes.

The individualized approach begins at the time of diagnosis with recognition of concomitant injuries to menisci, chondral surfaces, collateral ligaments, and capsular structures. From there, acknowledging patient goals is important. Nonoperative management can be considered for patients with a lower activity level and low-grade knee instability. However, nonoperative does not mean no treatment. Instead, the initial management consists of activity limitation, crutches until normal gait returns, control of swelling, and simple exercises for range of motion and quadriceps activation.[3] Supervised physical therapy is used for building lower extremity muscular strength and endurance, restoring knee range of motion, agility training, and eventual return to activities.[4,5] Functional knee braces are commonly used, and have been shown to decrease subjective instability and subsequent medial collateral ligament, meniscal, and osteochondral injuries.[6] Yet, clinical effectiveness remains controversial, and nonoperative management still remains inferior to surgical management in certain patient populations.[7]

A return to high-level pivoting sports is a common indication for operative management with ACLR. Patients' motivation and expectations are driving forces in the decision making for operative management.[8] Graft choice is individualized for the patient based on many factors including age, activity level, preoperative and intraoperative anatomic measurements, and sport. Each of the potential graft options, quadriceps tendon with or without bone block (QT), bone-patellar tendon-bone (BTB), hamstring tendons (HT), and allograft, has a role in the individualized, anatomic ACLR. Allograft is avoided in young, active patients due to a higher risk of failure.[9] HT and BTB remain popular choices worldwide. BTB may be avoided in patients with open physes, and those that participate heavily in kneeling exercises given the concern for postoperative anterior knee pain.[10] QT autograft has become an option growing in popularity. Given its broad and thick size, QT autograft is uniquely customizable to any native ACL footprint size.[11]

PRECISION ANTERIOR CRUCIATE LIGAMENT RECONSTRUCTION

Anatomic Anterior Cruciate Ligament Reconstruction and Concomitant Injuries

During the course of the last few decades, significant changes have been made in ACLR techniques, with the anatomic anteromedial (AM) portal approach replacing the more traditional nonanatomic transtibial drilling technique. As a result, anatomic ACLR has become the gold standard technique aiming to restore knee anatomy and stability by considering the ACL footprint. To ensure an anatomic ACLR, a checklist, "the anatomic ACL reconstruction scoring checklist (AARSC)" has been created.[12] This checklist includes steps such as proper tunnel placement, graft tensioning, and appropriate graft fixation, all of which have been shown to have an impact on the outcomes following an ACL surgery (**Table 1**). The checklist includes a total of 17 items with a maximum score of 19 points, where a score of 8 or higher has been defined as the threshold cutoff for anatomic ACLR.[13] Previous literature has further supported

Table 1
Anatomic anterior cruciate ligament reconstruction checklist by van Eck et al[12,13]

Item	Maximum Score
Individualization of the surgery to each patient	1
Use of a 30° arthroscope	1
Use of an accessory medial portal, in addition to medial and lateral portals	1
Direct visualization of the femoral ACL insertion site	1
Measuring the femoral ACL insertion site dimensions	1
Visualizing the lateral intercondylar ridge	1
Visualizing the lateral bifurcate ridge	1
Placing the femoral tunnel(s) in the femoral ACL insertion site	1
Transportal drilling of the femoral ACL tunnel(s)	1
Direct visualization of the tibial ACL insertion site	1
Measuring the ACL insertion site dimensions	1
Placing the tibial tunnel(s) in the tibial ACL insertion site	1
Documenting of femoral fixation method	1
Documenting of tibial fixation method	1
Documenting of knee flexion angle during femoral tunnel drilling	1
Documenting graft type	1
Documenting knee flexion angle during graft tensioning	1
Documentation used for ACL tunnel position	
Drawing, diagram, operative note, dictation, or clock face reference (0 points)	2
Arthroscopic radiographs 2D MRI, or 2D CT (1 point)	
3D MRI, 3D CT, or navigation (2 points)	

bbreviations: ACL, anterior cruciate ligament; CT, computer tomography; MRI, magnetic reso-ance imaging.

he use of the checklist by reporting improved long-term outcomes, such as a reduced isk of posttraumatic osteoarthritis after an anatomic ACLR compared with nonana-omically treated ACL injury.[14]

Because an ACL injury rarely occurs in isolation, it is important to consider the need or other concomitant procedures (**Table 2**). For instance, concomitant meniscal in-ıries as well as injuries to the medial collateral ligament (MCL) have been shown to lay a significant role in the postoperative course following ACLR. Lateral meniscal in-ıries have been reported to occur concomitantly with acute ACL injuries in 16% to 2% of the cases[23] and are further associated with decreased stability as well as ıcreased risk of revision ACLR.[24,25] Furthermore, lateral meniscal root tears have ound to be relatively common in ACL-injured knees and have good clinical outcomes vhen repaired in combination with ACLR.[26] Similar to the lateral meniscus, concom-ant medial meniscus tears inclusive ramp lesions are frequently observed.[27–29] leglecting these injuries has been shown to lead to poor outcomes, including early int degeneration and an increased risk of revision ACLR surgery.[23,30] Thus, repairing oncomitant meniscal injuries during ACLR has been shown to be crucial in achieving ptimal functional and subjective outcomes and further preventing later-term out-omes, such as OA.[23]

Concomitant MCL injuries are also common in the setting of ACL injuries, and the everity of the injury determines the treatment approach. Although low-grade MCL

Table 2
Treatment of concomitant pathologies in the setting of anterior cruciate ligament reconstruction

	Primary ACLR	Revision ACLR	Multiple Revision ACLR
Meniscal injury	Avoid resection Small, peripheral tears may be treated in situ[15]	High prevalence Look for repair Reconstruct in select cases	Repair Consider reconstruction
Meniscal root injury	15%–20% posterior lateral root injuries Repair Side-to-side suture may be preferred in cases of complex T shaped injuries/injuries located close to the intact tibial insertion[16] Transosseous technique is preferred in tibial-sided root injuries without multiligamentous reconstruction[16]	Commonly missed/chronic/avulsion Repair; consider centralization[17,18] Side-to-side suture may be preferred in cases of complex T shaped injuries/injuries located close to the intact tibial insertion[16] Transosseous technique is preferred in tibial-sided root injuries without multiligamentous reconstruction[16]	
Ramp lesion	Repair if unstable	Commonly missed, repair	
LET/ALLR	Preferred in the following settings[19–22]: Young pivoting sport athlete Hyperlaxity/knee hyperextension Increased PTS >12°, Anterolateral capsular injury	Perform, in no additional repairs done	
PLC	Repair/reconstruction if complete injury		
MCL	Repair if high grade tear AMRI—address if present with valgus laxity	Consider reconstruction if > 2.0 mm opening on stress fluoroscopy	
Sagittal malalignment	Consider if PTS >18° with history of previous contralateral ACLR	Consider ACW-HTO if PTS >15°	Consider ACW-HTO if PTS >12°
Coronal malalignment	Consider if varus malalignment >10°	Consider MOW-HTO Mild medial compartment osteoarthritis Varus malalignment >5° Concomitant meniscal deficiency	

This table presents authors' opinion at the time of this review, evidence may change with time.

Abbreviations: ACLR, anterior cruciate ligament reconstruction; ACW-HTO, anterior closing wedge high tibial osteotomy; ALLR, anterolateral ligament reconstruction; AMRI, anteromedial rotatory instability; LET, Lateral extra-articular tenodesis; MCL, medial collateral ligament; MOW-HTO, medial opening wedge high injuries may be managed nonsurgically, high-grade injuries or cases of persistent instability are recommended to be treated with either surgical repair or reconstruction. As a result, MCL deficiency has been reported as one of the most important risk factors for failure after ACLR owing to increased knee valgus instability along with increased anteromedial rotatory instability.[31–34] Furthermore, patients treated with combined MCL reconstruction and ACLR have shown high rates of return to sport (RTS) and improved patient outcomes, enhancing patient satisfaction and reducing the need for additional interventions.[35]

In certain instances, additional procedures such as lateral extra-articular tenodesis (LET) and high tibial osteotomies may be performed. Common indications for LET include patients with one or more of the following: younger individuals aged younger than 25 years with goals of returning to contact, pivoting sports, high-grade anterolateral rotatory laxity with grade 2 or higher pivot shift, generalized ligamentous laxity (Beighton score >4), knee hyperextension greater than 10°, lateral coronal plane laxity, increased posterior tibial slope greater than 12°, concomitant lateral meniscal deficiency, and MRI evidence of anterolateral capsular injury.[19–21] Furthermore, high tibial osteotomy may be indicated to correct coronal or sagittal plane malalignment. Medial opening wedge high tibial osteotomy and lateral closing wedge high tibial osteotomy are well-established treatment options in the setting of ACL deficiency with varus alignment, and anterior closing wedge high tibial osteotomy can be used in the revision ACLR setting to decrease posterior slope and improve clinical outcomes.[36] Thus, implementing these evidence-based steps in clinical settings can further contribute to improved patient-reported and long-term knee-related outcomes.

POSTOPERATIVE REHABILITATION

Postoperatively, rehabilitation should be designed with the goal of safely returning the patient to desired activity. Normally, protocols initiate immediate weight-bearing with graduated range of motion because evidence has associated these factors with reduced risk of knee pain.[37] A functional brace is prescribed only in the immediate postoperative period to allow for initial healing of skin incisions. The brace is discontinued as soon as the patient demonstrates return of protective quadriceps function.[38] Protocols should focus on closed chain exercises and muscle strengthening in the first 6 weeks. Open chain exercises should not be initiated before 6 weeks postoperatively because this is the time point associated with improvement in graft strength without increasing the risk of graft failure.[39–41]

OUTCOMES

Patient-reported Outcomes

Several patient reported outcome (PRO) measures have been used in the postoperative period to monitor patient's knee and activity-related function. The International Knee Documentation Committee is an 18 item patient-reported score evaluating knee-related symptoms (7 items), knee-related function (1 item), and participation in sport activities (10 items).[42] It was introduced in 1994 and has proven a quick and comprehensive assessment tool, which shows responsiveness to change following surgical interventions such as ACLR.[43] The Lysholm score, introduced in 1982, has been one of the most frequently used clinical outcome scales overtime aiming to evaluate knee-related symptoms, such as swelling, instability, pain, squatting, and locking.[44] The Knee Injury Osteoarthritis Outcomes Score (KOOS) is a 42-item patient-reported outcome scale, consisting of 5 subscales (pain, other symptoms, sports and recreational activities, quality of life, and activities of daily living), each of which are scaled from 0 to 100, where a higher score indicates a better outcome.[45] A specific version of the KOOS, KOOS-ACL, was later developed to assess outcomes in patients undergoing ACLR.[46] These outcomes among others can be used to monitor knee function in the preoperative and postoperative setting following ACLR. Measurement parameters such as Patient Acceptable Symptom State, Minimal Clinical Important Difference, Minimally Important Change, and Substantial Clinical Benefit can be administered to PROs in order to better compare changes between timepoints or different cohorts.

Finally, specific activity measures can be used to compare functional levels of patient preoperatively to postoperatively after ACLR. The Tegner activity score aims to provide a standardized method of determining level of sport or work before injury compared with post injury that is documentable on a numerical scale. It was first developed in 1985 for use in conjunction with the Lysholm knee scoring system.[47] The scale consists of one question scored 0 to 10, where 0 represents disability due to the knee problem and 10 represents participation in competitive sport at the national elite level. Answers in between comprise work at various levels of physical labor as well as sport participation at various competitive levels. Activity levels of 6 to 10 can only be achieved if the patient participates in recreational or competitive sport.[47] The Marx Activity Rating Scale was developed in 2001 to evaluate the activity level of patients with various knee conditions who participate in sports.[48] It focuses on 4 activity points: running, deceleration, cutting, and pivoting. Patients are asked to approximate how many times in the past 12 months they participated in the activity points at their healthiest and most active state within the past year. The 4 knee functions are rated on a 5-point frequency scale; scores are added to a maximum of 16. A higher score indicates more frequent participation.[48]

Return to Sport

Perhaps, one of the most important outcomes following ACLR in the athletic population is RTS. RTS testing protocols are designed to incorporate several domains include muscle strength recovery, hop tests, measures of quality of movement, and psychological confidence.[49] Muscle strength recovery may be measured by manual muscle testing or dynamometers,[50,51] and hop tests may consist of single hop for distance, triple hop for distance, tripe cross-over hop, and the 6-m timed hop.[52] In addition, movement quality assessments should be included as up to 60% of patients after ACLR may have abnormal landing kinematics in the operative leg compared with the nonoperative limb.[53] Finally, addressing psychological readiness to RTS is crucial because studies have revealed that up to 65% of patients cite a psychological reason for not returning to play, particularly with fear of reinjury.[54] The psychological readiness can be assessed by using ACL-Return to Sports after Injury Scale that is specifically developed to evaluate psychological readiness to RTS in patients with an ACL injury.[55,56]

RTS rates can vary significantly following ACLR, and accelerated rehabilitation programs have not been shown to speed RTS, with consistent RTS unusually occurring before 6 months.[57,58] Even further delayed RTS may be beneficial, with a 51% reduction in rerupture rates noted for every month RTS was delayed up to 9 months postoperatively.[59] Overall, clearance for RTS following ACLR must be a combined decision-making process that involves the surgeon, physical therapists, and patient, addressing not only the physical but the psychological readiness of the individual in order to promote the best outcomes. Finally, it is important to be aware of that RTS is a continuum and should occur gradually, along a dynamic continuum to decrease the risk of reinjuries and other complications.[60]

FUTURE CONSIDERATIONS

Precision ACLR is poised to revolutionize the field of orthopedic sports medicine, aiming to improve both functional and patient outcomes. Advancements in technology, treatment planning, and surgical techniques are expected to play an essential role in this process.

The integration of artificial intelligence (AI) and machine learning (ML) algorithms into preoperative planning as well as intraoperative and postoperative settings have been discussed to offer several possibilities in health-care settings.[61,62] Although these advanced tools are expected to allow clinicians to analyze patient-specific data on a more individualized level, such as patient demographical characteristics, imaging, and clinical data, they are also expected to help with combining and interpreting the data in innovative ways to provide surgeons a possibility of an individualized risk assessment.[61–65] The integration of AI is expected to enable clinicians to make more precise surgical decisions, including graft selection, addressing other concomitant injuries, and planning for extra-articular procedures, ultimately resulting in improved long-term outcomes for patients as well as cost savings and aid in value-based care.

Moreover, the development of robotics is likely to become an important part of precision ACLR. Thus, robotic-assisted surgery may help with improving surgical precision as well as guiding surgeons toward more accurate and reproducible procedures.[66,67] Similar to robotics used in arthroplasty today, the robotic platform could provide continuous feedback and ensure optimal graft placement through real-time imaging and navigation techniques and subsequently, reduce complications and improve overall surgical outcomes. Additionally, the future of precision ACLR is likely to involve advancements in regenerative medicine and tissue engineering,[68,69] including biomaterials, such as stem cells, scaffolds, and tissue-engineered grafts. These may further be used for ACLR to decrease comorbidity, costs, enhance graft healing, and ultimately improve patient long-term outcomes.

Finally, sustainability in orthopedic sports medicine surgery is likely to become a prominent topic of discussion. Because climate change continues to be an increasing concern, attention has been given to the operating rooms and their negative environmental impact, including increasing energy and resource utilization.[70] Future research is expected to focus on solutions to decrease the carbon footprint, incorporating measures, such as minimizing the use of single-use instruments and implementing appropriate recycling protocols, which are anticipated to play an essential role. Moreover, AI tools may have an important role is this. AI tools may allow more effective and less energy-consuming operating rooms by guiding the surgical planning and predicting operative duration,[71] subsequently, minimizing the use of unnecessary instruments and turnout time. This is ultimately expected to lead to smart operating rooms that are value-based and environment friendly, whereas still aiming to provide the same possibilities for high-quality health care as those operating rooms that we have today.

SUMMARY

In conclusion, precision ACLR refers to the individualized approach to prerehabilitation, surgery (including anatomy, bony morphology, and repair/reconstruction of concomitant injuries), postrehabilitation, and functional recovery. The future of precision ACLR is likely to involve the incorporation of AI and ML algorithms, along with innovations in robotic-assisted surgery as well as regenerative medicine. As these technologies continue to improve, orthopedic sports medicine is likely to experience a new era, marked by a paradigm shift toward more individualized and precise patient care.

CLINICS CARE POINTS

- Precision ACLR refers to the individualized approach to prerehabilitation, surgery (including anatomy, bony morphology, and repair/reconstruction of concomitant injuries), postrehabilitation, and functional recovery.
- The future of precision ACLR is likely to involve the incorporation of AI and ML algorithms, along with innovations in robotic-assisted surgery as well as regenerative medicine. As these technologies continue to improve, orthopedic sports medicine is likely to experience a new era, marked by a paradigm shift toward more individualized and precise patient care.

DISCLOSURE

V. Musahl reports educational grants, consulting fees, and speaking fees from Smith & Nephew plc, United Kingdom, educational grants from Arthrex and DePuy/Synthes, is a board member of the International Society of Arthroscopy, Knee Surgery and Orthopedic Sports Medicine (ISAKOS), and deputy editor-in-chief of Knee Surgery, Sports Traumatology, Arthroscopy (KSSTA).

REFERENCES

1. Fu FH, Nagai K. Editorial Commentary: The Anterior Cruciate Ligament Is a Dynamic Structure. Arthroscopy 2018;34(8):2476–7.
2. Hussein M, van Eck CF, Cretnik A, et al. Individualized anterior cruciate ligament surgery: a prospective study comparing anatomic single- and double-bundle reconstruction. Am J Sports Med 2012;40(8):1781–8.
3. Eitzen I, Moksnes H, Snyder-Mackler L, et al. A progressive 5-week exercise therapy program leads to significant improvement in knee function early after anterior cruciate ligament injury. J Orthop Sports Phys Ther 2010;40(11):705–21.
4. Chmielewski TL, Hurd WJ, Rudolph KS, et al. Perturbation training improves knee kinematics and reduces muscle co-contraction after complete unilateral anterior cruciate ligament rupture. Phys Ther 2005;85(8):740–9, discussion 750-744.
5. Swirtun LR, Jansson A, Renström P. The effects of a functional knee brace during early treatment of patients with a nonoperated acute anterior cruciate ligament tear: a prospective randomized study. Clin J Sport Med 2005;15(5):299–304.
6. Kocher MS, Sterett WI, Briggs KK, et al. Effect of functional bracing on subsequent knee injury in ACL-deficient professional skiers. J Knee Surg 2003;16(2):87–92.
7. Beard DJ, Davies L, Cook JA, et al. Rehabilitation versus surgical reconstruction for non-acute anterior cruciate ligament injury (ACL SNNAP): a pragmatic randomised controlled trial. Lancet 2022;400(10352):605–15.
8. Roessler KK, Andersen TE, Lohmander S, et al. Motives for sports participation as predictions of self-reported outcomes after anterior cruciate ligament injury of the knee. Scand J Med Sci Sports 2015;25(3):435–40.
9. Pallis M, Svoboda SJ, Cameron KL, et al. Survival comparison of allograft and autograft anterior cruciate ligament reconstruction at the United States Military Academy. Am J Sports Med 2012;40(6):1242–6.
10. Hardy A, Casabianca L, Andrieu K, et al. Complications following harvesting of patellar tendon or hamstring tendon grafts for anterior cruciate ligament reconstruction: Systematic review of literature. Orthop Traumatol Surg Res 2017;103(8s):S245–8.

11. Sheean AJ, Musahl V, Slone HS, et al. Quadriceps tendon autograft for arthroscopic knee ligament reconstruction: use it now, use it often. Br J Sports Med 2018;52(11):698–701.
12. van Eck CF, Gravare-Silbernagel K, Samuelsson K, et al. Evidence to support the interpretation and use of the Anatomic Anterior Cruciate Ligament Reconstruction Checklist. J Bone Joint Surg Am 2013;95(20):e153.
13. Fox MA, Engler ID, Zsidai BT, et al. Anatomic anterior cruciate ligament reconstruction: Freddie Fu's paradigm. J isakos 2023;8(1):15–22.
14. Rothrauff BB, Jorge A, de Sa D, et al. Anatomic ACL reconstruction reduces risk of post-traumatic osteoarthritis: a systematic review with minimum 10-year follow-up. Knee Surg Sports Traumatol Arthrosc 2020;28(4):1072–84.
15. Duchman KR, Westermann RW, Spindler KP, et al. The Fate of Meniscus Tears Left In Situ at the Time of Anterior Cruciate Ligament Reconstruction: A 6-Year Follow-up Study From the MOON Cohort. Am J Sports Med 2015;43(11):2688–95.
16. Bonasia DE, Pellegrino P, D'Amelio A, et al. Meniscal Root Tear Repair: Why, When and How? Orthop Rev 2015;7(2):5792.
17. Koga H, Muneta T, Watanabe T, et al. Two-Year Outcomes After Arthroscopic Lateral Meniscus Centralization. Arthroscopy 2016;32(10):2000–8.
18. Daney BT, Aman ZS, Krob JJ, et al. Utilization of Transtibial Centralization Suture Best Minimizes Extrusion and Restores Tibiofemoral Contact Mechanics for Anatomic Medial Meniscal Root Repairs in a Cadaveric Model. Am J Sports Med 2019;47(7):1591–600.
19. Getgood AMJ, Bryant DM, Litchfield R, et al. Lateral Extra-articular Tenodesis Reduces Failure of Hamstring Tendon Autograft Anterior Cruciate Ligament Reconstruction: 2-Year Outcomes From the STABILITY Study Randomized Clinical Trial. Am J Sports Med 2020;48(2):285–97.
20. Larson CM, Bedi A, Dietrich ME, et al. Generalized Hypermobility, Knee Hyperextension, and Outcomes After Anterior Cruciate Ligament Reconstruction: Prospective, Case-Control Study With Mean 6 Years Follow-up. Arthroscopy 2017; 33(10):1852–8.
21. Firth AD, Bryant DM, Litchfield R, et al. Predictors of Graft Failure in Young Active Patients Undergoing Hamstring Autograft Anterior Cruciate Ligament Reconstruction With or Without a Lateral Extra-articular Tenodesis: The Stability Experience. Am J Sports Med 2022;50(2):384–95.
22. Sonnery-Cottet B, Daggett M, Fayard J-M, et al. Anterolateral Ligament Expert Group consensus paper on the management of internal rotation and instability of the anterior cruciate ligament - deficient knee. J Orthop Traumatol 2017; 18(2):91–106.
23. Kopf S, Beaufils P, Hirschmann MT, et al. Management of traumatic meniscus tears: the 2019 ESSKA meniscus consensus. Knee Surg Sports Traumatol Arthrosc : official journal of the ESSKA 2020;28(4):1177–94.
24. Grassi A, Dal Fabbro G, Di Paolo S, et al. Medial and lateral meniscus have a different role in kinematics of the ACL-deficient knee: a systematic review. Journal of ISAKOS 2019;4(5):233–41.
25. Musahl V, Rahnemai-Azar AA, Costello J, et al. The Influence of Meniscal and Anterolateral Capsular Injury on Knee Laxity in Patients With Anterior Cruciate Ligament Injuries. Am J Sports Med 2016;44(12):3126–31.
26. Shekhar A, Tapasvi S, Williams A. Outcomes of Combined Lateral Meniscus Posterior Root Repair and Anterior Cruciate Ligament Reconstruction. Orthop J Sports Med 2022;10(3). 23259671221083318.

27. Cristiani R, van de Bunt F, Kvist J, et al. High prevalence of meniscal ramp lesions in anterior cruciate ligament injuries. Knee Surg Sports Traumatol Arthrosc 2023;31(1):316–24.
28. Erard J, Cance N, Shatrov J, et al. Delaying ACL reconstruction is associated with increased rates of medial meniscal tear. Knee Surg Sports Traumatol Arthrosc 2023;31(10):4458–66.
29. Kaarre J, Zsidai B, Winkler PW, et al. Different patient and activity-related characteristics result in different injury profiles for patients with anterior cruciate ligament and posterior cruciate ligament injuries. Knee Surg Sports Traumatol Arthrosc 2023;31(1):308–15.
30. Phillips M, Rönnblad E, Lopez-Rengstig L, et al. Meniscus repair with simultaneous ACL reconstruction demonstrated similar clinical outcomes as isolated ACL repair: a result not seen with meniscus resection. Knee Surg Sports Traumatol Arthrosc 2018;26(8):2270–7.
31. Ball S, Stephen JM, El-Daou H, et al. The medial ligaments and the ACL restrain anteromedial laxity of the knee. Knee Surg Sports Traumatol Arthrosc 2020;28(12):3700–8.
32. Ahn JH, Lee SH. Risk factors for knee instability after anterior cruciate ligament reconstruction. Knee Surg Sports Traumatol Arthrosc 2016;24(9):2936–42.
33. Svantesson E, Hamrin Senorski E, Alentorn-Geli E, et al. Increased risk of ACL revision with non-surgical treatment of a concomitant medial collateral ligament injury: a study on 19,457 patients from the Swedish National Knee Ligament Registry. Knee Surg Sports Traumatol Arthrosc 2019;27(8):2450–9.
34. Miyaji N, Holthof SR, Ball SV, et al. Medial Collateral Ligament Reconstruction for Anteromedial Instability of the Knee: A Biomechanical Study In Vitro. Am J Sports Med 2022;50(7):1823–31.
35. Wright ML, Coladonato C, Ciccotti MG, et al. Combined Anterior Cruciate Ligament and Medial Collateral Ligament Reconstruction Shows High Rates of Return to Activity and Low Rates of Recurrent Valgus Instability: An Updated Systematic Review. Arthrosc Sports Med Rehabil 2023;5(3):e867–79.
36. Klek M, Dhawan A. The Role of High Tibial Osteotomy in ACL Reconstruction in Knees with Coronal and Sagittal Plane Deformity. Curr Rev Musculoskelet Med 2019;12(4):466–71.
37. Shaw T, Williams MT, Chipchase LS. Do early quadriceps exercises affect the outcome of ACL reconstruction? A randomised controlled trial. Aust J Physiother 2005;51(1):9–17.
38. Tyler TF, McHugh MP, Gleim GW, et al. The effect of immediate weightbearing after anterior cruciate ligament reconstruction. Clin Orthop Relat Res 1998;357:141–8.
39. Fleming BC, Oksendahl H, Beynnon BD. Open- or closed-kinetic chain exercises after anterior cruciate ligament reconstruction? Exerc Sport Sci Rev 2005;33(3):134–40.
40. Heijne A, Fleming BC, Renstrom PA, et al. Strain on the anterior cruciate ligament during closed kinetic chain exercises. Med Sci Sports Exerc 2004;36(6):935–41.
41. Rehabilitation Predictors of Clinical Outcome Following Revision ACL Reconstruction in the MARS Cohort. J Bone Joint Surg Am 2019;101(9):779–86.
42. Irrgang JJ, Anderson AF, Boland AL, et al. Development and validation of the international knee documentation committee subjective knee form. Am J Sports Med 2001;29(5):600–13.

43. Irrgang JJ, Anderson AF, Boland AL, et al. Responsiveness of the International Knee Documentation Committee Subjective Knee Form. Am J Sports Med 2006;34(10):1567–73.
44. Lysholm J, Gillquist J. Evaluation of knee ligament surgery results with special emphasis on use of a scoring scale. Am J Sports Med 1982;10(3):150–4.
45. Roos EM, Roos HP, Lohmander LS, et al. Knee Injury and Osteoarthritis Outcome Score (KOOS)–development of a self-administered outcome measure. J Orthop Sports Phys Ther 1998;28(2):88–96.
46. Tremblay P, Getgood A, Bryant D, et al. Paper 75: Development and Validation of the KOOS-ACL: A Short-form Version of the KOOS for Young Patients with ACL Tears. Orthopaedic Journal of Sports Medicine 2022;10(7_suppl5). 2325967121S2325900638.
47. Tegner Y, Lysholm J. Rating systems in the evaluation of knee ligament injuries. Clin Orthop Relat Res 1985;198:43–9.
48. Marx RG, Stump TJ, Jones EC, et al. Development and evaluation of an activity rating scale for disorders of the knee. Am J Sports Med 2001;29(2):213–8.
49. Gokeler A, Dingenen B, Hewett TE. Rehabilitation and Return to Sport Testing After Anterior Cruciate Ligament Reconstruction: Where Are We in 2022? Arthrosc Sports Med Rehabil 2022;4(1):e77–82.
50. Greenberg EM, Greenberg ET, Albaugh J, et al. Rehabilitation Practice Patterns Following Anterior Cruciate Ligament Reconstruction: A Survey of Physical Therapists. J Orthop Sports Phys Ther 2018;48(10):801–11.
51. Lynch AD, Logerstedt DS, Grindem H, et al. Consensus criteria for defining 'successful outcome' after ACL injury and reconstruction: a Delaware-Oslo ACL cohort investigation. Br J Sports Med 2015;49(5):335–42.
52. Logerstedt DS, Scalzitti D, Risberg MA, et al. Knee Stability and Movement Coordination Impairments: Knee Ligament Sprain Revision 2017. J Orthop Sports Phys Ther 2017;47(11):A1–47.
53. Welling W, Benjaminse A, Seil R, et al. Altered movement during single leg hop test after ACL reconstruction: implications to incorporate 2-D video movement analysis for hop tests. Knee Surg Sports Traumatol Arthrosc 2018;26(10):3012–9.
54. Nwachukwu BU, Adjei J, Rauck RC, et al. How Much Do Psychological Factors Affect Lack of Return to Play After Anterior Cruciate Ligament Reconstruction? A Systematic Review. Orthop J Sports Med 2019;7(5). 2325967119845313.
55. Webster KE, Feller JA. Development and Validation of a Short Version of the Anterior Cruciate Ligament Return to Sport After Injury (ACL-RSI) Scale. Orthop J Sports Med 2018;6(4). 2325967118763763.
56. Webster KE, Feller JA, Lambros C. Development and preliminary validation of a scale to measure the psychological impact of returning to sport following anterior cruciate ligament reconstruction surgery. Phys Ther Sport 2008;9(1):9–15.
57. Beynnon BD, Uh BS, Johnson RJ, et al. Rehabilitation after anterior cruciate ligament reconstruction: a prospective, randomized, double-blind comparison of programs administered over 2 different time intervals. Am J Sports Med 2005;33(3):347–59.
58. Chen JL, Allen CR, Stephens TE, et al. Differences in mechanisms of failure, intraoperative findings, and surgical characteristics between single- and multiple-revision ACL reconstructions: a MARS cohort study. Am J Sports Med 2013;41(7):1571–8.
59. Grindem H, Snyder-Mackler L, Moksnes H, et al. Simple decision rules can reduce reinjury risk by 84% after ACL reconstruction: the Delaware-Oslo ACL cohort study. Br J Sports Med 2016;50(13):804–8.

60. Meredith SJ, Rauer T, Chmielewski TL, et al. Return to sport after anterior cruciate ligament injury: Panther Symposium ACL Injury Return to Sport Consensus Group. Knee Surg Sports Traumatol Arthrosc 2020;28(8):2403–14.
61. Ko S, Pareek A, Ro DH, et al. Artificial intelligence in orthopedics: three strategies for deep learning with orthopedic specific imaging. Knee Surg Sports Traumatol Arthrosc 2022;30(3):758–61.
62. Lu Y, Pareek A, Wilbur RR, et al. Understanding anterior shoulder instability through machine learning: new models that predict recurrence, progression to surgery, and development of arthritis. Orthop J Sports Med 2021;9(11). 23259671211053326.
63. Johnson QJ, Jabal MS, Arguello AM, et al. Machine learning can accurately predict risk factors for all-cause reoperation after ACLR: creating a clinical tool to improve patient counseling and outcomes. Knee Surg Sports Traumatol Arthrosc 2023.
64. Lu Y, Forlenza E, Wilbur RR, et al. Machine-learning model successfully predicts patients at risk for prolonged postoperative opioid use following elective knee arthroscopy. Knee Surg Sports Traumatol Arthrosc 2022;30(3):762–72.
65. Bayliss L, Jones LD. The role of artificial intelligence and machine learning in predicting orthopaedic outcomes. Bone & Joint Journal 2019;101-B(12):1476–8.
66. Guo N, Wang T, Wei M, et al. An ACL reconstruction robotic positioning system based on anatomical characteristics. Int J Adv Rob Syst 2020;17(1). 1729881419886160.
67. Ding G, Yang G, Zhang J, et al. Feasibility and accuracy of orthopaedic surgical robot system for intraoperative navigation to locate bone tunnel in anterior cruciate ligament reconstruction. Int J Med Robot 2022;18(2):e2354.
68. Cengiz IF, Pereira H, de Girolamo L, et al. Orthopaedic regenerative tissue engineering en route to the holy grail: disequilibrium between the demand and the supply in the operating room. Journal of Experimental Orthopaedics 2018;5(1):14.
69. Costa JB, Pereira H, Espregueira-Mendes J, et al. Tissue engineering in orthopaedic sports medicine: current concepts. Journal of ISAKOS 2017;2(2):60–6.
70. Engler ID, Curley AJ, Fu FH, et al. Environmental Sustainability in Orthopaedic Surgery. J Am Acad Orthop Surg 2022;30(11):504–11.
71. Miller LE, Goedicke W, Crowson MG, et al. Using Machine Learning to Predict Operating Room Case Duration: A Case Study in Otolaryngology. Otolaryngol Head Neck Surg 2023;168(2):241–7.

Moving?

Make sure your subscription moves with you!

To notify us of your new address, find your **Clinics Account Number** (located on your mailing label above your name), and contact customer service at:

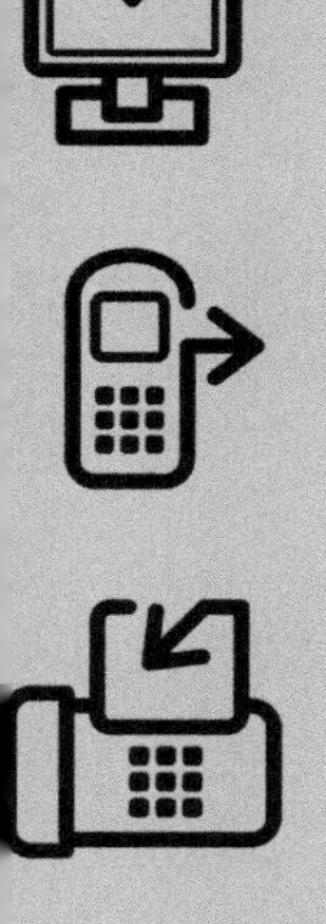

Email: journalscustomerservice-usa@elsevier.com

800-654-2452 **(subscribers in the U.S. & Canada)**
314-447-8871 **(subscribers outside of the U.S. & Canada)**

Fax number: 314-447-8029

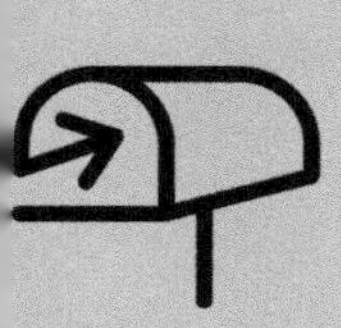

Elsevier Health Sciences Division
Subscription Customer Service
3251 Riverport Lane
Maryland Heights, MO 63043

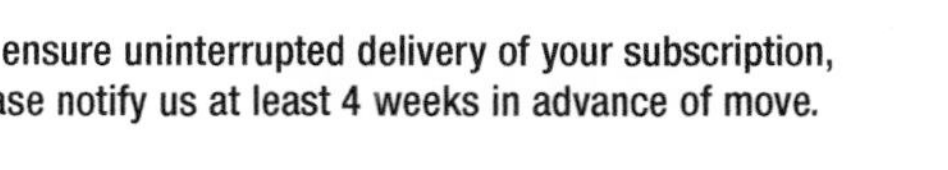

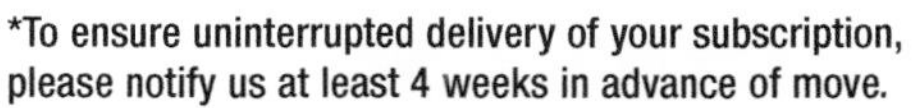

*To ensure uninterrupted delivery of your subscription, please notify us at least 4 weeks in advance of move.

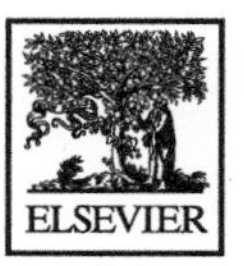

Printed and bound by CPI Group (UK) Ltd, Croydon, CR0 4YY

08/05/2025

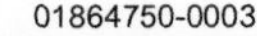

01864750-0003